The NEW ENGLAND
JOURNAL *of* MEDICINE

Clinical Practice

EDITED BY

CAREN G. SOLOMON, M.D., M.P.H.,
& JEFFREY M. DRAZEN, M.D.

McGraw-Hill
Medical Publishing Division

New York   Chicago   San Francisco   Lisbon   London   Madrid
Mexico City   Milan   New Delhi   San Juan   Seoul   Singapore   Sydney   Toronto

Clinical Practice

1234567890 DOC/DOC 09876

ISBN 0-07-147161-8

This book is printed on acid-free paper.

The editors wish to thank the editorial, production, and publishing staffs of the Journal for their cheerful diligence in producing this volume. Their work was accomplished in the face of the unrelenting demands of a weekly publication.

CLINICAL PRACTICE

Contents

Each of these *Clinical Practice* features begins with a case vignette highlighting a common clinical problem. Evidence supporting various strategies is then presented, followed by review of areas of uncertainty and, when they exist, formal guidelines. The article ends with the author's clinical recommendations.

CONTRIBUTORS

Shannon M. Bates, MD, MSc
McMaster University Medical Centre
Hamilton, Ontario, Canada

John P. Bilezikian, MD
College of Physicians and Surgeons
Columbia University
New York, NY

Lieve Brochez, MD, PhD
Ghent University Hospital
Ghent, Belgium

Blase A. Carabello, MD
Baylor College of Medicine
Houston, TX

Allen S. Craig, MD
Vanderbilt University School of Medicine
Nashville, TN

Kathryn M. Edwards, MD
Vanderbilt University School of Medicine
Nashville, TN

Joann G. Elmore, MD, MPH
University of Washington School of Medicine
Seattle, WA

Suzanne W. Fletcher, MD, MSc
Harvard Medical School
Boston, MA

Theodore M Freeman, MD, FACP, FACAAI,
FAAAAI
Private Practice
San Antonio, TX

Donald H. Gilden, MD
University of Colorado Health Sciences Center
Denver, CO

Jeffrey S. Ginsberg, MD
McMaster University
Hamilton, Ontario, Canada

LTC Robert V. Gibbons, MD, MPH
Armed Forces Research Institute for Medical Sciences
Bangkok, Thailand

Laszlo Hegedüs, MD, DSc
Odense University Hospital
Odense, Denmark

Erik L. Hewlett, MD
University of Virginia School of Medicine
Charlottesville, VA

Matthew Kalady, MD
Cleveland Clinic
Cleveland, OH

Jeffrey N. Katz, MD, MS
Harvard Medical School
Brigham and Women's Hospital
Boston, MA

Jean Marie Naeyaert, MD, PhD
Ghent University Hospital
Ghent, Belgium

Richard L. Page, MD
University of Washington School of Medicine
Seattle, WA

Theodore N. Pappas, MD
Duke University
Durham, NC

Barbara L. Parry, MD
University of California, San Diego
La Jolla, CA

Erik K. Paulson, MD
Duke University Medical Center
Durham, NC

Jeffrey F. Peipert, MD, MPH
Brown Medical School
Providence, RI

Catherine M. Piontek, MD
Interlink Healthcare Communications
Lawrenceville, NJ

Frank C. Powell, FRCPI
Mater M Hospital
Dublin, Ireland

Marsha D. Rappley, MD
Michigan State University
East Lansing, MI

Nancy A. Rigotti, MD
Harvard Medical School
Boston, MA

Charles E. Rupprecht, VMD, MS, PhD
Centers for Disease Control & Prevention
Atlanta, GA

Hugh A. Sampson, MD
Mount Sinai School of Medicine
New York, NY

William Schaffner, MD
Vanderbilt University School of Medicine
Nashville, TN

Shonni J. Silverberg, MD
College of Physicians and Surgeons
Columbia University
New York, NY

Barry P. Simmons, MD
Harvard Medical School
Brigham and Women's Hospital
Boston, MA

Andrew F. Stewart, MD
University of Pittsburgh School of Medicine
Pittsburgh, PA

James K. Stoller, MD, MS
Cleveland Clinic Lerner College of Medicine
of Case Western Reserve University
Cleveland, OH

Morton N. Swartz, MD
Harvard Medical School
Boston, MA

Mary Tinetti, MD
Yale University School of Medicine
New Haven, CT

Anthony Toft, MD
Royal Infirmary
Edinburgh, Scotland

Carolyn Westhoff, MD
College of Physicians and Surgeons
Columbia University
New York, NY

Katherine L. Wisner, MD, MS
University of Pittsburgh Medical Center
Pittsburgh, PA

Preface

The Clinical Practice series was introduced in the *New England Journal of Medicine* in 2001 to help meet the information needs of clinicians who want to remain up to date on a wide variety of problems commonly encountered in practice. Articles in this biweekly series review clinical problems at the interface of primary and specialty care in a concise, easily recognized format. Each article begins with a brief case vignette to highlight the major clinical question or questions to be covered. Subsequent sections include: "The Clinical Problem" (Who is at risk? How common is the condition?), "Strategies and Evidence" (What are the data to support particular approaches?), "Areas of Uncertainty" (What are major gaps in our current knowledge?), "Guidelines" (What do professional organizations recommend?), and finally, "Summary and Conclusions" (What would the author(s) recommend with respect to the diagnosis or treatment of the patient outlined in the vignette?). Simply put, each article is a structured "curbside consult" about a patient with a well-defined clinical problem.

Recognizing that data are lacking to guide the "optimal" approach to many clinical problems that physicians must manage, the experts who author these articles are asked to not only make clear where rigorous data are or are not available, but also to provide recommendations based on their assessment of the literature and their personal experience where rigorous data are lacking.

This book includes selected Clinical Practice articles previously published in the *New England Journal of Medicine.* Topics covered include those in cardiology, pulmonary medicine, dermatology, women's health, psychiatry, infectious disease, allergy–immunology, and gastroenterology. In cases where there have been clinically meaningful changes in the area covered by the article since publication, authors have provided a short update to their article.

We have created this collection to provide an easy way to access this clinical resource. We anticipate that once you have scanned the book, you will use it as a reference as you encounter problems similar to the ones outlined in the chapters. We hope that you will find the material of value in your care of patients.

CAREN G. SOLOMON, M.D., M.P.H.
Deputy Editor
The New England Journal of Medicine
Assistant Professor of Medicine
Harvard Medical School
Brigham and Women's Hospital

JEFFREY M. DRAZEN, M.D.
Editor-in-Chief
The New England Journal of Medicine
Distinguished Parker B. Francis
   Professor of Medicine
Harvard Medical School

Subclinical Hyperthyroidism

ANTHONY D. TOFT, M.D.

A 67-year-old woman presents with palpitations and is found to be in atrial fibrillation at a rate of 120 beats per minute. The only other finding on physical examination is a goiter, which is known to be long-standing. Echocardiography shows neither valvular disease nor left ventricular systolic dysfunction. The serum thyrotropin concentration is less than 0.05 mU per liter, and the serum total triiodothyronine and free thyroxine concentrations are in the normal range. Should the thyroid dysfunction be treated?

THE CLINICAL PROBLEM

The combination of an undetectable serum thyrotropin concentration, as measured by an assay with a threshold of detection that is 0.1 mU per liter or less, and normal serum triiodothyronine and thyroxine concentrations (usually at the upper end of the normal range) is known as subclinical hyperthyroidism. This condition reflects the fact that before clinical features of thyrotoxicosis are apparent, the thyrotrophs usually respond to minor increments in thyroid hormone concentrations, which remain within the normal range, by switching off the production and secretion of thyrotropin.[1] An absence of symptoms was once part of the definition of subclinical hyperthyroidism, but we now understand that subtle symptoms or signs of thyrotoxicosis may be present. Subclinical hyperthyroidism is classified as endogenous in patients with thyroid hormone production associated with nodular thyroid disease or underlying Graves' disease; it is classified as exogenous in those with undetectable serum thyrotropin concentrations as a result of treatment with levothyroxine. Not all patients with undetectable serum thyrotropin concentrations and normal thyroxine and triiodothyronine concentrations have subclinical hyperthyroidism, and this combination of findings can be associated with various other conditions (Table 1).

Multinodular goiter is usually palpable, if not visible, and may be sufficiently large to cause compressive complications. Imaging with technetium-99m pertechnetate or iodine-123 generally shows "hot" (functioning) nodules and is particularly useful for detecting a single, impalpable, autonomously functioning adenoma. Most patients who present with

Table 1. Patterns of Thyroid Function Associated with a Suppressed Serum Thyrotropin Concentration and a Thyroid Hormone Concentration That May Be Normal.

Condition or Factor	Triiodothyronine		Thyroxine	
	Free	Total	Free	Total
Endogenous subclinical hyperthyroidism (associated with Graves' disease or nodular goiter)*	Upper end of normal range	Upper end of normal range	Upper end of normal range	Upper end of normal range
Exogenous subclinical hyperthyroidism (associated with levothyroxine therapy)	Normal	Normal	Upper end of normal range or elevated	Upper end of normal range or elevated
Nonthyroidal illness	Normal, low, or elevated†	Normal or low	Normal, low, or elevated‡	Normal, low, or elevated§
Drug therapy¶				
Dopamine	Normal	Normal	Normal	Normal
Corticosteroids	Normal	Normal	Normal	Normal
Amiodarone	Normal	Normal	Usually elevated but may be at upper end of normal range	Usually elevated but may be at upper end of normal range
Central hypothyroidism	Normal or low	Normal or low	Low end of normal range or low	Low end of normal range or low

* Subclinical hyperthyroidism may also be noted during the hyperthyroid phase of subacute, silent, or postpartum thyroiditis.
† In patients with nonthyroidal illness, the concentration of free triiodothyronine may be found to be elevated if a particular commercial assay system (Vitros ECi, Ortho Clinical Diagnostics) is used.
‡ The value depends on both the severity of the illness and the method of measurement used.
§ The value depends on the type and severity of the illness.
¶ Thyroid-function test results in patients with nonthyroidal illness may be influenced by concomitant drug therapy.

multinodular goiter have been aware of thyroid enlargement for several years, and they may have undergone partial thyroidectomy. The so-called simple, diffuse goiter observed in patients in their late teens and 20s tends to progress to a more obvious, multinodular goiter at around 40 years of age. As the goiter increases in size and as the autonomous nodules become larger and more numerous, subclinical or overt hyperthyroidism is increasingly present.[2]

Underlying Graves' disease may be present if a patient has a family history of the disorder or has other organ-specific autoimmune diseases, such as type 1 diabetes mellitus, vitiligo, pernicious anemia, myasthenia gravis, or Addison's disease, or if the patient has diffuse goiter, ophthalmopathy, or pretibial myxedema. Thyroid imaging with isotope methods shows an even distribution, and the results in patients with early-stage Graves' disease are likely to be similar to those in normal persons. The presence of thyrotropin-receptor antibodies in serum is diagnostic of Graves' disease, irrespective of the clinical findings, but the antibodies are absent in approximately 5 to 20 percent of patients with hyperthyroid Graves' disease, depending on the assay used,[3] and almost certainly in a greater proportion of those with subclinical hyperthyroidism.

STRATEGIES AND EVIDENCE

The issue of screening for thyroid disease in patients with few or no symptoms was discussed in a recent article in the *Journal*.[4] In view of the relatively high prevalence of unrecognized hypothyroidism in older adults, especially women, an expert panel of the American Thyroid Association has recommended routine screening of adults for thyroid disease by measurement of serum thyrotropin.[5] In hospital practice, thyroid-function testing has become almost routine. Such screening will inevitably identify patients with undetectable serum thyrotropin concentrations but normal thyroxine and triiodothyronine concentrations, although the prevalence of such findings is low. In one study, for example, involving 1210 patients over the age of 60 years who were seen at a single general practice in the United Kingdom and who were not taking thyroxine, serum thyrotropin concentrations were undetectable in 16 patients (1.3 percent).[6] During one year of follow-up, thyrotoxicosis developed in only one patient, and serum thyrotropin concentrations returned to normal in two patients. In some patients, the thyrotropin concentration may have been undetectable because of a transient nonthyroidal disorder or because of drug therapy for such a disorder.

The estimated rate of progression from subclinical to overt hyperthyroidism in patients with multinodular goiter is 5 percent each year,[7] and it may be significantly higher with the administration of iodine as a dietary supplement in areas where goiter is endemic, or with the use of the antiarrhythmic drug amiodarone, which contains iodine. Progression to prolonged overt hyperthyroidism in patients with underlying Graves' disease is probably less common, given the relapsing and remitting nature of Graves' disease and the eventual development of hypothyroidism in some patients.

If screening or the investigation of goiter shows that a patient has subclinical hyperthyroidism, should it be treated? Other than regular monitoring, the options for managing subclinical hyperthyroidism are the same as those for managing overt hyperthyroidism: the administration of antithyroid drugs (in patients with Graves' disease only) or iodine-131. Although iodine-131 uptake is likely to be lower in patients with subclinical hyperthyroidism than in those with overt hyperthyroidism, there is no evidence that a dose that is therapeutic in the second group is less effective in the first. Partial thyroidectomy would be indicated for a large multinodular goiter that caused mediastinal compression. One reason to treat subclinical hyperthyroidism is to prevent the development of overt hyperthyroidism. Prevention of atrial fibrillation and prevention of osteoporosis are the other chief potential benefits of treatment, but how good is the evidence of these preventive effects?

Atrial Fibrillation

The best evidence that subclinical hyperthyroidism is a risk factor for the development of atrial fibrillation comes from the Framingham Study.[8] A cohort of 2007 persons 60 years of age or older was followed for 10 years, and the development of atrial fibrillation was analyzed in relation to the initial concentration of serum thyrotropin. Among the 61 subjects with a thyrotropin concentration of less than 0.1 mU per liter and a normal serum thyroxine concentration at the outset, atrial fibrillation developed in 13, of whom an unspecified number were taking thyroxine. The relative risk of atrial fibrillation in this group of 61 subjects was 3.1 as compared with those who had a normal serum thyrotropin concentration (0.4 to 5.0 mU per liter); the risk was similar when the patients who were taking thyroxine were excluded from the analysis. A low but detectable serum thyrotropin concentration (0.1 to 0.4 mU per liter) was not associated with an increased risk of atrial fibrillation.

Assuming that antithyroid therapy would reduce the risk of dysrhythmia to that in the general population, 4.2 cases of subclinical hyperthyroidism would need to be treated to prevent 1 case of atrial fibrillation over a period of 10 years.[9] There is only limited evidence that established atrial fibrillation in patients with subclinical hyperthyroidism reverts spontaneously or after cardioversion once the serum thyrotropin concentration has been normalized with antithyroid therapy.[10]

Thyrotoxic atrial fibrillation is commonly considered a risk factor for systemic embolism, but the reported risk has ranged from negligible to 40 percent — extremes that do not reflect clinical experience. Even a risk of 10 percent probably represents an overestimate, since it is based on data obtained at a time when accurate tests of thyroid function were not widely available[11] and when an early diagnosis of hyperthyroidism was less likely than it is now. However, the available data suggest that among patients with atrial fibrillation that is unrelated to rheumatic heart disease, those with thyrotoxicosis have a higher rate of embolism than do patients without the condition. The risk of systemic embolism in patients with atrial fibrillation complicating subclinical hyperthyroidism is not known.

Osteoporosis

Frank hyperthyroidism is a recognized risk factor for osteoporosis, but the effects of subclinical hyperthyroidism on bone mineral density are less well defined. The increased bone turnover that is characteristic of Graves' disease persists during treatment with antithyroid drugs if serum thyrotropin concentrations remain suppressed, despite normal concentrations of thyroid hormones.[12] In two cross-sectional studies of patients with subclinical hyperthyroidism due to multinodular goiter, there was statistically and clinically significantly lower bone mineral density at the femoral neck and radius than in age-matched controls.[13,14] Whether these changes are associated with an increased rate of fracture is not known. More impressive are the reports that postmenopausal women with subclinical hyperthyroidism due to multinodular goiter have a 2 percent loss of bone mineral density each year, which can be reversed by treatment that restores serum thyrotropin concentrations to the normal range.[15,16]

A large meta-analysis of patients with exogenous subclinical hyperthyroidism showed that bone loss was greater among postmenopausal women with this condition than among those without it.[17] However, the validity of these results is questionable, since the study also found increased bone loss in premenopausal women who were receiving levothyroxine replacement therapy and who had normal serum thyrotropin concentrations. Furthermore, the increased risk of fracture reported in older women taking thyroid hormones disappears when those with a history of hyperthyroidism are excluded.[18] The evidence that exogenous subclinical hyperthyroidism is a risk factor for osteoporosis is therefore inconclusive.[19,20]

Other Considerations

Other abnormalities have been linked to both endogenous and exogenous subclinical hyperthyroidism. There is evidence that patients with subclinical hyperthyroidism due to multinodular goiter have increased left ventricular mass, increased systolic function, and impaired diastolic function, but the clinical significance of these observations is not known.[21] Impairment of the quality of life, as assessed with the use of a questionnaire, was also reported in these patients.[21] Whether normalization of the serum thyrotropin concentration improves these measures is uncertain. An increased risk of dementia and Alzheimer's disease was recently reported among patients with endogenous subclinical hyperthyroidism who were 55 years of age or older, particularly if antibodies against thyroid peroxidase were present[22]; this finding requires confirmation.

Patients receiving long-term suppressive therapy with levothyroxine have been reported to have diminished cardiac reserve and exertional capacity.[23] However, similar abnormalities were abolished by reducing the dose of levothyroxine to a level that was still associated with subclinical hyperthyroidism.[24] Short-term studies of small numbers of patients with exogenous subclinical hyperthyroidism have found changes in target-organ function — e.g., an increase in the nocturnal heart rate and an altered ratio of diurnal urinary sodium excretion to nocturnal excretion. These changes are similar to but less marked than those in overt hyperthyroidism[25] but may not be sustained in the long term.[26]

AREAS OF UNCERTAINTY

The natural history of subclinical hyperthyroidism remains unclear. Furthermore, the evidence that endogenous or exogenous subclinical hyperthyroidism is a risk factor for osteoporosis and atrial fibrillation is not definitive. However, it would be surprising if the complications of overt hyperthyroidism were not seen, albeit at a reduced frequency, in a condition that is effectively the mildest form of thyrotoxicosis; such complications are more likely to occur in patients with multinodular goiter, since the biochemical abnormality is persistent and the age of affected persons puts them at increased risk for bone loss or ischemic or structural heart disease.

The issue is further complicated by confusion over the meaning of subclinical hyperthyroidism, which is sometimes used to describe elevated serum thyroxine concentrations in patients who are taking thyroxine as replacement therapy. The inclusion of patients with wide ranges of thyroid-function test results and ratios of thyroxine to triiodothyronine may explain, at least in part, the disparate results of studies of target-organ function.

GUIDELINES

In its 1995 consensus statement on the treatment of patients with hyperthyroidism and hypothyroidism, the American Thyroid Association does not mention subclinical hyperthyroidism.[27] However, the association does state that in patients taking levothyroxine as replacement therapy, the dose should be adjusted to achieve clinical euthyroidism, with normal serum concentrations of both thyroxine and thyrotropin.[28] In statements issued in 1996 and 1998, respectively, the Royal College of Physicians of London[29] and the American College of Physicians[9] concluded that there is no agreement about the benefits of detecting and treating endogenous subclinical hyperthyroidism or about whether it causes excess morbidity. The statement of the American College of Physicians was based on a meta-analysis of available data. In contrast, the American Association of Clinical Endocrinologists[30] concluded that subclinical hyperthyroidism associated with goiter requires treatment in most cases.

RECOMMENDATIONS

In the absence of clinical signs of thyroid disease, and even after additional investigations such as isotope uptake and imaging and measurement of the thyrotropin-receptor antibody concentration, it may be difficult to decide whether the pattern seen on thyroid-function tests is a consequence of nonthyroidal illness and concomitant medication, underlying autonomous thyroid function, or the initial phase of thyroiditis. In such circumstances, thyroid-function tests should be repeated after eight weeks; a normal or elevated serum thyrotropin concentration at this time suggests recovery from nonthyroidal illness or the hypothyroid phase of thyroiditis. If the initial pattern persists, the choice should be made between a trial of antithyroid drugs and close clinical follow-up.

Exogenous Subclinical Hyperthyroidism

The dose of thyroxine should normally be reduced in patients with exogenous subclinical hyperthyroidism, excluding those with prior thyroid cancer, in whom thyrotropin suppression may be desired. The dose can usually be reduced abruptly to a more appropriate level. For example, in a symptomatic patient who has a markedly elevated serum free thyroxine concentration and a triiodothyronine concentration at the high end of the normal range while taking 250 μg of levothyroxine daily, it would be appropriate to reduce the dose to 150 μg daily and to retest thyroid function at a follow-up visit. The thyrotropin concentration may remain suppressed for six to eight weeks or more in patients with previous overreplacement of levothyroxine.

Although most patients feel well when thyroid function is normalized, a minority of patients have a sense of well-being only when taking a suppressive dose of levothyroxine.[31] In the absence of apparent complications of excess thyroid hormone, which would clearly warrant a dose reduction (Table 2), I would consider a slightly supratherapeutic dose acceptable as long as the serum triiodothyronine concentration remained well within the normal range.[29]

Endogenous Subclinical Hyperthyroidism

In many patients with endogenous subclinical hyperthyroidism who do not have nodular thyroid disease or complications of excess thyroid hormone, treatment is unnecessary, but thyroid-function tests should be performed every six months, with the recognition that the serum triiodothyronine concentration may become elevated before the serum thyrox-

---

Table 2. Indications for Reducing the Dose of Thyroxine in Patients with Exogenous Subclinical Hyperthyroidism.

New atrial fibrillation, angina, or cardiac failure

Accelerated loss of bone density

Oligomenorrhea, amenorrhea, or infertility

Nonspecific symptoms such as tiredness, hyperdefecation, and palpitations

Borderline high serum triiodothyronine concentration

ine concentration does. In patients with questionable symptoms, such as fatigue, I would use the empirical approach of a six-month trial with an antithyroid drug at a low dose, such as methimazole at a daily dose of 5 to 10 mg initially, and if this approach was effective, I would consider ablative therapy with iodine-131. To treat a woman who wanted to become pregnant, propylthiouracil at a dose of 50 mg twice a day would be more appropriate, because aplasia cutis congenita, a rare scalp defect, has been linked to the use of methimazole during pregnancy. The management of hyperthyroidism during pregnancy is beyond the scope of this review, but it would require extremely close monitoring and use of the lowest possible dose of propylthiouracil.[32] In older patients with atrial fibrillation or osteoporosis that could have been caused or exacerbated by the mild excess of thyroid hormone, ablative therapy with iodine-131 is the best initial option.

Treatment of patients with subclinical hyperthyroidism due to nodular thyroid disease is more routinely justified, given the expected progression to overt hyperthyroidism. The patient described in the vignette has both goiter and atrial fibrillation, two findings that warrant therapy. In the case of atrial fibrillation, I would first administer an antithyroid drug such as methimazole in order to restore the serum thyrotropin concentration to a normal value as quickly as possible. I would also administer warfarin because of the risk of systemic embolism, even though there are no data from controlled studies of anticoagulant therapy in patients with thyrotoxic atrial fibrillation. Careful monitoring of the dose is essential, since patients with overt hyperthyroidism and, presumably to a lesser degree, those with subclinical hyperthyroidism are more sensitive than euthyroid patients to the anticoagulant effects of warfarin. If sinus rhythm is not restored within four months after the normalization of the serum thyrotropin concentration, cardioversion should be performed.[33] The definitive treatment would be an ablative dose of iodine-131. In the case described, and in similar cases, this approach is warranted for several reasons: the potential contribution of subclinical hyperthyroidism to the development of osteoporosis, the low incidence of hypothyroidism after iodine-131 therapy in patients with multinodular goiter (6 percent at one year at my institution, as compared with 75 percent in patients with Graves' disease), the possibility of loss to follow-up and the attendant worsening of symptoms if treatment is withheld in favor of continued observation, and the likely cosmetic benefit of up to a 50 percent reduction in the size of the goiter at one to two years.[34,35]

This article first appeared in the August 16, 2001, issue of the New England Journal of Medicine.

REFERENCES

1.
Snyder PJ, Utiger RD. Inhibition of thyrotropin response to thyrotropin-releasing hormone by small quantities of thyroid hormones. J Clin Invest 1972;51:2077-84.
2.
Berghout A, Wiersinga WM, Smits NJ, Touber JL. Interrelationships between age, thyroid volume, thyroid nodularity, and thyroid function in patients with sporadic nontoxic goiter. Am J Med 1990;89:602-8.
3.
Costagliola S, Morgenthaler NG, Hoermann R, et al. Second generation assay for thyrotropin receptor antibodies has superior diagnostic sensitivity for Graves' disease. J Clin Endocrinol Metab 1999;84:90-7.
4.
Cooper DS. Subclinical hypothyroidism. N Engl J Med 2001;345:260-5.
5.
Ladenson PW, Singer PA, Ain KB, et al. American Thyroid Association guidelines for detection of thyroid dysfunction. Arch Intern Med 2000;160:1573-5.
6.
Parle JV, Franklyn JA, Cross KW, Jones SC, Sheppard MC. Prevalence and follow-up of abnormal thyrotrophin (TSH) concentrations in the elderly in the United Kingdom. Clin Endocrinol (Oxf) 1991;34:77-83.

7.
Wiersinga WM. Subclinical hypothyroidism and hyperthyroidism.I. Prevalence and clinical relevance. Neth J Med 1995;46:197-204.
8.
Sawin CT, Geller A, Wolf PA, et al. Low serum thyrotropin concentrations as a risk factor for atrial fibrillation in older patients. N Engl J Med 1994;331:1249-52.
9.
Helfand M, Redfern CC. Screening for thyroid disease: an update. Ann Intern Med 1998;129:144-58. [Erratum, Ann Intern Med 1999;130:246.]
10.
Forfar JC, Feek CM, Miller HC, Toft AD. Atrial fibrillation and isolated suppression of the pituitary-thyroid axis: response to specific antithyroid therapy. Int J Cardiol 1981;1:43-8.
11.
Staffurth JS, Gibberd MC, Fui SNG. Arterial embolism in thyrotoxicosis with atrial fibrillation. Br Med J 1977;2:688-90.
12.
Kumeda Y, Inaba M, Tahara H, et al. Persistent increase in bone turnover in Graves' patients with subclinical hyperthyroidism. J Clin Endocrinol Metab 2000;85:4157-61.
13.
Mudde AH, Reijnders FJL, Kruseman AC. Peripheral bone density in women with untreated multinodular goitre. Clin Endocrinol (Oxf) 1992;37:35-9.

14.
Földes J, Tarjan G, Szathmari M, Varga F, Krasznai I, Horvath CS. Bone mineral density in patients with endogenous subclinical hyperthyroidism: is this thyroid status a risk factor for osteoporosis? Clin Endocrinol (Oxf) 1993;39:521-7.
15.
Mudde AH, Houben AJHM, Nieuwenhuijzen Kruseman AC. Bone metabolism during anti-thyroid drug treatment of endogenous subclinical hyperthyroidism. Clin Endocrinol (Oxf) 1994;41:421-4.
16.
Faber J, Jensen IW, Petersen L, Nygaard B, Hegedus L, Siersbaek-Nielsen K. Normalization of serum thyrotrophin by means of radioiodine treatment in subclinical hyperthyroidism: effect on bone loss in postmenopausal women. Clin Endocrinol (Oxf) 1998;48:285-90.
17.
Uzzan B, Campos J, Cucherat M, Nony P, Boissel JP, Perret GY. Effects on bone mass of long term treatment with thyroid hormones: a meta-analysis. J Clin Endocrinol Metab 1996;81:4278-89.
18.
Cummings SR, Nevitt MC, Browner WS, et al. Risk factors for hip fracture in white women. N Engl J Med 1995;332:767-73.
19.
Toft AD. Thyroxine therapy. N Engl J Med 1994;331:174-80. [Erratum, N Engl J Med 1994;331:1035.]
20.
Franklyn JA, Betteridge J, Daykin J, et al. Long-term thyroxine treatment and bone mineral density. Lancet 1992;340:9-13.

21.
Biondi B, Palmieri EA, Fazio S, et al. Endogenous subclinical hyperthyroidism affects quality of life and cardiac morphology and function in young and middle-aged patients. J Clin Endocrinol Metab 2000;85:4701-5.
22.
Kalmijn S, Mehta KM, Pols HA, Hofman A, Drexhage HA, Breteler MM. Subclinical hyperthyroidism and the risk of dementia: the Rotterdam Study. Clin Endocrinol (Oxf) 2000;53:733-7.
23.
Biondi B, Fazio S, Cuocolo A, et al. Impaired cardiac reserve and exercise capacity in patients receiving long-term thyrotropin suppressive therapy with levothyroxine. J Clin Endocrinol Metab 1996;81:4224-8.
24.
Mercuro G, Panzuto MG, Bina A, et al. Cardiac function, physical exercise capacity, and quality of life during long-term thyrotropin-suppressive therapy with levothyroxine: effect of individual dose tailoring. J Clin Endocrinol Metab 2000;85:159-64.
25.
Bell GM, Todd WTA, Forfar JC, et al. End-organ responses to thyroxine therapy in subclinical hypothyroidism. Clin Endocrinol (Oxf) 1985;22:83-9.
26.
Nyström E, Lundberg P-A, Petersen K, Bengtsson C, Lindstedt G. Evidence for a slow tissue adaptation to circulating thyroxine in patients with chronic L-thyroxine treatment. Clin Endocrinol (Oxf) 1989;31:143-50.

27.
Singer PA, Cooper DS, Levy EG, et al. Treatment guidelines for patients with hyperthyroidism and hypothyroidism. JAMA 1995;273:808-12.

28.
Surks MI, Chopra IJ, Mariash CN, Nicoloff JT, Solomon DH. American Thyroid Association guidelines for use of laboratory tests in thyroid disorders. JAMA 1990;263:1529-32.

29.
Vanderpump MP, Ahlquist JA, Franklyn JA, Clayton RN. Consensus statement for good practice and audit measures in the management of hypothyroidism and hyperthyroidism. BMJ 1996;313:539-44.

30.
American Association of Clinical Endocrinologists releases clinical guidelines for thyroid disease. Am Fam Physician 1995;51:679-80.

31.
Carr D, McLeod DT, Parry G, Thornes HM. Fine adjustment of thyroxine replacement dosage: comparison of the thyrotrophin releasing hormone test using a sensitive thyrotrophin assay with measurement of free thyroid hormones and clinical assessment. Clin Endocrinol (Oxf) 1988;28:325-33.

32.
Haddow JE, Palomaki GE, Allan WC, et al. Maternal thyroid deficiency during pregnancy and subsequent neuropsychological development of the child. N Engl J Med 1999;341:549-55.

33.
Nakazawa HK, Sakurai K, Hamada N, Momotani N, Ito K. Management of atrial fibrillation in the post-thyrotoxic state. Am J Med 1982;72:903-6.

34.
Hegedus L, Hansen BM, Knudsen N, Hansen JM. Reduction of size of thyroid with radioactive iodine in multinodular non-toxic goitre. BMJ 1988;297:661-2.

35.
Le Moli R, Wesche MFT, Tiel-Van Buul MMC, Wiersinga WM. Determinants of longterm outcome of radioiodine therapy of sporadic non-toxic goitre. Clin Endocrinol (Oxf) 1999;50:783-9

Treatment of Tobacco Use and Dependence

NANCY A. RIGOTTI, M.D.

A 66-year-old woman with stable angina and a history of depression smokes 25 cigarettes daily. She would like to stop smoking but is concerned about weight gain. She has tried to quit several times on her own without success. What should her physician recommend?

THE CLINICAL PROBLEM

Tobacco use is the leading preventable cause of death in the United States, responsible for more than 400,000 deaths annually, or 1 of every 5 deaths.[1] Half of regular smokers die prematurely of a tobacco-related disease.[1] The potential health benefits of smoking cessation are substantial. Cessation reduces the risk of tobacco-related diseases, slows the progression of established tobacco-related diseases, and increases life expectancy, even when smokers stop smoking after the age of 65 years or after the development of a tobacco-related disease.[2]

An estimated 70 percent of smokers see a physician each year, providing physicians with substantial opportunity to influence smoking behavior.[3] However, that opportunity presents challenges, as the case vignette illustrates. Many patients continue to smoke despite knowing about or experiencing the health consequences of tobacco use. Some who try to quit repeatedly fail. Most mistakenly believe that stopping smoking requires only willpower and are unaware that effective treatments are available. To help smokers, physicians must be familiar with the spectrum of effective therapies. They must also appreciate that tobacco use has complex physiological and psychological determinants and understand that changing any behavior is a gradual process. Smoking is best regarded as a chronic disease that requires a long-term management strategy, rather than a quick fix.[3]

Currently, 23.5 percent of U.S. adults (25.7 percent of men and 21.5 percent of women) smoke cigarettes.[4] Nearly all smokers acknowledge that tobacco use is harmful to health but underestimate the magnitude of their own risk. Few know the full spectrum of health risks.[2,5] For many smokers, the risk of future disease does not outweigh the current perceived benefits of smoking or barriers to cessation. Yet 70 percent of smokers report that they want to quit.[2] Approximately one third of smokers try to stop smoking each year, but only 20 percent of them seek help.[2,6] Fewer than 10 percent of smokers who attempt to quit on their own are successful over the long term.[2,3] Smokers have a higher rate of success when they seek help with quitting.[6] Even then, several attempts are often required before long-term abstinence is achieved.[2]

The chief physiological obstacle to quitting is the addictive nature of nicotine. Nicotine causes tolerance and physical dependence. When tobacco use is stopped, there is a withdrawal syndrome characterized by irritability, anger, impatience, restlessness, difficulty concentrating, insomnia, increased appetite, anxiety, and depressed mood.[7] Symptoms of nicotine withdrawal are nonspecific, vary widely in intensity and duration, and are not correctly identified by smokers. Symptoms begin a few hours after the last cigarette, peak two to three days later, and wane over a period of several weeks or months.

Psychological factors also contribute to the difficulties that smokers have when they try to quit. Tobacco use is a learned behavior. Cigarettes become part of a smoker's daily routine, associated with events, such as finishing a meal, that become cues that trigger the desire to smoke. Smokers also use cigarettes to handle stress and negative emotions such as anger or anxiety. To stop smoking, a smoker must learn new coping skills and break old patterns, an incremental process in which attempts to quit often end in the resumption of smoking until abstinence is achieved.

STRATEGIES AND EVIDENCE

Two approaches have strong evidence of efficacy for smoking cessation: pharmacotherapy and counseling.[3,8,9] Each is effective by itself, but the two in combination achieve the highest rates of smoking cessation. The efficacy of a treatment correlates with its intensity, but even brief interventions by physicians during an office visit promote smoking cessation.

Interventions by Physicians

Randomized, controlled trials conducted in primary care practices demonstrate that a physician's advice to stop smoking increases the rates of smoking cessation among patients by approximately 30 percent.[8] Providing a brief period of counseling (three minutes or less) is more effective than simply advising the patient to quit and doubles the cessation rate, as compared with no intervention. Effective interventions have a common approach[3] (Figure 1). Optimal implementation requires support from the health care system to bolster the efforts of individual physicians.[8,10] Office-based systems that document every patient's smoking status before the patient sees the physician and remind

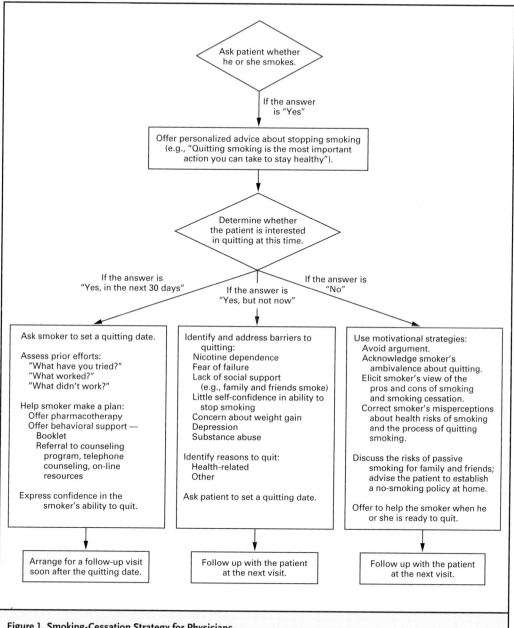

Figure 1. Smoking-Cessation Strategy for Physicians.

This strategy uses the five steps (the "five A's") recommended in Public Health Service guidelines[3]: ask, advise, assess, assist, and arrange follow-up.

the physician to address the use of tobacco by patients who smoke triple the likelihood that a physician will intervene.[8]

Counseling

Counseling about smoking cessation can be delivered effectively in person or by telephone.[8,9] Group or individual counseling is effective when it is provided by trained counselors and includes repeated contacts over a period of at least four weeks.[8] The efficacy of this approach increases as the amount of time spent with the patient increases.[8] Cognitive behavioral methods form the core of most counseling programs. Typically, smokers learn to identify smoking cues, then use cognitive and behavioral methods to break the link between the cues and smoking. They also learn strategies for coping with stress, managing symptoms of nicotine withdrawal, and once they quit, preventing relapse, such as anticipating tempting situations and rehearsing coping strategies.

Smoking-counseling strategies are also summarized in pamphlets and booklets, audiotapes, videotapes, and computer programs. Written self-help material has negligible efficacy when used alone but may augment other interventions.[8,9] Self-help material is more effective when its content is tailored to an individual patient's specific concerns or readiness to change.[8,9]

Pharmacotherapy

The Food and Drug Administration (FDA) has approved five products for smoking cessation: sustained-release bupropion and four nicotine-replacement products (gum, a transdermal patch, a nasal spray, and a vapor inhaler) (Table 1).[11] Each has demonstrated efficacy in randomized double-blind trials, approximately doubling the long-term (one-year) rates of abstinence, as compared with placebo.[8,9,11] Most clinical trials combine drug therapy with counseling; typical rates of smoking cessation are 40 to 60 percent at the end of drug treatment and 25 to 30 percent at one year.[8] Few randomized, controlled trials have directly compared one drug with another. Nortriptyline and clonidine have also been found to aid smoking cessation, but they have not been approved by the FDA for this indication.[8]

Nicotine-Replacement Therapy   Nicotine-replacement therapy provides an alternative form of nicotine to relieve symptoms of withdrawal in a smoker who is abstaining from tobacco use. The pharmacokinetic properties of available products differ, but none deliver nicotine to the circulation as fast as does inhaling cigarette smoke[11] (Figure 2). The patch provides a relatively stable, fixed dose of nicotine over a period of 16 or 24 hours. The other products have a more rapid onset and a shorter duration of action, allowing

Table 1. Drugs Used for Smoking Cessation.

Product	Daily Dose	Duration of Treatment	Common Side Effects	Advantages	Disadvantages
Nicotine-replacement therapy					
Transdermal patch*			Skin irritation, insomnia	Provides steady level of nicotine; easy to use; unobtrusive; available without prescription	User cannot adjust dose if craving occurs; nicotine released more slowly than in other products
24 hr (e.g., Nicoderm CQ)	7-, 14-, or 21-mg patch worn for 24 hr†	8 wk			
16 hr (e.g., Nicotrol)	15-mg patch worn for 16 hr	8 wk			
Nicotine polacrilex gum (Nicorette)* 2 mg (<25 cigarettes/day) 4 mg (≥25 cigarettes/day)	1 piece/hr (<24 pieces/day)	8–12 wk	Mouth irritation, sore jaw, dyspepsia, hiccups	User controls dose; oral substitute for cigarettes; available without prescription	Proper chewing technique needed to avoid side effects and achieve efficacy‡; user cannot eat or drink while chewing the gum; can damage dental work; difficult for denture wearers to use
Vapor inhaler (Nicotrol Inhaler)*	6–16 cartridges/day (delivered dose, 4 mg/cartridge)	3–6 mo	Mouth and throat irritation, cough	User controls dose; hand-to-mouth substitute for cigarettes	Frequent puffing needed; device visible when used
Nasal spray (Nicotrol NS)*	1–2 doses/hr (1 mg total; 0.5 mg in each nostril) (maximum, 40 mg/day)	3–6 mo	Nasal irritation; sneezing, cough, teary eyes	User controls dose; offers most rapid delivery of nicotine and the highest nicotine levels of all nicotine-replacement products	Most irritating nicotine-replacement product to use§; device visible when used
Non-nicotine therapy					
Sustained-release bupropion (Zyban or Wellbutrin SR)*	150 mg/day for 3 days, then 150 mg twice a day¶	7–12 wk (up to 6 mo to maintain abstinence)	Insomnia, dry mouth, agitation	Easy to use (pill), no exposure to nicotine	Increases risk of seizure (≤0.1 percent)
Nortriptyline‖	75–100 mg/day**	12 wk	Dry mouth, sedation, dizziness	Easy to use (pill), no exposure to nicotine	Side effects common; should be used cautiously in patients with coronary heart disease
Clonidine‖	0.1–0.3 mg twice a day	3–10 wk	Dry mouth, sedation, dizziness	No exposure to nicotine	Side effects limit use

* This product has been approved by the Food and Drug Administration as a smoking-cessation aid. The Public Health Service clinical guidelines also recommend it as a first-line drug for smoking cessation.[8]

† The starting dose is 21 mg per day unless the smoker weighs less than 45.5 kg (100 lb) or smokes fewer than 10 cigarettes per day, in which case the starting dose is 14 mg per day. The starting dose should be maintained for four weeks, after which the dose should be decreased every week until it is stopped.

‡ The user should chew the gum slowly until he or she experiences a distinct taste, indicating that nicotine is being released. The user should then place the gum between cheek and gum until the taste disappears to allow the nicotine to be absorbed through oral mucosa. The sequence should be repeated for 30 minutes before the gum is discarded. Acidic beverages (such as coffee and soft drinks) reduce the absorption of nicotine and should be avoided for 30 minutes before and during chewing.

§ Tolerance develops to local side effects during the first week of use.

¶ Treatment should be started one week before the quitting date.

‖ This agent has not been approved by the Food and Drug Administration as a smoking-cessation aid. The Public Health Service clinical guidelines recommend it as a second-line drug for smoking cessation.[8]

**Treatment should be started 10 to 28 days before the quitting date at a dose of 25 mg per day, and the dose should be increased as tolerated.

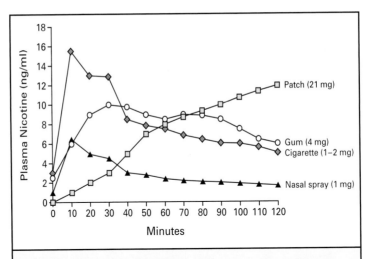

Figure 2. Plasma Nicotine Levels after a Smoker Has Smoked a Cigarette, Received Nicotine Nasal Spray, Begun Chewing Nicotine Gum, or Applied a Nicotine Patch.

The amount of nicotine in each product is given in parentheses. The pattern produced by the use of the nicotine inhaler (not shown) is similar to that for nicotine gum. Modified from Garrett et al.[12]

the user to adjust the dose of nicotine. Blood nicotine levels peak 5 to 10 minutes after the administration of nicotine nasal spray, 20 minutes after the user begins chewing nicotine gum or uses a vapor inhaler, and 2 to 4 hours after the application of a nicotine patch. The nicotine gum and the inhaler have similar pharmacokinetic properties since in both the nicotine is absorbed through the oral mucosa.

The use of all nicotine-replacement products increases the long-term rates of smoking cessation and relieves cravings for nicotine and the symptoms of nicotine withdrawal. In meta-analyses of placebo-controlled trials, the nicotine patch doubled the long-term smoking-cessation rate. The use of nicotine gum increases cessation rates by 50 to 70 percent.[8,9] For heavy smokers (those who smoke at least 25 cigarettes per day), the gum that contains 4 mg of nicotine per piece is more effective than that containing 2 mg per piece. Fewer studies have assessed the nasal spray and the vapor inhaler, but in meta-analyses both products doubled the cessation rates, as compared with placebo inhaler.

One randomized, controlled trial directly compared the four nicotine-replacement products.[13] The efficacy of each product was similar at week 12 of follow-up, but the rates of compliance varied, being highest for the patch, intermediate for the gum, and lowest for the vapor inhaler and the nasal spray. Studies consistently report higher rates of smoking cessation when nicotine-replacement therapy is combined with counseling, although the former is effective even when used alone.[8,9,11] Different nicotine-replacement products can be combined safely. In some studies, combining the nicotine patch with gum, inhaler, or nasal spray was more efficacious than the use of any of these products alone.[8,9,14]

The safety of nicotine-replacement products is underscored by the fact that the patch and gum, initially sold only by prescription, are now available without a prescription. Although nicotine's hemodynamic effects increase the myocardial workload, nicotine-replacement therapy is safe in patients with cardiovascular disease, including stable angina.[15,16] The safety of nicotine-replacement therapy has not been studied in patients with unstable angina or in those who have had a myocardial infarction within two weeks before treatment, but the risk of cardiac complications should be lower than with smoking. Unlike smoking, nicotine-replacement therapy does not increase the coagulability of blood or expose a patient to carbon monoxide or oxidizing gases that damage endothelium.[17] The side effects of these products vary according to the manner in which nicotine is administered (Table 1).

Non-Nicotine Therapy   Bupropion, an antidepressant with dopaminergic and noradrenergic activity, was efficacious for smoking cessation when combined with counseling in randomized, controlled trials.[18,19] The efficacy of bupropion when accompanied by minimal levels of psychosocial support, as occurs in medical practice, is unknown. Like nicotine-replacement therapy, treatment with bupropion doubles smoking-cessation rates as compared with placebo treatment.[8,9,11] Bupropion lowers the threshold for seizure and is contraindicated in patients who are at risk for seizures. The risk of seizure associated with the use of bupropion is 0.1 percent or less.[8,9] In one randomized, placebo-controlled trial that directly compared bupropion alone or in combination with the nicotine patch,[19] bupropion produced a significantly higher rate of abstinence at one year than either the nicotine patch or placebo. Treatment with both bupropion and the nicotine patch was safe but did not lead to significantly higher cessation rates than did treatment with bupropion alone (36 percent and 30 percent, respectively). Nonetheless, many clinicians use the combination for smokers who are very dependent on nicotine.

Nortriptyline was effective for smoking cessation in two small studies that used 75 to 100 mg daily for three months, starting 10 to 28 days before the quitting date.[20,21] No other antidepressant has had demonstrated efficacy for use in smoking cessation in a published trial,[8,9] nor are there data to support the use of anxiolytic agents for smoking cessation.[8,9] Treatment with clonidine reduces the symptoms of nicotine withdrawal and has been effective for smoking cessation, but the high frequency of adverse effects limits its use.[8,9]

Other Methods

Hypnosis and acupuncture have also been suggested as therapies for smoking cessation. However, few controlled trials of hypnosis have been conducted,[8,9] and acupuncture was found to be ineffective in randomized trials.[8,9]

Weight Gain after Smoking Cessation

Weight gain averages 2.3 to 4.5 kg (5 to 10 lb) after smoking cessation and is thus a concern for many smokers who are contemplating quitting, especially women.[2,22] Large weight gains (more than 13 kg [29 lb]) are uncommon, but are more likely in women, nonwhites, and heavy smokers than in other groups.[23] A large weight gain does not negate the benefits of smoking cessation, but this point rarely comforts smokers who are concerned about their weight. In one study, a weight-management program did not avert post-cessation weight gain.[24] Vigorous exercise reduced weight gain and increased abstinence rates in one trial.[25] Whether moderate physical activity has similar benefits is unknown, but exercise has sufficient merits on its own to be recommended routinely. Bupropion and, in some studies, nicotine gum (but not the nicotine patch) temporarily reduced weight gain after smoking cessation, but only while the drug was being administered.[17,22]

AREAS OF UNCERTAINTY

Most treatment studies have been conducted in healthy adults who were motivated to stop smoking. Effective treatment for adolescent smokers, for smokers who are not interested in quitting smoking, or for those who repeatedly fail to quit is unclear. For smokers who are reluctant to attempt cessation, experts recommend "motivational interviewing," a counseling technique developed to help people prepare for a change in behavior.[26] The counselor builds empathy by acknowledging a smoker's ambivalence about stopping smoking, supports the smoker's autonomy with respect to making a responsible decision, and bolsters a smoker's self-confidence so that he or she can make a change. The technique is promising and reasonable, but it has not yet been proved to increase cessation rates.

Characteristics associated with a low rate of successful treatment include coexisting psychiatric conditions (current or past depression or schizophrenia), alcohol or substance abuse, strong nicotine dependence, lack of social support for quitting (e.g., a spouse who smokes), and a low level of confidence in one's ability to quit.[8,9] The optimal treatment for such persons is also not known. Most experts advise the use of more intensive treatments for longer periods.

Current and past major depression are more common in smokers than nonsmokers.[27] Smokers with a history of depression who attempt to quit smoking not only have lower rates of success but also have more depressive symptoms during nicotine withdrawal and a greater risk of recurrent depression after cessation than do smokers with no history of depression.[28] The optimal treatment for smokers with current or past depression is uncertain, but they may require longer and more intensive treatment.[9] Bupropion and nortriptyline are effective in smokers with a history of depression.[8,9] Nicotine-replacement therapy may also be effective in such patients.[29,30] Psychological support appears to be important.[31]

GUIDELINES

Two sets of clinical-practice guidelines based on independent, systematic reviews of the evidence were released in 2000. The Public Health Service's *Treating Tobacco Use and Dependence* (available at http://www.surgeongeneral.gov/tobacco)[8] updated a 1996 clinical-practice guideline issued by the Agency for Health Care Policy and Research.[32] The guidelines issued by Britain's Health Education Authority draw on systematic reviews by the Cochrane Collaboration's Tobacco Addiction Review group (available at http://www.cochrane.org/cochrane/revabstr).[9,33,34] The 1996 guidelines of the Preventive Services Task Force are consistent with newer guidelines except that they do not address newer types of pharmacotherapy (available at http://www.odphp.osophs.dhhs.gov/pubs/guidecps).[35] In 2001, the Task Force on Community Preventive Services of the Centers for Disease Control and Prevention released evidence-based guidelines for interventions at the level of the health care system (available at http://www.thecommunityguide.org).[10] The rate at which physicians provide advice on smoking cessation to their patients is now a standard measure for assessing the quality of care delivered by U.S. health plans.[36]

Guidelines consistently recommend that physicians assess and record patients' smoking status; advise smokers to quit; assess their readiness to do so; and assist smokers by offering support, pharmacotherapy (a nicotine-replacement product or bupropion), and referrals to cessation resources. Health care delivery systems (including hospitals) are directed to identify patients' smoking status, offer smoking-cessation services, and document these actions. The Public Health Service guidelines urge health insurers to cover all recommended treatments, including counseling and pharmacotherapy.[8]

CONCLUSIONS AND RECOMMENDATIONS

There is broad agreement, based on strong evidence, about what constitutes effective treatment of tobacco use and dependence. Physicians should routinely identify patients' smoking status and readiness to quit, advise and assist smokers to quit, and offer pharmacotherapy to help them quit (Figure 1).[8] There is insufficient evidence to determine whether nicotine-replacement products or bupropion is superior. Current guidelines and most experts regard them as roughly equivalent.[8,9,11] The choice of pharmacotherapy (Table 1) should take the patient's preferences and past experiences into consideration, unless one agent is contraindicated. A general approach is to start with a single agent and add a second if the smoker has severe withdrawal symptoms, cravings, or difficulty maintaining abstinence. Nicotine-replacement products can safely be combined with one another and with bupropion. Drugs are most effective when accompanied by counseling, whether delivered in person or by telephone. The addition of pharmacotherapy to counseling doubles the cessation rate.[11] Counseling is also effective by itself and should not be neglected.

The case vignette highlights common challenges facing physicians who treat smokers. The patient has repeatedly failed to quit smoking on her own, she has coexisting medical and psychiatric conditions, and she is concerned about gaining weight if she does quit smoking.[37] Often, smokers who repeatedly fail to quit have never received effective treatments (especially counseling) or have used pharmacotherapy incorrectly. Such patients may also have coexisting psychiatric conditions or substance abuse. When a smoker has a history of depression, careful screening for symptoms of depression is warranted before and during treatment.

In the case of the woman described in the clinical vignette, intensive treatment combining counseling with one or more drugs is warranted; bupropion may be a good choice, since it has proved effective in depressed patients. Strong symptoms of nicotine withdrawal should be expected but can be relieved by pharmacotherapy. The use of two or more products may be necessary. Even though she has stable angina, the patient can safely use either nicotine-replacement therapy or bupropion. She may reduce her risk of weight gain after smoking cessation by participating in a program of moderate exercise and by using bupropion, nicotine gum, or both.

Smoking is a chronic problem, like hypertension or hyperlipidemia, that requires long-term management.[3] Assistance with smoking cessation is a cost-effective intervention that is underused by physicians and inadequately covered by many health insurers.[38,39] For physicians and health care systems alike, the challenge is implementing effective treatment in routine medical practice.

Supported by a Mid-Career Investigator Award in Patient-Oriented Research from the National Heart, Lung, and Blood Institute (HL04440).

This article first appeared in the February 14, 2002, issue of the New England Journal of Medicine.

REFERENCES

1.
Tobacco use — United States, 1900–1999. MMWR Morb Mortal Wkly Rep 1999;48:986-93. [Erratum, MMWR Morb Mortal Wkly Rep 1999;48:1027.]

2.
Department of Health and Human Services. The health benefits of smoking cessation: a report of the Surgeon General. Washington, D.C.: Government Printing Office, 1990. (DHHS publication no. (CDC) 90-8416.)

3.
A clinical practice guideline for treating tobacco use and dependence: a US Public Health Service report. JAMA 2000;283:3244-54.

4.
Cigarette smoking among adults — United States, 1999. MMWR Morb Mortal Wkly Rep 2001;50:869-73.

5.
Ayanian JZ, Cleary PD. Perceived risks of heart disease and cancer among cigarette smokers. JAMA 1999;281:1019-21.

6.
Zhu SH, Melcer T, Sun J, Rosbrook B, Pierce JP. Smoking cessation with and without assistance: a population-based analysis. Am J Prev Med 2000;18:305-11.

7.
Diagnostic and statistical manual of mental disorders, 4th ed.: DSM-IV. Washington, D.C.: American Psychiatric Association, 1994.

8.
Fiore MC, Bailey WC, Cohen SJ, et al. Treating tobacco use and dependence. Rockville, Md.: Department of Health and Human Services, Public Health Service, 2000. (Also available at http://www.surgeongeneral.gov/tobacco.)

9.
Lancaster T, Stead L, Silagy C, Sowden A. Effectiveness of interventions to help people stop smoking: findings from the Cochrane Library. BMJ 2000;321:355-8.

10.
Recommendations regarding interventions to reduce tobacco use and exposure to environmental tobacco smoke. Am J Prev Med 2001;20:Suppl:10-5. (Also available at http://www.thecommunityguide.org.)

11.
Hughes JR, Goldstein MG, Hurt RD, Schiffman S. Recent advances in the pharmacotherapy of smoking. JAMA 1999;281:72-6.

12.
Garrett BE, Rose CA, Henningfield JE. Tobacco addiction and pharmacological interventions. Expert Opin Pharmacother 2001;2:1548.

13.
Hajek P, West R, Foulds J, Nilsson F, Burrows S, Meadow A. Randomized comparative trial of nicotine polacrilex, a transdermal patch, nasal spray, and an inhaler. Arch Intern Med 1999;159:2033-8.

14.
Bohadana A, Nilsson F, Rasmussen T, Martinet Y. Nicotine inhaler and nicotine patch as a combination therapy for smoking cessation: a randomized, double-blind, placebo-controlled trial. Arch Intern Med 2000;160:3128-34.

15.
Joseph AM, Norman SM, Ferry LH, et al. The safety of transdermal nicotine as an aid to smoking cessation in patients with cardiac disease. N Engl J Med 1996;335:1792-8.

16.
Working Group for the Study of Transdermal Nicotine in Patients with Coronary Artery Disease. Nicotine replacement therapy for patients with coronary artery disease. Arch Intern Med 1994;154:989-95.

17.
Benowitz NL, Gourlay SG. Cardiovascular toxicity of nicotine: implications for nicotine replacement therapy. J Am Coll Cardiol 1997;29:1422-31.

18.
Hurt RD, Sachs DPL, Glover ED, et al. A comparison of sustained-release bupropion and placebo for smoking cessation. N Engl J Med 1997;337:1195-202.

19.
Jorenby DE, Leischow SJ, Nides MA, et al. A controlled trial of sustained-release bupropion, a nicotine patch, or both for smoking cessation. N Engl J Med 1999;340:685-91.

20.
Prochazka AV, Weaver MJ, Keller RT, Fryer GE, Licari PA, Lofaso D. A randomized trial of nortriptyline for smoking cessation. Arch Intern Med 1998;158:2035-9.

21.
Hall SM, Reus VI, Muñoz RF, et al. Nortriptyline and cognitive-behavioral therapy in the treatment of cigarette smoking. Arch Gen Psychiatry 1998;55:683-90.

22.
Rigotti NA. Treatment options for the weight-conscious smoker. Arch Intern Med 1999;159:1169-71.

23.
Williamson DF, Madans J, Anda RF, Kleinman JC, Giovino GA, Byers T. Smoking cessation and severity of weight gain in a national cohort. N Engl J Med 1991;324:739-45.

24.
Hall SM, Tunstall CD, Vila KL, Duffy J. Weight gain prevention and smoking cessation: cautionary findings. Am J Public Health 1992;82:799-803.

25.
Marcus BH, Albrecht AE, King TK, et al. The efficacy of exercise as an aid for smoking cessation in women: a randomized controlled trial. Arch Intern Med 1999;159:1229-34.

26.
Miller WR, Rollnick S. Motivational interviewing: preparing people to change addictive behavior. New York: Guilford Press, 1991.

27.
Lasser K, Boyd JW, Woolhandler S, Himmelstein DU, McCormick D, Bor DH. Smoking and mental illness: a population-based prevalence study. JAMA 2000;284:2606-10.

28.
Glassman AH, Helzer JE, Covey LS, et al. Smoking, smoking cessation, and major depression. JAMA 1990;264:1546-9.

29.
Kinnunen T, Doherty K, Militello FS, Garvey AJ. Depression and smoking cessation: characteristics of depressed smokers and effects of nicotine replacement. J Consult Clin Psychol 1996;64:791-8.

30.
Stapleton JA, Russell MA, Feyerabend C, et al. Dose effects and predictors of outcome in a randomized trial of transdermal nicotine patches in general practice. Addiction 1995;90:31-42.

31.
Hall SM, Munoz RF, Reus VI, et al. Mood management and nicotine gum in smoking treatment: a therapeutic contact and placebo-controlled study. J Consult Clin Psychol 1996; 64:1003-9.

32.
The Agency for Health Care Policy and Research. Smoking cessation clinical practice guideline. JAMA 1996;275:1270-80.

33.
West R, McNeill A, Raw M. Smoking cessation guidelines for health professionals: an update. Thorax 2000;55:987-99.

34.
Raw M, McNeill A, West R. Smoking cessation guidelines for health professionals: a guide to effective smoking cessation interventions for the health care system. Thorax 1998;53: Suppl 5:S1-S19.

35.
Preventive Services Task Force. Guide to clinical preventive services: report of the U.S. Preventive Services Task Force. 2nd ed. Baltimore: Williams & Wilkins, 1996.

36.
The state of managed care quality, 2000. Washington, D.C.: National Committee for Quality Assurance, 2000:28.

37.
Rigotti NA. A 36-year-old woman who smokes cigarettes. JAMA 2000;284:741-9.

38.
Cromwell J, Bartosch WJ, Fiore MC, Hasselblad V, Baker T. Cost-effectiveness of the clinical practice recommendations in the AHCPR guideline for smoking cessation. JAMA 1997;278:1759-66.

39.
Thorndike AN, Rigotti NA, Stafford RS, Singer DE. National patterns in the treatment of smokers by physicians. JAMA 1998;279:604-8.

Aortic Stenosis

BLASE A. CARABELLO, M.D.

A 60-year-old man is evaluated for a heart murmur. He jogs 3 mi (5 km) per day and is asymptomatic. Physical examination reveals a delayed carotid upstroke, a 3/6 late-peaking systolic ejection murmur that radiates to the neck, and a single S_2. An echocardiogram shows normal systolic function and a heavily calcified aortic valve. The patient's peak Doppler transvalvular gradient is 64 mm Hg, with a mean gradient of 50 mm Hg. His calculated valve area is 0.7 cm². How should this patient be treated?

THE CLINICAL PROBLEM

Aortic stenosis is the most common cardiac-valve lesion in the United States. Two factors account for its common occurrence: approximately 1 to 2 percent of the population is born with a bicuspid aortic valve, which is prone to stenosis; and aortic stenosis develops with age, and the population is aging.

The clinician is usually first alerted to the presence of aortic stenosis by the finding of a systolic ejection murmur at the right upper sternal border that radiates to the neck. Clues that the disease is at least moderate in severity are peaking of the murmur late in systole, palpable delay of the carotid upstroke, and a soft single second heart sound, because the aortic component of S_2 disappears when the valve no longer opens or closes well.

Although once thought of as a degenerative lesion, calcific aortic stenosis has many features in common with coronary disease.[1] Both conditions are more common in men, older persons, and patients with hypercholesterolemia, and both derive in part from an active inflammatory process.[2]

Aortic stenosis is distinguished from aortic sclerosis by the degree of valve impairment. In aortic sclerosis, the valve leaflets are abnormally thickened, but obstruction to outflow is minimal, whereas in aortic stenosis, the functional area of the valve has decreased enough to cause measurable obstruction of outflow. Little hemodynamic disturbance occurs as the valve area is reduced from the normal 3 to 4 cm² to 1.5 to 2 cm². However, as shown in Table 1, an additional reduction in the valve area from half its normal size to

Table 1. Relation of the Aortic-Valve Area to the Mean Gradient.*

Aortic-Valve Area	Mean Gradient
cm^2	$mm\ Hg$
4	1.7
3	2.9
2	6.6
1	26
0.9	32
0.8	41
0.7	53
0.6	73
0.5	105

*Data were derived with the Gorlin formula: aortic-valve area =

$$\frac{cardiac\ output \div (systolic\ ejection\ period \times heart\ rate)}{44.3\ \sqrt{mean\ gradient}}$$

where the cardiac output was assumed to be 6 liters per minute, the systolic ejection period was assumed to be 0.33 second, and the heart rate was assumed to be 80 beats per minute.

one quarter of its normal size produces severe obstruction to flow and a progressive pressure overload on the left ventricle. The concentric hypertrophy that develops in response to this overload is both adaptive and maladaptive. Whereas the increased muscle mass allows the ventricle to generate the increased force necessary to propel blood past the obstruction, the hypertrophied myocardium has decreased coronary blood flow reserve[3] (even in the presence of normal epicardial coronary arteries) and can also cause both diastolic and systolic left ventricular dysfunction, producing the symptoms of congestive heart failure.[4,5] The obvious question for the physician is when is the optimal time for clinical intervention? Although aortic stenosis often coexists with other valvular diseases, this review focuses on isolated aortic stenosis.

STRATEGIES AND EVIDENCE

There is no effective medical therapy for severe aortic stenosis; aortic stenosis is a mechanical obstruction to blood flow that requires mechanical correction. In children with congenital aortic stenosis, the valve leaflets are merely fused, and balloon valvotomy may offer substantial benefit.[6] In adults with calcified valves, however, balloon valvot-

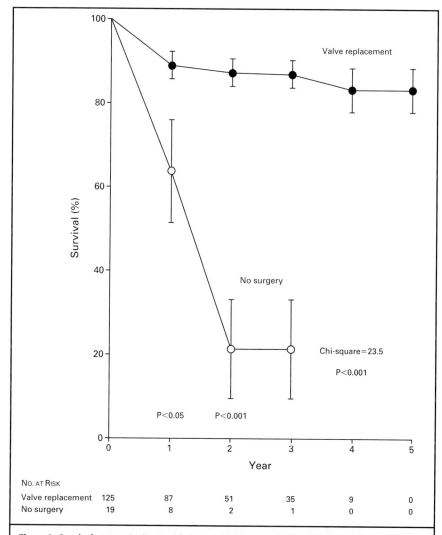

Figure 1. Survival among Patients with Severe Symptomatic Aortic Stenosis Who Underwent Valve Replacement and Similar Patients Who Declined to Undergo Surgery.

The overall and individual P values are shown, as is the overall chi-square value. Reprinted from Schwarz et al.[11] with the permission of the publisher.

omy only temporarily relieves symptoms and does not prolong survival.[7] Thus, the intervention required in adults, other than standard prophylactic antibiotics against infective endocarditis,[8] is the replacement of the valve. The risks of replacing that valve must be weighed against the risks of delaying the procedure. The procedure can usually be delayed until symptoms develop.[9,10] Studies of aortic stenosis uniformly demonstrate that once angina, syncope, dyspnea, or other symptoms of heart failure develop and are found to be due to aortic stenosis, the patient's life span is drastically shortened unless the valve is replaced (Figure 1). Of the 35 percent of patients with aortic stenosis who present with angina, half will die within five years in the absence of aortic-valve replacement. Of the 15 percent of patients who present with syncope, half will die within three years, and of the 50 percent of patients who present with dyspnea, half will die within two years, unless the aortic valve is replaced. In contrast, 10-year age-corrected rates of survival among patients who have undergone aortic-valve replacement approach the rate in the normal population.[11,12]

The striking contrast between the excellent prognosis after aortic-valve replacement and the dismal prognosis in the absence of replacement in symptomatic patients makes the presence or absence of symptoms the crucial factor with respect to management. In general, the clinician can be confident that, in a given patient, the symptoms are due to aortic stenosis if the mean aortic-valve gradient exceeds 50 mm Hg or if the aortic-valve area is no larger than 1 cm^2. I will use these as criteria for severe disease, although there is no universally accepted definition that relies on valve area or gradient.

AREAS OF UNCERTAINTY

Management of Severe Asymptomatic Aortic Stenosis

There is overwhelming evidence that patients with severe aortic stenosis who become symptomatic require prompt aortic-valve replacement. Conversely, asymptomatic patients, even those with severe disease, generally have an excellent prognosis without aortic-valve replacement. Unfortunately, approximately 1 to 2 percent of asymptomatic patients die suddenly or have a very rapid rate of progression to the symptomatic state and then to sudden death.[9,10,13,14] Thus, the question arises whether patients with severe asymptomatic aortic stenosis should undergo aortic-valve replacement to protect them from sudden death. Although some experts advocate this approach, this strategy exposes the entire group of asymptomatic patients with severe aortic stenosis to the risk of perioperative and valve-related complications and death. Even in the best of circumstances, the surgical mortality rate is approximately 1 percent and the risk of a valve-related complication (including thromboembolism; bleeding during therapy with anticoagulants; deterioration of the prosthetic valve, requiring reoperation; and infective endocarditis) is 1 percent per year.[15]

Echocardiography and exercise testing may identify asymptomatic patients who are likely to benefit from surgery. Otto et al.[16] found that patients with asymptomatic aortic stenosis whose peak transaortic blood flow velocity exceeded 4 m per second (a peak gradient of 64 mm Hg) had a risk of becoming symptomatic and requiring aortic-valve replacement of 70 percent within two years. None of the patients in this moderate-sized series died suddenly, and all underwent exercise testing.

Although exercise testing is unwarranted and dangerous in patients with symptomatic aortic stenosis, it has proved safe in patients with moderate-to-severe asymptomatic aortic stenosis.[16,17] A preliminary report suggests that exercise testing may identify some patients with latent symptoms or exercise-induced hemodynamic instability, facilitating timely aortic-valve replacement. In a study of 58 asymptomatic patients,[18] 21 had symptoms for the first time during the exercise test. Most likely, these patients had failed to recognize the symptoms previously or had not engaged in activities that would have precipitated symptoms. Although patients with asymptomatic aortic stenosis can exercise safely under a physician's scrutiny, it seems most unwise to permit patients with moderate-to-severe aortic stenosis to engage in vigorous, unmonitored exercise in view of the limitations imposed by left ventricular hypertrophy on coronary blood flow.

Treatment of the Patient with a Low Gradient and Reduced Ejection Fraction

In patients with left ventricular dysfunction who have a substantial transvalvular gradient (a mean gradient of more than 40 mm Hg), the outcome of surgery is excellent despite the presence of a reduced ejection fraction preoperatively.[19] In these patients, the excessive afterload generated by the obstructing valve is a prime contributor to the left ventricular dysfunction. Once the obstruction is removed and the afterload is reduced, left ventricular function returns to or approaches normal.

Patients with a reduced ejection fraction and a small transvalvular gradient (less than 30 mm Hg)[19,20] have a high operative risk, and only half such patients are alive three to four years after surgery.[21] The poor outcome in these patients is related to the presence of both severely depressed myocardial contractility and the excessive afterload.[19]

Although the overall prognosis for this group of patients is poor, some patients in this category, presumably those with severe valve obstruction, benefit from surgery.[21,22] In other patients, the calculated valve area may be severely reduced because cardiomyopathy inhibits the left ventricle from completely opening a mildly but not a severely stenotic valve. The presence of low output may lead clinicians to the false conclusion that the valve is severely stenotic (aortic pseudostenosis).[23-25] The best method for distinguishing these two conditions is to increase cardiac output during Doppler echocardiography or cardiac catheterization and to use the new data to recalculate the valve area. In the case of pseudostenosis, increased output causes a large increase in the calculated valve area, often to more than 1 cm^2. In this group of patients, valve replacement is unlikely to be beneficial. Conversely, patients in whom increased cardiac output produces a substantial increase in gradient have a true outflow obstruction and may benefit from surgery. Patients with a low gradient who have no response to inotropic stimulation have a poor outcome, presumably because the myocardial damage is so far advanced.[26]

Safety of Cardiac Surgery in Patients with Mild-to-Moderate Aortic Stenosis

Controversy also exists regarding the optimal approach to patients with mild-to-moderate aortic stenosis (as indicated by a transvalvular gradient in the range of 10 to 30 mm Hg and a valve area of more than 1 cm^2) who require cardiac surgery for some other cause, usually coronary revascularization. Concomitant aortic-valve replacement increases the risk of both perioperative death and complications related to the prosthetic valve. However, if the native valve is left in place, aortic stenosis may progress so rapidly that another cardiac surgery is required despite the fact that the bypass grafts are functioning normally.[27] Unfortunately, there is wide individual variability in the rate of disease progression,[27-29] virtually precluding prognostication of the course of a given patient. Concomitant aortic-valve replacement is considered unwise if it is likely to increase the gradient even further.

Safety of Noncardiac Surgery in Patients with Severe Asymptomatic Aortic Stenosis

On the basis of a small number of adverse events, one study indicated that noncardiac surgery posed an increased risk among patients with aortic stenosis.[30] However, O'Keefe et al. examined the course of 48 patients with severe aortic stenosis who underwent noncardiac surgery[31] and found that there were no complications in the 25 patients who had local anesthesia and only one complication in the 23 patients who received general anesthesia. Thus, although intraoperative hemodynamics must be closely monitored during noncardiac surgery in patients with asymptomatic aortic stenosis, there is no apparent need for concomitant aortic-valve intervention.

Ability to Slow or Halt Progression of the Valve Lesion

As noted above, the lesion of aortic stenosis shares many features with coronary disease. Although recent data suggest that hydroxymethylglutaryl coenzyme A reductase inhibitors (referred to as "statins") can retard the progression of aortic stenosis,[32] in my opinion it is a bit too early to begin prescribing statins for this purpose.

> **Table 2.** Recommendations for the Use of Aortic-Valve Replacement in Patients with Aortic Stenosis.
>
> **Aortic-valve replacement indicated**
>
> Patients with severe aortic stenosis and any of its classic symptoms (angina, syncope, or dyspnea)
>
> Patients with severe aortic stenosis who are undergoing coronary-artery bypass surgery
>
> Patients with severe aortic stenosis who are undergoing surgery on the aorta or other heart valves
>
> **Aortic-valve replacement possibly indicated**
>
> Patients with only moderate aortic stenosis who require coronary-artery bypass surgery or surgery on the aorta or other heart valves
>
> Asymptomatic patients with severe aortic stenosis and at least one of the following: an ejection fraction of no more than 0.50, hemodynamic instability during exercise (e.g., hypotension), or ventricular tachycardia*

* Aortic-valve replacement is not indicated to prevent sudden death in asymptomatic patients who have none of the findings listed.

GUIDELINES

Guidelines for the use of valve replacement in patients with aortic stenosis are provided in Table 2. In 1998 the American Heart Association and American College of Cardiology issued guidelines for the treatment of valvular heart disease (available at http://www.americanheart.org).[8] These guidelines recommend the use of standard antibiotic prophylaxis against infective endocarditis. Doppler echocardiography is recommended for the initial diagnosis and assessment of the severity of aortic stenosis and the function and hemodynamics of the left ventricle, as well as for the reevaluation of patients whose symptoms and signs are changing and of patients known to have severe asymptomatic aortic stenosis.

CONCLUSIONS AND RECOMMENDATIONS

Doppler echocardiography is indicated for the initial evaluation in all patients suspected of having aortic stenosis, as well as in patients with established disease if symptoms develop or physical signs change. The development of angina, syncope, or dyspnea in a patient with severe aortic stenosis constitutes a grave medical condition, requiring prompt aortic-valve replacement. For patients with severe asymptomatic disease, such as the patient described in the clinical vignette, the presence of an aortic-jet velocity of at least 4 m per second on Doppler echocardiography indicates the need for close scrutiny. I routinely recommend exercise

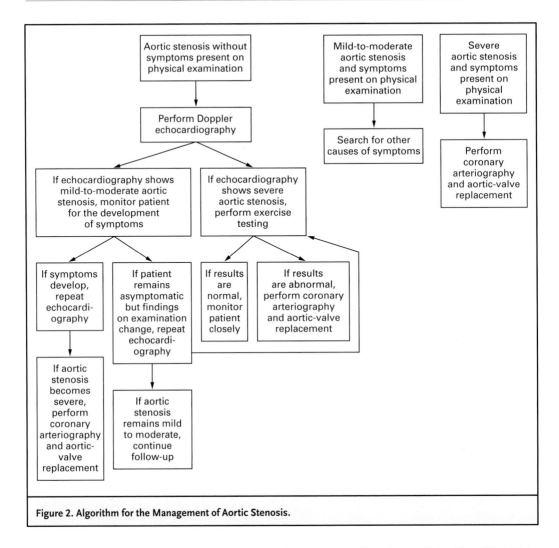

Figure 2. Algorithm for the Management of Aortic Stenosis.

testing in this group (but never in symptomatic patients), since it may help identify which of these patients are at high enough risk to warrant undergoing surgery (Figure 2).

The postoperative prognosis of patients with a reduced ejection fraction is good if the mean transvalvular pressure gradient exceeds 40 mm Hg. Thus, a low ejection fraction alone should never be an absolute contraindication to surgery. However, the prognosis of patients with a low gradient and a low ejection fraction is worse. For such patients I recommend hemodynamic manipulation in the catheterization or echocardiographic laboratory to help determine which patients are more likely to benefit from surgery.

Preliminary evidence indicates that patients who have moderate aortic stenosis (as indicated by a gradient of more than 20 mm Hg and a valve area of less than 1.2 cm^2) but who require heart surgery for other diseases should probably undergo concomitant aortic-valve replacement. Further study of this approach is required.

This article first appeared in the February 28, 2002, issue of the New England Journal of Medicine.

REFERENCES

1.
Otto CM, Kuusisto J, Reichenbach DD, Gown AM, O'Brien KD. Characterization of the early lesion of "degenerative" valvular aortic stenosis: histological and immunohistochemical studies. Circulation 1994;90:844-53.

2.
Otto CM, Lind BK, Kitzman DW, Gersh BJ, Siscovick DS. Association of aortic-valve stenosis with cardiovascular mortality and morbidity in the elderly. N Engl J Med 1999;341:142-7.

3.
Marcus ML, Doty DB, Hiratzka LF, et al. Decreased coronary reserve: a mechanism for angina pectoris in patients with aortic stenosis and normal coronary arteries. N Engl J Med 1982;307:1362-7.

4.
Hess OM, Ritter M, Schneider J, Grimm J, Turina M, Krayenbuehl HP. Diastolic stiffness and myocardial structure in aortic valve disease before and after valve replacement. Circulation 1984;69:855-65.

5.
Huber D, Grimm J, Koch R, Krayenbuehl HP. Determinants of ejection performance in aortic stenosis. Circulation 1981;64:126-34.

6.
McCrindle BW. Independent predictors of immediate results of percutaneous balloon aortic valvotomy in children. Am J Cardiol 1996;77:286-93.

7.
Otto CM, Mickel MC, Kennedy JW, et al. Three-year outcome after balloon aortic valvuloplasty: insights into prognosis of valvular aortic stenosis. Circulation 1994;89:642-50.

8.
ACC/AHA Guidelines for the management of patients with valvular heart disease: a report of the American College of Cardiology/American Heart Association Task Force on Practice Guidelines (Committee on Management of Patients with Valvular Heart Disease). J Am Coll Cardiol 1998;32:1486-588.

9.
Ross J Jr, Braunwald E. Aortic stenosis. Circulation 1968;38:Suppl V:V-61–V-67.

10.
Pellikka PA, Nishimura RA, Bailey KR, Tajik AJ. The natural history of adults with asymptomatic, hemodynamically significant aortic stenosis. J Am Coll Cardiol 1990;15:1012-7.

11.
Schwarz E, Baumann P, Manthey J, et al. The effect of aortic valve replacement on survival. Circulation 1982;66:1105-10.

12.
Lindblom D, Lindblom U, Qvist J, Lundstrom H. Long-term relative survival rates after heart valve replacement. J Am Coll Cardiol 1990;15:566-73.

13.
Kelly TA, Rothbart RM, Cooper CM, Kaiser DL, Smucker ML, Gibson RS. Comparison of outcome of asymptomatic to symptomatic patients older than 20 years of age with valvular aortic stenosis. Am J Cardiol 1988;61:123-30.

14.
Pellikka PA, Nishimura RA, Bailey KR, et al. Natural history of 610 adults with asymptomatic hemodynamically significant aortic stenosis over prolonged follow-up. J Am Coll Cardiol 2001;37:Suppl A:489A. abstract.

15.
Thai HM, Gore JM. Prosthetic heart valves. In: Alpert JS, Dalen JE, Rahimtoola SH, eds. Valvular heart disease. 3rd ed. Philadelphia: Lippincott Williams & Wilkins, 2000:393-407.

16.
Otto CM, Burwash IG, Legget ME, et al. Prospective study of asymptomatic valvular aortic stenosis: clinical, echocardiographic, and exercise predictors of outcome. Circulation 1997;95:2262-70.

17.
Linderholm H, Osterman G, Teien D. Detection of coronary artery disease by means of exercise ECG in patients with aortic stenosis. Acta Med Scand 1985;218:181-8.

18.
Goldman L, Caldera DL, Nussbaum SR, et al. Multifactorial index of cardiac risk in noncardiac surgical procedures. N Engl J Med 1977;297:845-50.

19.
Carabello BA, Green LH, Grossman W, Cohn LH, Koster JK, Collins JJ Jr. Hemodynamic determinants of prognosis of aortic valve replacement in critical aortic stenosis and advanced congestive heart failure. Circulation 1980;62:42-8.

20.
Lund O. Preoperative risk evaluation and stratification of long-term survival after valve replacement for aortic stenosis: reasons for earlier operative intervention. Circulation 1990;82:124-39.

21.
Connolly HM, Oh JK, Schaff HV, et al. Severe aortic stenosis with low transvalvular gradient and severe left ventricular dysfunction: result of aortic valve replacement in 52 patients. Circulation 2000;101:1940-6.

22.
Brogan WC III, Grayburn PA, Lange RA, Hillis LD. Prognosis after valve replacement in patients with severe aortic stenosis and a low transvalvular pressure gradient. J Am Coll Cardiol 1993;21:1657-60.

23.
Cannon JD Jr, Zile MR, Crawford FA Jr, Carabello BA. Aortic valve resistance as an adjunct to the Gorlin formula in assessing the severity of aortic stenosis in symptomatic patients. J Am Coll Cardiol 1992;20:1517-23.

24.
deFilippi CR, Willett DL, Brickner ME, et al. Usefulness of dobutamine echocardiography in distinguishing severe from nonsevere valvular aortic stenosis in patients with depressed left ventricular function and low transvalvular gradients. Am J Cardiol 1995;75:191-4.

25.
Burwash IG, Pearlman AS, Kraft CD, Miyake-Hull C, Healy NL, Otto CM. Flow dependence of measures of aortic stenosis severity during exercise. J Am Coll Cardiol 1994;24:1342-50.

26.
Monin JL, Monchi M, Gest V, Duval-Moulin AM, Dubois-Rande JL, Gueret P. Aortic stenosis with severe left ventricular dysfunction and low transvalvular pressure gradients: risk stratification by low-dose dobutamine echocardiography. J Am Coll Cardiol 2001;37:2101-7.

27.
Faggiano P, Aurigemma GP, Rusconi C, Gaasch WH. Progression of valvular aortic stenosis in adults: literature review and clinical implications. Am Heart J 1996;132:408-17.

28.
Otto CM, Pearlman AS, Gardner CL. Hemodynamic progression of aortic stenosis in adults assessed by Doppler echocardiography. J Am Coll Cardiol 1989;13:545-50.

29.
Nestico PF, DePace NL, Kimbiris D, et al. Progression of isolated aortic stenosis: analysis of 29 patients having more than 1 cardiac catheterization. Am J Cardiol 1983;52:1054-8.

30.
Das P, Rimington H, McGrane K, Chambers J. The value of treadmill exercise testing in apparently asymptomatic aortic stenosis. J Am Coll Cardiol 2001;37:Suppl A:489A. abstract.

31.
O'Keefe JH Jr, Shub C, Rettke SR. Risk of noncardiac surgical procedures in patients with aortic stenosis. Mayo Clin Proc 1989;64:400-5.

32.
Novaro GM, Tiong IY, Pearce GL, Lauer MS, Sprecher DL, Griffin BP. Effect of hydroxymethylglutaryl coenzyme A reductase inhibitors on the progression of calcific aortic stenosis. Circulation 2001;104:2205-9.

ADDENDUM

Since publication of this article, additional data from newly added, prospectively enrolled patients with aortic stenosis, low ejection fractions (less than 0.30), and low transvalvular gradients (less than 30 mm Hg) have indicated that those patients with inotropic reserve (i.e., those who are able to increase their forward output by at least 20 percent) benefit more from aortic-valve replacement than do similar patients treated medically, and that these patients have a much better outcome after surgery than do patients without inotropic reserve.[1]

In addition, a recent analysis[2] demonstrated that among patients under 70 years of age with mild-to-moderate aortic stenosis undergoing coronary-artery bypass graft surgery, survival was better in those who also underwent concomitant aortic-valve replacement, provided that they had a transvalvular gradient of more than 25 mm Hg.

The threshold transvalvular gradient at which valve replacement was associated with improved survival increased by 1 to 2 mm Hg per year, so that by the age of 80, the transvalvular gradient above which combined aortic and coronary surgery appeared warranted was 40 mm Hg.

A recently published randomized trial of patients with mild-to-moderate aortic stenosis found no benefit of statins in retarding disease progression.[3]

1. Monin JL, Quere JP, Monchi M, et al. Low-gradient aortic stenosis: operative risk stratification and predictors for long-term outcome: a multicenter study using dobutamine stress hemodynamics. Circulation 2003;108:319-24.
2. Smith WT IV, Ferguson TB Jr, Ryan T, Landolfo CK, Peterson ED. Should coronary artery bypass graft surgery patients with mild or moderate aortic stenosis undergo concomitant aortic valve replacement? A decision analysis approach to the surgical dilemma. J Am Coll Cardiol 2004;44:1241-7.
3. Cowell SJ, Newby DE, Prescott RJ, et al. A randomized trial of intensive lipid-lowering therapy in calcific aortic stenosis. N Engl J Med 2005;352:2389-97.

Acute Exacerbations of Chronic Obstructive Pulmonary Disease

JAMES K. STOLLER, M.D.

A 68-year-old former heavy smoker with a history of chronic obstructive pulmonary disease (COPD) presents to the emergency room with a two-day history of worsened dyspnea and increased purulence and volume of phlegm. Chest radiography shows hyperinflation and no acute infiltrates. Measurement of arterial blood gases while the patient is breathing room air shows acute respiratory acidosis. How should this patient be treated?

THE CLINICAL PROBLEM

COPD, which is characterized by a fixed obstruction of the airway caused by emphysema, chronic bronchitis, or both, is a common and growing clinical problem that is responsible for a substantial worldwide health burden.[1-6] COPD affects 16.4 million persons in the United States and at least 52 million worldwide, and it accounted for 2.74 million deaths in 2000.[2,3] In the United States, COPD is now the fourth leading cause of death[2-4] and is the only leading cause of death for which the mortality rate is currently increasing. COPD has been estimated to account for more than 16 million office visits and 500,000 hospitalizations annually in the United States. Costs attributable to this condition totaled $30.4 billion in 1995, with $14.7 billion spent directly on health care.[2,3,7]

Acute exacerbations of COPD are variously defined but are characterized by worsened dyspnea and increased volume of phlegm, purulence of phlegm, or both. They are often accompanied by hypoxemia and worsened hypercapnia.[8-10] Available series data suggest that patients have such exacerbations regularly (e.g., median rates of 2.4 and 3 episodes per year in two recent series[10,11]). Furthermore, active smokers have more frequent exacerbations than nonsmokers; stopping smoking can reduce the frequency by approximately one third.[12] Data reported in 1996 on 1016 patients who were hospitalized for acute exacerbations,[13] half of whom required intensive care, demonstrated an in-hospital mortality rate of 11 percent, and six-month and one-year mortality rates of 33 percent and 43 percent, respectively. Those who survived the first hospitalization had a 50 percent rate of rehospitalization within six months after discharge.

STRATEGIES AND EVIDENCE

Overview

The optimal treatment of an outpatient with an acute exacerbation of COPD involves diagnostic assessment and use of bronchodilators, systemic corticosteroids, and antibi-

Table 1. Some Commonly Used Medications for Acute Exacerbations of Chronic Obstructive Pulmonary Disease.

Drug	Mode of Delivery	Dose	Frequency
Bronchodilators			
Beta-adrenergic agonist			
Albuterol	Metered-dose inhaler	100–200 µg	4 times daily
	Nebulizer	0.5–2.0 mg	4 times daily
	Pill	4 mg	Twice daily
Fenoterol	Metered-dose inhaler	12–24 µg	Twice daily
Metaproterenol	Nebulizer	0.1–0.2 mg	4 times daily
	Pill	10–20 mg	3 to 4 times daily
Terbutaline	Metered-dose inhaler	400 µg	4 times daily
	Subcutaneous injection	0.2–0.25 mg	Every 15–30 min (maximum, two times)
	Pill	2.5–5 mg	4 times daily
Anticholinergic agent			
Ipratropium bromide*	Metered-dose inhaler	18–36 µg	4 times daily
	Nebulizer	0.5 mg	4 times daily
Methylxanthines			
Aminophylline†	Intravenous	0.9 mg/kg of body weight/hr	Infusion
Theophylline	Pill (sustained-release preparations)	150–450 mg‡	Twice daily
Corticosteroids			
Methylprednisolone succinate (for inpatients)§	Infusion, then	125 mg	Every 6 hours for 3 days, then
	Pill	60 mg	Daily for 4 days
		40 mg	Daily for 4 days
		20 mg	Daily for 4 days
Prednisone (for outpatients)	Pill	30–60 mg	Daily for 5 to 10 days, for example,
		40 mg	Daily for 2 days
		30 mg	Daily for 2 days
		20 mg	Daily for 2 days and
		10 mg	Daily for 2 days
Limited-spectrum antibiotics¶			
Trimethoprim–sulfamethoxazole	Pill	160 mg and 800 mg	Twice daily for 5 to 10 days
Amoxicillin	Pill	250 mg	4 times daily for 5 to 10 days
Doxycycline	Pill	100 mg	2 tablets first day, then 1 tablet/day for 5 to 10 days

* Quaternary ammonium anticholinergic agents (e.g., ipratropium, glycopyrrolate) are preferred to tertiary ammonium compounds (e.g., atropine) because they have fewer side effects.
† Aminophylline is sometimes administered after a loading dose; the dose should be determined on the basis of serum levels of theophylline.
‡ The dose varies among and within patients.
§ Recommendations are according to Saint et al.[14]
¶ According to Anthonisen et al.,[8] all should be 10-day courses.

otics; for patients who are sick enough to be hospitalized, oxygen and mechanical ventilation may also be used. The types and dosages of some commonly used medications for an acute exacerbation of COPD are presented in Table 1.

Diagnostic Assessment

For patients assessed in the emergency department or hospital, chest radiography is recommended because it reveals abnormalities that prompt a change in short-term treatment in 16 percent[15] to 21 percent[16] of cases. Spirometry is infrequently performed in hospitalized patients with acute exacerbations of COPD,[13] although observational studies of patients in the emergency department suggest that a forced expiratory volume in one second (FEV$_1$) that is less than 40 percent of the predicted value has a sensitivity of 96 percent for predicting relapse or the need for hospitalization[17]; hypercapnia is unlikely when the FEV$_1$ exceeds 35 percent of the predicted value.[18]

Oxygen

Although it has been relatively unstudied (perhaps because of its evident benefit), supplemental oxygen should be included in the initial therapy for a flare of COPD associated with hypoxemia; oxygen is usually administered by nasal cannula or through a face mask equipped to control the inspired oxygen fraction. Target oxygen saturation values are 90 to 92 percent, with corresponding target values for partial pressure of arterial oxygen (PaO$_2$) of 60 to 65 mm Hg. These targets ensure near-maximal hemoglobin saturation while lessening the likelihood of the hypercapnia that can accompany the use of supplemental oxygen.[19] Although the cause of such hypercapnia can be multifactorial, increased inhomogeneity of ventilation and perfusion accompanied by increased dead-space ventilation appears to be more important than decreased alveolar ventilation caused by the suppression of the hypoxic drive.

Bronchodilators

Substantial evidence shows that both inhaled beta-adrenergic agonists (for example, albuterol, fenoterol, metaproterenol, and terbutaline) and anticholinergic agents (including ipratropium bromide and glycopyrrolate) can improve airflow during acute exacerbations of COPD. Specifically, the administration of a bronchodilator can increase the FEV$_1$ and the forced vital capacity (FVC) by 15 to 29 percent over a period of 60 to 120 minutes.[20-23] Beta-adrenergic agonists have not been shown to be superior to anticholinergic agents.[7,20-23] Factors such as the time to peak effect (which is slightly more rapid with beta-adrenergic agonists) and the frequency of adverse effects (which are generally fewer and milder with ipratropium bromide) may influence the choice of agent for a given patient.

Data from randomized clinical trials have not shown a benefit of the combined use of beta-adrenergic agonists and anticholinergic agents over therapy with either class alone. A recent meta-analysis[22] supports a strategy of initial use of an inhaled anticholinergic agent, with subsequent addition of a beta-adrenergic agonist only if it is needed despite the use of maximal doses of the anticholinergic medication. However, this approach remains controversial.

The benefits of using a methylxanthine drug such as aminophylline as an additional bronchodilator remain unclear. In three randomized, controlled trials,[7,20,24-26] the addition of intravenous aminophylline did not result in improvements on tests of pulmonary function, produce apparent clinical benefit, or reduce the likelihood of a return to the emergency department during the succeeding week. Furthermore, aminophylline was associated with an increased rate of adverse effects, especially nausea and vomiting.[25] However, in one study, patients treated with aminophylline in the emergency department had a hospitalization rate that was 70 percent lower than that in a control group.[24]

Equivalent bronchodilation appears to be achieved with the use of metered-dose inhalers or nebulizers.[27] Because metered-dose inhalers cost less than nebulizers, but are frequently ineffective during respiratory distress, it is reasonable to initiate therapy with nebulizers and then switch to metered-dose inhalers when clinically feasible.[7,28]

Antibiotics

Bacterial infection may contribute to acute exacerbations of COPD. Two recent meta-analyses of 11 randomized, placebo-controlled trials of antibiotics for acute exacerbations of COPD support their use when there is purulent sputum.[14,20] Pooled data from six trials that evaluated peak expiratory flow rates showed a mean increase in the peak expiratory flow rate of 10.75 liters per minute, in contrast to the decrease in peak expiratory flow rate that has been observed during an acute flare.[11] In the largest trial from which the results are available, symptoms resolved within 21 days in 68 percent of the patients who received antibiotics, as compared with 55 percent of those given placebo.[8]

Antibiotics appear to be most useful in patients with severe exacerbations. For example, in a randomized trial involving 173 patients who were assigned to a 10-day course of doxycycline, trimethoprim–sulfamethoxazole, or amoxicillin,[8] patients with more severe exacerbations (as assessed in terms of worsened dyspnea and the purulence and volume of phlegm) received greater benefit from treatment than those with milder exacerbations.

Although concern about resistant flora has prompted some to advocate the initial use of broader-spectrum antibiotics, there have been no definitive studies supporting the first-line use of newer, more expensive antibiotics. Gram's staining of sputum has generally not been useful,[8] and sputum culture has generally been reserved for patients with no response to initial empirical therapy directed at the common causal pathogens (e.g., *Streptococcus pneumoniae*, *Moraxella catarrhalis*, and *Haemophilus influenzae*). Without definitive data regarding the optimal duration of therapy, most clinicians prescribe courses of 5 to 10 days.

Corticosteroids

Several randomized, placebo-controlled trials[7,19] have demonstrated that systemic corticosteroids accelerate improvement in airflow, gas exchange, and symptoms and reduce the rate of treatment failure. In the largest of these trials,[29] 271 hospitalized veterans were randomly assigned to receive a 3-day course of intravenous methylprednisolone (125 mg every six hours) or placebo, and the recipients of corticosteroids were further assigned to have the dose of oral prednisone tapered over the course of either 15 days or 8 weeks. Patients who received corticosteroids had an FEV_1 that was slightly but significantly higher (by 0.1 liter) than that in the placebo group on day 1. Other benefits associated with corticosteroid use were a lower rate of treatment failure at 30 and 90 days and a shorter hospital stay. The difference in FEV_1 between the corticosteroid group and the placebo group was no longer significant at 2 weeks, and outcomes were no better with an 8-week course of corticosteroids than with a 15-day course.

The optimal duration of corticosteroid therapy for an acute exacerbation of COPD remains uncertain, but recent data support a course of 5 to 10 days.[30-32] Specifically, in a randomized trial comparing oral prednisolone (a two-week regimen of 30 mg per day) with placebo, the FEV_1 improved through day 5 more in the corticosteroid group than in the placebo group.[30] In a more recent study comparing a 3-day regimen with a 10-day regimen of intravenous methylprednisolone in hospitalized patients,[31] improvements in FEV_1 and PaO_2 were evident after 3 days of therapy, but the 10-day course was associated with greater improvement in FEV_1, FVC, and PaO_2, as well as with more rapid resolution of symptoms. No difference was observed in the rate of recurrence at six months.

Noninvasive Positive-Pressure Ventilation

Enhancing ventilation by unloading fatigued ventilatory muscles is an important treatment goal in the case of an acute exacerbation of COPD that is complicated by respiratory failure. In six of seven randomized, controlled trials of positive-pressure ventilation without intubation, patients who received this type of therapy had better outcomes than those who did

Table 2. Recommendations by Professional Societies Regarding the Management of Acute Exacerbations of Chronic Obstructive Pulmonary

Variable	British Thoracic Society[6]	American College of Chest Physicians and American College of Physicians–American Society of Internal Medicine[18-20]
Date of statement	1997	2001
Type of statement	Consensus	Evidence-based systematic review
Diagnostic testing	Recommended for patients being admitted: chest radiography, arterial blood gases, complete blood count, electrolytes, blood urea nitrogen, electrocardiography, and FEV_1, peak flow, or both; sputum culture and sensitivity	Recommended for patients admitted from emergency department: chest radiography Not recommended: spirometry
Bronchodilator therapy	Recommended: For outpatients: beta-adrenergic agonists, anticholinergic agents, or both For inpatients: beta-adrenergic agonists and anticholinergic agents; add IV aminophylline if no response	Recommended: anticholinergic agent in maximal dose as first-line agent; then add beta-adrenergic agonist Not recommended: methylxanthines
Bronchodilator delivery	For outpatients: metered-dose inhaler (with instruction) For inpatients: nebulizer	Insufficient evidence for a preferred delivery device
Antibiotics	Recommended for moderate or severe exacerbations: oral route; "common" antibiotic (e.g., tetracycline, amoxicillin) as first-line agent; broader-spectrum cephalosporin or macrolide if no response	Optimal duration of therapy unclear
Corticosteroids	Not recommended for outpatients unless already receiving, known response, or failure to achieve response to increased bronchodilator dose Recommended for inpatients: e.g., 30 mg of prednisone daily for 7 to 14 days	Recommended for patients not receiving long-term oral corticosteroids: systemic corticosteroids for up to 2 wk
Supplemental oxygen	Recommended: to achieve PaO_2 ≥50 mm Hg without pH <7.26; initial treatment with face mask with FIO_2 ≤0.28	Recommended
Chest physiotherapy and clearance of secretions	Not recommended	Not recommended
Mucokinetic drugs	Not recommended	Not recommended
Mechanical ventilation	Recommended: when pH <7.26 and no response to other treatment; initial trial of NIPPV, IV doxapram, or both	Recommended: NIPPV in severe exacerbations
Other	Diuretics for raised jugular venous pressure and peripheral edema	

*GOLD denotes the Global Initiative for Chronic Obstructive Lung Disease (a joint panel of the National Heart, Lung, and Blood Institute and the World Health Organization), FEV_1 forced expiratory volume in one second, IV intravenous, PaO_2 partial pressure of arterial oxygen, FIO_2 fraction of inspired oxygen, $PaCO_2$ partial pressure of arterial carbon dioxide, SaO_2 arterial oxygen saturation, and NIPPV noninvasive positive-pressure ventilation.

Disease.*		
European Respiratory Society[5]	American Thoracic Society[1]	GOLD[2]
1995	1995	2001
Consensus	Consensus	Evidence-based review
Recommended for hospitalized patients: FEV_1, arterial blood gases, chest radiography, complete blood count, sputum Gram's stain and culture, electrolytes, electrocardiography	Recommended: determine the cause of exacerbation; sputum culture in severe exacerbations, if condition has worsened despite use of antibiotics, or for residents of a nursing home	Recommended: chest radiography, electrocardiography, arterial blood gases, sputum culture and sensitivity testing (if no response to initial antibiotics), electrolytes, hematocrit
Recommended: beta-adrenergic agonists, anticholinergic agents, or both in increased dose or frequency; consider IV aminophylline in severe exacerbations	Recommended: beta-adrenergic agonist as first-line agent, possibly in combination with anticholinergic agent; IV aminophylline if aerosol therapy cannot be given or proves inadequate	Recommended: beta-adrenergic agonist as first-line agent; add anticholinergic agent if prompt response not evident; consider oral or IV methylxanthine in severe exacerbation
Metered-dose inhaler can generally achieve good response; some patients prefer nebulizer during exacerbations	No preference	Not discussed
Recommended: 7-to-14-day course of inexpensive antibiotic (e.g., amoxicillin or tetracycline)	Recommended for abnormal mucus: "simple" antibiotic (e.g., doxycycline or amoxicillin) unless severe exacerbation, in which case consider extended-spectrum penicillin or cephalosporin	Recommended with increased sputum volume and purulence: choice should reflect local sensitivity for Streptococcus pneumoniae, Haemophilus influenzae, and Moraxella catarrhalis
Recommended: 0.4–0.6 mg/kg/day of oral corticosteroids for outpatients; IV for severe exacerbation in hospitalized patients	Recommended: reassess use after 1–2 wk	Recommended: 30–40 mg of oral or IV prednisolone per day for 10–14 days
Recommended: to raise PaO_2 ≥60 mm Hg without raising $PaCO_2$ by ≥10 mm Hg	Recommended: to raise PaO_2 just above 60 mm Hg	Recommended: target PaO_2 >60 mm Hg or SaO_2 >90%; measure arterial blood gases 30 min after the initiation of oxygen
Recommended: coughing to clear sputum; physiotherapy at home	Recommended for hospitalized patients with ≥25 ml of sputum/day	Manual or mechanical chest percussion and postural drainage possibly beneficial for patients with lobar atelectasis or >25 ml of sputum/day; facilitate sputum clearance by stimulating coughing
Mucokinetic drugs	Not recommended	Not discussed
Mechanical ventilation	Recommended: when criteria met (e.g., ample experience, adequate staffing, hemo dynamic stability, patient awake without copious secretions)	Recommended when ≥2 of the following present: severe dyspnea with accessory muscle use or paradoxical abdominal motion; pH, 7.30–7.35, and $PaCO_2$, 45–60 mm Hg; respiratory rate >25
Other		Diet; low-molecular-weight heparin; fluids

not.[33-35] Benefits included lower rates of intubation, lower in-hospital mortality rates, accelerated symptomatic and physiological improvement, and shorter hospital stays.

Noninvasive positive-pressure ventilation[33,36-38] should be considered when there is a need for ventilatory assistance, as indicated by such symptoms as worsened dyspnea, acute respiratory acidosis, and worsened oxygenation (e.g., a ratio of PaO_2 to the fraction of inspired oxygen of less than 200). Patients unlikely to benefit from noninvasive positive-pressure ventilation include those with respiratory arrest, medical instability (e.g., hypotensive shock or uncontrolled cardiac ischemia), an inability to protect the airway, excessive secretions, agitation or uncooperativeness, or conditions that preclude the placement of a mask or the achievement of a proper fit. Although there has been some concern to the contrary, management of noninvasive positive-pressure ventilation does not require more of health care providers' time and does not cost more than the treatment of intubated patients.[36-40]

AREAS OF UNCERTAINTY

Better methods are needed to encourage smoking cessation, since smoking is a key causative factor in COPD. More attention to detecting and treating alpha$_1$-antitrypsin deficiency is also needed.[41] In addition, standards are needed for the definition of an acute exacerbation of COPD and for the stratification of risk. The optimal bronchodilator regimen and route of delivery remain uncertain, especially with the advent of new drugs (e.g., tiotropium). The role of broader-spectrum antibiotics and guidelines for their use, and the indications for noninvasive positive-pressure ventilation, especially outside the intensive care unit, remain to be defined.

GUIDELINES

Five sets of guidelines for managing acute exacerbations of COPD have been issued by five widely recognized professional societies and health organizations since 1994: the European Respiratory Society,[5] the British Thoracic Society,[6] the American Thoracic Society,[1] a joint panel of the American College of Chest Physicians and the American College of Physicians–American Society of Internal Medicine,[20-22] and a joint panel of the National Heart, Lung, and Blood Institute and the World Health Organization (known as the Global Initiative for Chronic Obstructive Lung Disease, or GOLD).[2] These guidelines, summarized in Table 2, are similar in many respects; most (including those proposed by GOLD) endorse a short course of systemic corticosteroids and antibiotics for severe exacerbations and the use of noninvasive ventilation for exacerbations complicated by acute ventilatory failure. Unlike some of the guidelines, those from GOLD favor beta-adrenergic agonists as first-line bronchodilator therapy, recommend adding an anticholinergic agent if there is no response to the beta-adrenergic agonist, and endorse consideration of a methylxanthine drug.

SUMMARY AND RECOMMENDATIONS

My approach to treating the patient with an acute exacerbation of COPD is as follows. For patients who present to the emergency department or who are deemed sick enough to be hospitalized, diagnostic assessment includes chest radiography and, if the patient's distress or somnolence prompts concern about acute respiratory acidemia, measurement of arterial blood gases. Initial therapy includes supplemental oxygen, usually through a face mask to ensure an oxyhemoglobin saturation, measured by pulse oximetry, of 90 to 92 percent. For both inpatients and outpatients, combined bronchodilator therapy should be used, with ipratropium bromide and albuterol administered every four to six hours initially; nebulizers are recommended whenever the patient's distress level raises doubt about the effective use of a metered-dose inhaler. As the condition improves and the distress level is reduced, metered-dose inhalers can be used in place of nebulizers. Since many patients do not use their inhalers appropriately, spacer devices should be prescribed and appropriate techniques should be reviewed.

On the basis of data from a randomized trial,[8] a 10-day course of a narrow-spectrum antibiotic (e.g., trimethoprim–sulfamethoxazole, doxycycline, or amoxicillin) should be prescribed when there is increased dyspnea and increased purulence and volume of phlegm. Sputum staining and cultures are reserved for cases that are refractory to antibiotic therapy. Oral systemic corticosteroids are prescribed both for outpatients (tapering over the course of eight days, beginning with 40 mg per day and decreasing the dose by 10 mg every other day) and for inpatients (Table 1).[29] Given the lack of evidence to support the usefulness of chest physiotherapy or mucokinetic drugs, neither of these should be routinely prescribed.

For eligible patients with acute respiratory acidemia, bilevel noninvasive positive-pressure ventilation should be implemented for multiple-hour stretches, with occasional interruption, during the first several days of hospitalization. Such ventilation is initially administered in the intensive care unit to ensure close monitoring and ready access to intubation and mechanical ventilation, should the trial of noninvasive positive-pressure ventilation fail.

For patients who present for the first time with an exacerbation of underlying COPD, recovery from the acute episode provides an opportunity to discuss smoking cessation, to explore the possibility of alpha$_1$-antitrypsin deficiency, to vaccinate the patient against pneumococcus and influenza, and to consider referral to a pulmonary rehabilitation program. For patients who require hospitalization, an outpatient follow-up visit should be scheduled for four to eight weeks after hospital discharge. Spirometry should be performed after the administration of a bronchodilator, and the patient's need for supplemental oxygen both while at rest and during activity should be reassessed. Bronchodilator therapy should be continued over the long term, with the addition of an inhaled corticosteroid reserved for patients in whom the obstruction of airflow has been demonstrated to be reversible (e.g., those who have an increase of at least 12 percent and 200 ml in the FEV$_1$ after the use of a bronchodilator) and patients who have frequent exacerbations.

Given this approach, the short-term treatment of the patient described in the vignette should include admission to the hospital because of acute respiratory acidemia, and the administration of a combination of bronchodilators, a limited-spectrum antibiotic, and intravenous corticosteroids. Unless there is rapid reversal of acidemia, bilevel noninvasive positive-pressure ventilation should be initiated.

This article first appeared in the March 28, 2002, issue of the New England Journal of Medicine.

REFERENCES

1.
American Thoracic Society. Standards for the diagnosis and care of patients with chronic obstructive pulmonary disease. Am J Respir Crit Care Med 1995;152: Suppl:S77-S121. (Also available at http://www. thoracic.org.)

2.
Pauwels RA, Buist AS, Calverley PMA, Jenkins CR, Hurd SS. Global strategy for the diagnosis, management, and prevention of chronic obstructive pulmonary disease: NHLBI/WHO Global Initiative for Chronic Obstructive Lung Disease (GOLD) Workshop summary. Am J Respir Crit Care Med 2001;163:1256-76. (Also available at http:// www.goldcopd.com.)

3.
Fact sheet: chronic obstructive pulmonary disease (COPD). New York: American Lung Association, January 2001. (Accessed January 31, 2006, at http://www. lungusa.org/pub/minority/ copd_00.html.)

4.
Statistical abstract of the United States, 2000. Washington, D.C.: Census Bureau, 2000:91.

5.
Siafakas NM, Vermeire P, Pride NB, et al. Optimal assessment and management of chronic obstructive pulmonary disease (COPD). Eur Respir J 1995;8:1398-420.

6.
The COPD Guidelines Group of the Standards of Care Committee of the BTS. BTS guidelines for the management of chronic obstructive pulmonary disease. Thorax 1997;52:Suppl 5:S1-S28.

7.
Sherk PA, Grossman RF. The chronic obstructive pulmonary disease exacerbation. Clin Chest Med 2000;21:705-21.

8.
Anthonisen NR, Manfreda J, Warren CPW, Hershfield ES, Harding GK, Nelson NA. Antibiotic therapy in exacerbations of chronic obstructive pulmonary disease. Ann Intern Med 1987;106:196-204.

9.
Rodriguez-Roisin R. Toward a consensus definition for COPD exacerbations. Chest 2000;117:Suppl 2:398S-401S.

10.
Seemungal TAR, Donaldson GC, Bhowmik A, Jeffries DJ, Wedzicha JA. Time course and recovery of exacerbations in patients with chronic obstructive pulmonary disease. Am J Respir Crit Care Med 2000;161:1608-13.

11.
Seemungal TAR, Donaldson GC, Paul EA, Bestall JC, Jeffries DJ, Wedzicha JA. Effect of exacerbation on quality of life in patients with chronic obstructive pulmonary disease. Am J Respir Crit Care Med 1998;157:1418-22.

12.
Kanner RE, Anthonisen NR, Connett JE. Lower respiratory illnesses promote FEV1 decline in current smokers but not ex-smokers with mild chronic obstructive pulmonary disease: results from the Lung Health Study. Am J Respir Crit Care Med 2001;164:358-64.

13.
Connors AF Jr, Dawson NV, Thomas C, et al. Outcomes following acute exacerbation of severe chronic obstructive lung disease. Am J Respir Crit Care Med 1996;154:959-67. [Erratum, Am J Respir Crit Care Med 1997;155:386.]

14.
Saint S, Bent S, Vittinghoff E, Grady D. Antibiotics in chronic obstructive pulmonary disease exacerbations: a meta-analysis. JAMA 1995;273:957-60.

15.
Emerman CL, Cydulka RK. Evaluation of high-yield criteria for chest radiography in acute exacerbation of chronic obstructive pulmonary disease. Ann Emerg Med 1993;22:680-4.

16.
Tsai TW, Gallagher EJ, Lombardi G, Gennis P, Carter W. Guidelines for the selective ordering of admission chest radiography in adult obstructive airway disease. Ann Emerg Med 1993;22:1854-8.

17.
Emerman CL, Effron D, Lukens TW. Spirometric criteria for hospital admission of patients with acute exacerbation of COPD. Chest 1991;99:595-9.

18.
Emerman CL, Connors AF, Lukens TW, Effron D, May ME. Relationship between arterial blood gases and spirometry in acute exacerbations of chronic obstructive pulmonary disease. Ann Emerg Med 1989;18:523-7.

19.
Aubier M, Murciano D, Milic-Emili J, et al. Effects of administration of O_2 on ventilation and blood gases in patients with chronic obstructive pulmonary disease during acute respiratory failure. Am Rev Respir Dis 1980;122:747-54.

20.
McCrory DC, Brown C, Gelfand SE, Bach PB. Management of exacerbations of COPD: a summary and appraisal of the published evidence. Chest 2001;119:1190-209.

21.
Bach PB, Brown C, Gelfand SE, McCrory DC. Management of exacerbations of chronic obstructive pulmonary disease: a summary and appraisal of published evidence. Ann Intern Med 2001;134:600-20.

22.
Snow V, Lascher S, Mottur-Pilson C. Evidence base for management of acute exacerbations of chronic obstructive pulmonary disease. Ann Intern Med 2001;134:595-9.

23.
Ferguson GT. Recommendations for the management of COPD. Chest 2000;117: Suppl:23S-28S.

24.
Wrenn K, Slovis CM, Murphy F, Greenberg RS. Aminophylline therapy for acute bronchospastic disease in the emergency room. Ann Intern Med 1991;115:241-7.

25.
Rice KL, Leatherman JW, Duane PG, et al. Aminophylline for acute exacerbations of chronic obstructive pulmonary disease: a controlled trial. Ann Intern Med 1987;107:305-9.

26.
Seidenfeld JJ, Jones WN, Moss RE, Tremper J. Intravenous aminophylline in the treatment of acute bronchospastic exacerbations of chronic obstructive pulmonary disease. Ann Emerg Med 1984;13:248-52.

27.
Turner MO, Patel A, Ginsburg S, FitzGerald JM. Bronchodilator delivery in acute airflow obstruction — a meta-analysis. Arch Intern Med 1997;157:1736-44.

28.
Stoller JK, Lange PA. Inpatient management of chronic obstructive pulmonary disease. Respir Care Clin N Am 1998;4:425-38.

29.
Niewoehner DE, Erbland ML, Deupree RH, et al. Effect of systemic glucocorticoids on exacerbations of chronic obstructive pulmonary disease. N Engl J Med 1999;340:1941-7.

30.
Davies L, Angus RM, Calverley PM. Oral corticosteroids in patients admitted to hospital with exacerbation of chronic obstructive pulmonary disease: a prospective randomised controlled trial. Lancet 1999;354:456-60.

31.
Sayiner A, Aytemur ZA, Cirit M, Unsal I. Systemic glucocorticoids in severe exacerbations of COPD. Chest 2001;119:726-30.

32.
Stanbrook MB, Goldstein RS. Steroids for acute exacerbtions of COPD: how long is enough? Chest 2001;119:675-6.

33.
Mehta S, Hill NS. Noninvasive ventilation. Am J Respir Crit Care Med 2001;163:540-77.

34.
Keenan SP, Kernerman PD, Cook DJ, Martin CM, McCormack D, Sibbald WJ. Effect of noninvasive positive-pressure ventilation on mortality in patients admitted with acute respiratory failure: a meta-analysis. Crit Care Med 1997;25:1685-92.

35.
Plant PK, Owen JL, Elliott MW. Early use of non-invasive ventilation for acute exacerbations of chronic obstructive pulmonary disease on general respiratory wards: a multicentre randomised controlled trial. Lancet 2000;355:1931-5.

36.
International consensus conferences in intensive care medicine: noninvasive positive pressure ventilation in acute respiratory failure. Am J Respir Crit Care Med 2001;163:283-91.

37.
American Association for Respiratory Care. Consensus Conference IV (noninvasive positive pressure ventilation): preamble and consensus statement. Respir Care 1997;42:362-9.

38.
Clinical indications for noninvasive positive pressure ventilation in chronic respiratory failure due to restrictive lung disease, COPD, and nocturnal hypoventilation — a consensus conference report. Chest 1999;116:521-34.

39.
Kramer N, Meyer TJ, Meharg J, Cece RD, Hill NS. Randomized, prospective trial of noninvasive positive pressure ventilation for acute exacerbations of COPD. Am J Respir Crit Care Med 1995;151:1799-806.

40.
Nava S, Evangelisti I, Rampulla C, Campagnoni ML, Fracchia C, Rubini F. Human and financial costs of noninvasive mechanical ventilation in patients affected by COPD and acute respiratory failure. Chest 1997;111:1631-8.

41.
Stoller JK. Clinical features and natural history of severe alpha 1-antitrypsin deficiency: Roger S. Mitchell Lecture. Chest 1997;111: Suppl:123S-128S.

Addendum

Since publication of this article, data have been published suporting the benefits of early treatment of acute exacerbations of chronic obstructive pulmonary disease (COPD).[1] In an observational study of 128 patients with COPD and a history of frequent exacerbations, earlier initiation of therapy with oral antibiotics, systemic corticosteroids, or both was associated with faster recovery. Moreover, patients who did not seek treatment for acute exacerbations, as compared with patients who did seek treatment, had poorer recovery health-related quality of life and were more likely to be hospitalized. Although these results could be confounded by unknown factors influencing patients' care-seeking behavior, they support early initiation of therapy for acute exacerbations of COPD.

Another important observation is that use of the long-acting anticholinergic drug tiotropium lessens the risk of having an acute exacerbation of COPD or of being hospitalized for it.[2-4] Specifically, in three different randomized, controlled trials comparing tiotropium with placebo,[2] ipratropium,[3] and salmeterol,[4] treatment with tiotropium improved outcomes. As compared with placebo, tiotropium reduced the proportion of patients having one or more acute exacerbations of COPD in a year, the yearly incidence of exacerbations, the number of hospitalizations for exacerbations, and the time from initiation of treatment to the first exacerbation.[2] As compared with ipratropium, tiotropium reduced the likelihood of having an acute exacerbation of COPD and the number of exacerbations.[3] Finally, as compared with salmeterol, tiotropium reduced the number of hospitalizations for acute exacerbations of COPD, although there was no significant difference in the number of exacerbations.[4]

1. Wilkinson TM, Donaldson GC, Hurst JR, Seemungal TA, Wedzicha J. Early therapy improves outcomes of exacerbations of chronic obstructive pulmonary disease. Am J Respir
Crit Care Med 2004;169:1298-303.
2. Casaburi R, Mahler DA, Jones PW, et al. A long-term evaluation of once-daily inhaled tiotropium in chronic obstructive pulmonary disease. Eur Respir J 2002;19:217-24.
3. Vincken W, van Noord JA, Greefhorst AP, et al. Improved health outcomes in patients with COPD during 1 yr's treatment with tiotropium. Eur Respir J 2002;19:209-16.
4. Brusasco V, Hodder R, Miravitlles M, Korducki L, Towse L, Kesten S. Health outcomes following treatment for six months with once daily tiotropium compared with twice daily salmeterol in patients with COPD. Thorax 2003;58:399-404.

Peanut Allergy

HUGH A. SAMPSON, M.D.

A 19-year-old woman is brought to the emergency room because of the acute onset of dyspnea, wheezing, vomiting, and generalized flushing. She has well-controlled asthma as well as a history of atopic dermatitis as an infant and urticaria after ingesting peanut butter at the age of five years. According to friends she ate a chocolate-chip cookie from a vending machine in her college dormitory just before the symptoms developed. The list of ingredients on the cookie wrapper does not include peanuts. Nevertheless, how should this patient's condition be treated?

THE CLINICAL PROBLEM

In a patient with asthma, the acute onset of severe bronchospasm in the absence of earlier signs of asthma must always raise the suspicion of anaphylaxis. Food allergy affects about 6 to 8 percent of children younger than four years of age and about 2 percent of the U.S. population beyond the first decade of life.[1] Food allergy is the leading cause of anaphylaxis treated in hospital emergency departments in the United States and many westernized countries. Food allergy accounts for about 30,000 anaphylactic reactions, 2000 hospitalizations, and 200 deaths each year in the United States.[2] Allergies to peanuts and tree nuts account for the majority of fatal and near-fatal anaphylactic reactions.[3,4] A national survey indicated that about 1.1 percent of Americans, or 3 million people, are allergic to peanuts, tree nuts, or both.[5] Ironically, despite an increasing public awareness of food allergy, most patients are ill prepared to deal with anaphylactic reactions.[6] In a recent series, over 80 percent of patients who died from allergic reactions to food were not given appropriate information to avoid accidental food-induced reactions or self-injectable epinephrine to manage them.[4]

Food-induced anaphylaxis is primarily a clinical diagnosis and is often mistaken for severe status asthmaticus or an acute cardiovascular event. People who have life-threatening reactions usually have asthma and frequently have a history of atopy, including atopic dermatitis and food allergy as young children.[7] Symptoms may develop within minutes to a few hours after ingestion of the food, and in life-threatening cases, symptoms include severe bronchospasm. Although similar to anaphylaxis due to other causes, early symptoms of food-induced anaphylaxis often include oral pruritus and "tingling," pharyngeal pruritus and a sensation of tightening of the airways, colicky abdominal pain, nausea and vomiting, and cutaneous flushing, urticaria, and angioedema. Progressive respiratory symptoms, hypotension, and dysrhythmias typically develop in fatal and near-fatal cases. Obstructive laryngeal edema is uncommon, and cutaneous symptoms may be absent in severe cases. Surveys of fatal and near-fatal reactions suggest that a delay in the initiation of therapy such as injectable epinephrine is associated with a poorer prognosis, although about 10 percent of patients who receive epinephrine early still die.[3,4] Biphasic reactions have been noted in up to one third of patients with fatal or near-fatal reactions. These patients seem to have fully recovered when severe bronchospasm suddenly recurs; the recurrence is typically more refractory to standard therapy and often requires intubation and mechanical ventilation. The mechanism underlying this phenomenon is unknown, but it appears to be more common when therapy is initiated late and symptoms at presentation are more severe. Secondary pneumothoraxes are a fairly common consequence of the high airway pressures generally required to overcome the obstruction.

Although the relative epidemic of peanut allergy appears to be a phenomenon of the past two decades, peanuts were first cultivated in South America about 2000 to 3000 B.C., and the practice has spread throughout the world.[8] After the Civil War, peanuts became increasingly popular throughout the United States. America now ranks third only to China and India in peanut production, with over 40 percent of the U.S. peanut crop consumed as peanut butter. Whereas the per capita consumption of peanuts in China is similar to that of the United States,[9] peanut allergy is extremely rare in China.[10] In addition, the prevalence of peanut allergy appears to be rising in the United States and other westernized countries. In a population-based study of three-year-olds in the United Kingdom, the prevalence of sensitization to peanuts increased from 1.3 percent to 3.2 percent from 1989 to 1995.[11] In a cohort of American children referred for the evaluation of moderate-to-severe atopic dermatitis between 1990 and 1994, the prevalence of allergic reactivity to peanuts was nearly twice as high as that in a similar group evaluated between 1980 and 1984.[12] Data from the third National Health and Nutrition Examination Survey (collected from 1988 to 1994) indicated that about 6 percent of Americans have serologic evidence of sensitivity to peanuts (i.e., the presence of IgE antibodies specific for peanut proteins),[13] although the majority of these people will not have an allergic reaction when they eat peanuts.

There appears to be something unique about the peanut that is not shared by other members of the legume family or most other food proteins. The three major allergenic

---

Table 1. Approach to Patients with Peanut Allergy.

Patient education

Avoidance of peanut proteins
Recognition of early signs of anaphylaxis
Early treatment of allergic symptoms (anaphylaxis) with injectable epinephrine (EpiPen Autoinjector) and oral liquid
    diphenhydramine (the most easily absorbed form)

Treatment of acute reaction*

By patient and family members
    Injection of epinephrine, depending on patient's history and symptoms
    Administration of oral liquid diphenhydramine (1 mg/kg of body weight; maximum, 75 mg)
    Transport to emergency facility
By emergency personnel
    Administration of supplemental oxygen and airway management
    Administration of intramuscular epinephrine (0.01 ml of a 1:1000 dilution/kg every 10 to
       20 minutes as needed; maximum, 0.3 to 0.5 ml) or intravenous epinephrine in patients with
       severe hypotension (0.5 to 5 μg/min to maintain blood pressure)
    Administration of intravenous fluids
    Administration of oral, intramuscular, or intravenous H_1-receptor antagonist (e.g., diphenhydramine, 1 mg/kg;
       maximum, 75 mg)
    Treatment with oral prednisone (1 to 2 mg/kg; maximum, 75 mg) or intravenous methylprednisolone (2 mg/kg; maxi-
       mum, 250 mg)
    Administration of nebulized albuterol (1.25 to 2.5 mg every 20 minutes as needed or continuously with monitoring)
    Use of H_2-receptor antagonist (e.g., for adults: 4 to 5 mg of ranitidine/kg orally; maximum, 300 mg; 50 mg intramus-
       cularly or intravenously every 6 to 8 hr; for children: 1.5 mg/kg intramuscularly or intravenously; maximum, 50 mg)

Follow-up

Treatment with oral H_1-receptor antagonist for 3 days: cetirizine (patients weighing less than 30 kg, 5 mg/day; patients
    weighing at least 30 kg, 10 mg/day), fexofenadine (patients younger than 12 years of age, 30 mg twice a day; patients
    at least 12 years of age, 60 mg twice a day), or loratadine (patients younger than 6 years of age, 5 mg/day; patients
    at least 6 years of age, 10 mg/day)
Treatment with oral prednisone (1 mg/kg/day; maximum, 75 mg) for 3 days
Referral for evaluation by allergist if patient has not previously been evaluated

---

* Treatment varies depending on the patient's symptoms.

---

proteins in peanuts are Ara h 1, 2, and 3.[14] Although other legumes contain similar proteins and most patients with peanut allergy have IgE antibodies against these proteins, fewer than 15 percent of such patients react to other members of the legume family.[15] In addition, other legumes rarely provoke severe anaphylactic reactions or result in a lifelong allergy. However, in 25 to 35 percent of patients with peanut allergy, an allergic reaction to tree nuts (such as walnuts, cashews, and pistachios) will develop even though tree nuts are from a different botanical family.[16]

STRATEGIES AND EVIDENCE

Diagnosis

A physician who knows about food allergies should evaluate any person who is thought to have had an adverse reaction to peanuts. The evaluation should include a careful history-taking, skin-prick tests, radioallergosorbent tests, and possibly, an oral food challenge. Patients who have had unequivocal symptoms of allergy after the isolated ingestion of a peanut product (especially if they occur on more than one occasion) and who have evidence of peanut-specific IgE antibodies (a positive skin-prick test or radioallergosorbent test) do not usually need to undergo oral peanut challenges to establish the diagnosis. The use of a radioallergosorbent test to quantify the level of peanut-specific serum IgE antibodies can be diagnostic, since patients with peanut-specific serum IgE levels of at least 15 kU per liter have a likelihood of an allergic reaction of 95 percent or greater if they ingest peanuts.[17] In the absence of a conflicting history, these patients may be given a diagnosis of peanut allergy and do not need to undergo a food challenge. In persons who have peanut-specific serum IgE antibody levels of less than 15 kU per liter and no clear-cut history of peanut-induced symptoms, a physician-supervised food challenge is necessary to make a definitive diagnosis. The double-blind, placebo-controlled challenge is considered the gold standard for diagnosing food allergy, but less rigorous challenges are often adequate if they are performed by a physician with experience in food allergies and the treatment of anaphylaxis. Such challenges may lead to severe anaphylactic symptoms and so should be conducted only in a hospital setting by an experienced specialist.

Peanut allergy generally develops at an early age and, unlike many other food allergies in children, is often a lifelong disorder. In a registry of 4685 patients with peanut allergy, the first reaction to peanuts occurred at a median age of 14 months.[18] Infants who have peanut allergy tend to have more severe allergic reactions as they get older. However, recent studies suggest that about 20 percent of young infants who have allergic reactions to peanuts will outgrow their allergy, especially if they have low levels of peanut-specific serum IgE antibodies in infancy (less than 5 kU per liter).[19] Therefore, children with low levels of peanut-specific IgE antibodies should be reevaluated periodically to determine whether they have outgrown their allergy. A conversion of the skin-prick test from positive to negative generally indicates that a patient has outgrown his or her peanut allergy. However, skin-prick tests often remain positive for many years in children who have outgrown their peanut allergy and are therefore not as useful as the measurement of peanut-specific IgE antibodies for assessing clinical reactivity.

The diagnosis of an acute allergic reaction is based on clinical symptoms and a history of exposure to an allergen. Laboratory studies are not helpful in distinguishing food-induced anaphylaxis from severe asthma, since serum β-tryptase levels, a hallmark of mast-cell activation that is associated with anaphylactic reactions, usually remain normal in patients with food-induced anaphylaxis.[3,20]

Management

Currently, treatment of peanut allergy consists of teaching patients and their families how to avoid the accidental ingestion of peanuts, how to recognize early symptoms of an allergic reaction, and how to manage the early stages of an anaphylactic reaction (Table 1).[21] Patients must learn to check all food labels for the presence of peanuts and to avoid high-risk situations, such as foods served in buffets and ice-cream parlors and unlabeled candies and desserts. Although most patients with peanut allergy avoid ingesting peanut oil, highly processed oils — acid-extracted, heat-distilled oils — do not contain peanut protein and can be safely consumed by such patients.[22] However, cold-pressed or extruded peanut oils contain peanut protein and many induce allergic reactions.

Although considerable educational material is available through organizations such as the Food Allergy and Anaphylaxis Network (telephone number, 1-800-929-4040; Web site, http://www.foodallergy.org), inadvertent exposure as a result of peanut contamination of equipment used in the manufacture of various products, inadequate food labeling, cross-contamination of food during cooking in restaurants (e.g., the use of the same pan to cook foods containing peanuts and foods without peanuts),[23] and unanticipated exposures (e.g., the inhalation of peanut dust in airplanes[24]) result in an allergic reaction every three to five years in the average patient with peanut allergy.[16] Consequently, such patients must be given a written emergency plan (one is available at the Food Allergy and Anaphylaxis Network Web site) and appropriate doses of liquid diphenhydramine and self-injectable epinephrine (e.g., EpiPen Autoinjector, Dey) so that therapy can be initiated in case they accidentally eat peanuts. Patients who have an allergic reaction to peanuts that requires the use of epinephrine should always go to a local emergency room for follow-up in case they have persistent refractory symptoms or a biphasic response.

Patients who have an anaphylactic reaction to peanuts should be treated aggressively with intramuscular epinephrine[25]; oral, intramuscular, or intravenous histamine H_1- and H_2-receptor antagonists; oxygen; inhaled albuterol; and systemic corticosteroids. Because over 90 percent of biphasic responses occur within four hours after the initial reaction, patients should be observed for at least four hours before being discharged from the emergency department.[3] The administration of corticosteroids does not appear to reduce the risk of a biphasic response. A subsequent three-day course of oral prednisone (1 mg per kilogram of body weight per day; maximum, 75 mg per day) and an antihistamine is often recommended, although there are no studies demonstrating that this practice decreases the risk of recurrent symptoms.

Cause of the Increasing Prevalence of Peanut Allergy

The cause of the rising prevalence of peanut allergy and the reasons this increase appears to be confined to westernized countries remain uncertain. In addition to theories regarding the general increase in the prevalence of allergic disease worldwide over the past several decades,[26] a number of factors have been suggested to account for the apparent increase in prevalence. The growing demand for highly nutritional, "quick-energy" foods has made the peanut a staple of the American diet. Breast-feeding is increasingly common, and peanut products have increasingly been promoted as excellent nutritional sources for pregnant and lactating women. In one registry of patients with peanut allergy, about 85 percent had been breast-fed and more than 70 percent had had their first allergic reaction after their first apparent contact with peanuts. Since reactions require previous exposure for sensitization and since IgE antibodies do not cross the placenta, these findings suggest that peanut protein was encountered in utero or through breast milk.[24,27] In a French study of 54 infants who were less than 11 days of age and 71 who were 17 days to 4 months of age, 8 percent had a positive skin-prick test for peanuts.[10] Another study found that mothers of children with peanut allergy ate more peanuts during pregnancy, but not during lactation, than mothers of children with an allergy to milk or eggs.[28]

Given the immaturity of the immune system at birth, food allergies are more likely to develop during the first few years of life.[1] The majority of American children are exposed to peanuts (e.g., peanut butter) in the first year of life, and virtually all have been exposed by their second birthday.[29] In countries where peanut butter is rarely eaten, such as Denmark and Norway, peanut allergy is much less common.

Differences in the way peanuts are prepared may also contribute to the increasing prevalence of peanut allergy as well as to variations in the rates of peanut allergy among countries. Most peanuts in the United States are dry-roasted, including peanuts that are made into peanut butter, whereas peanuts in China are typically boiled or fried. The higher temperatures required for dry-roasting increase the allergenicity of the three major peanut proteins more than do the lower temperatures used for boiling or frying.[9] Although genetics plays a part in the development of peanut allergy,[30] the prevalence of peanut allergy is similar among the children of Chinese immigrants to the United States and the children of native-born Americans.

Therapy for Peanut Allergy

Unlike traditional immunotherapy for allergic reactions to inhalants and bee stings, injections of peanut extracts have an unacceptable risk–benefit ratio.[31] However, novel therapeutic agents are being investigated for the treatment of peanut allergy.[32] One approach being evaluated in phase 1 and 2 trials is monthly injections of humanized recombinant anti-IgE antibodies, which may reduce the levels of IgE bound to mast cells and basophils sufficiently to prevent the activation of allergic responses, at least to small amounts of peanut protein. Another approach uses engineered (mutant) recombinant peanut proteins, in which substitutions of critical amino acids within the IgE-binding epitopes prevent the activation of IgE-mediated reactions, for traditional desensitizing immunotherapy. Both engineered recombinant proteins and a series of overlapping peptides comprising T-cell epitopes of peanut reversed sensitivity to peanuts in a murine model of peanut-induced anaphylaxis without triggering IgE-mediated acute reactions.[32] However, the clinical usefulness of these approaches has not been established.

GUIDELINES

Both the American Academy of Asthma, Allergy and Immunology and the American Academy of Pediatrics have published guidelines on the management of food-induced anaphylaxis.[33,34] Patients, as well as the parents and caregivers of children with peanut allergy, must be educated to avoid accidentally ingesting peanuts, learn to recognize early signs of an allergic reaction, and learn to medicate themselves as soon as symptoms develop. All patients with peanut allergy should be given a written emergency plan and adequate doses of liquid diphenhydramine and self-injectable epinephrine for use in case they accidentally ingest peanuts. School and day-care personnel must also be educated to provide a safe environment for children with peanut allergy[35] and to recognize and treat food-induced reactions. In the event of an allergic reaction to peanuts, especially if epinephrine is used, patients should be taken to the nearest emergency room where they can be treated further and observed for at least four hours.

Whether peanut allergy can be prevented remains in question. Nonetheless, the Department of Health in the United Kingdom (and many allergists in the United States) recommends that mothers from "high-risk" families (those with a history of atopy) avoid eating peanuts during pregnancy and lactation and that they not give their infants peanut products for the first three years of life.[36]

CONCLUSIONS AND RECOMMENDATIONS

Food allergy — and peanut allergy in particular — has become a major health concern in the United States and many other westernized countries. Pending further information, it is probably wise to encourage mothers from families with a history of atopy to avoid eating peanuts during pregnancy and lactation and to avoid introducing peanut proteins to their offspring for the first three years of life. Children in whom an allergy to milk or eggs develops during the first year of life should also avoid peanuts, since other food allergies will develop in about one third of them. Any person suspected of having had an allergic reaction to peanuts should be evaluated by a specialist knowledgeable in this area. Since about one third of patients with peanut allergy are also allergic to at least one tree nut,[16] patients who have had an anaphylactic reaction to peanuts should be evaluated for nut allergy. Children younger than five years of age who are allergic to peanuts should avoid all nuts because of the risk of developing new nut sensitivities and the difficulty children in this age group have accurately identifying peanut-containing products. Physicians must teach their patients appropriate avoidance strategies and to recognize early signs of an allergic reaction and provide them with emergency plans and appropriate medications in case of an accidental peanut ingestion. Child-care facilities and schools must develop appropriate plans to protect children with peanut allergy and initiate treatment in case of an accidental ingestion. Restaurants and other public eating establishments and airlines need to be more cognizant of the needs of people with peanut allergy. Mandatory food-labeling laws and manufacturing practices should be enacted to prevent the inadvertent ingestion of mislabeled or contaminated products.[37]

If an accidental ingestion occurs, as apparently occurred in the patient described in the clinical vignette, intramuscular epinephrine and liquid diphenhydramine should be given immediately (Table 1). The patient should be brought to an emergency department as quickly as possible and treated with epinephrine, antihistamines, supplemental oxygen, intravenous fluids, nebulized albuterol, and corticosteroids, as appropriate. Because of the risk of a biphasic reaction, the patient should be observed for at least four hours before being discharged and should then be given a short course of prednisone and an antihistamine.

Dr. Sampson reports having received research support from Pharmacia–Upjohn.

This article first appeared in the April 25, 2002, issue of the New England Journal of Medicine.

REFERENCES

1.
Sampson HA. Food allergy.
1. Immunopathogenesis and
clinical disorders. J Allergy
Clin Immunol 1999;103:717-
28.
2.
Yocum MW, Butterfield JH,
Klein JS, Volcheck GW,
Schroeder DR, Silverstein
MD. Epidemiology of ana-
phylaxis in Olmsted County:
a population-based study.
J Allergy Clin Immunol
1999;104:452-6.
3.
Sampson HA, Mendelson L,
Rosen JP. Fatal and near-
fatal anaphylactic reactions
to food in children and
adolescents. N Engl J Med
1992;327:380-4.
4.
Bock SA, Munoz-Furlong A,
Sampson HA. Fatalities due
to anaphylactic reactions to
foods. J Allergy Clin Immunol 2001;107:191-3.
5.
Sicherer SH,
Munoz-Furlong A,
Burks AW, Sampson HA.
Prevalence of peanut and
tree nut allergy in the US
determined by a random
digit dial telephone survey.
J Allergy Clin Immunol
1999;103:559-62.
6.
Gold MS, Sainsbury R. First
aid anaphylaxis manage-
ment in children who were
prescribed an epinephrine
autoinjector device (EpiPen).
J Allergy Clin Immunol
2000;106:171-6.
7.
Sampson HA. Fatal food-
induced anaphylaxis. Allergy
1998;53:Suppl:125-30.

8.
Saavedra-Delgado A. The
many faces of the peanut.
Allergy Proc 1989;10:291-4.
9.
Beyer K, Morrow E, Li XM,
et al. Effects of cooking
methods on peanut allergenicity. J Allergy Clin Immunol 2001;107:1077-81.
10.
Hatahet R, Kirch F, Kanny G,
Moneret-Vautrin DA. Sen-
sibilisation aux allergènes
d'arachide chez les nourris-
sons de moins de quatre mois:
à propos de 125 observations.
Rev Fr Allergol Immunol Clin
1994;34:377-81.
11.
Grundy J, Bateman BJ,
Gant C, Matthews SM,
Dean TP, Arshad SH. Peanut
allergy in three year old
children — a population
based study. J Allergy Clin
Immunol 2001;107:Suppl:
S231. abstract.
12.
Sampson HA. Managing
peanut allergy. BMJ
1996;312:1050-1.
13.
Chiu L, Sampson HA,
Sicherer SH. Estimation of
the sensitization rate to peanut by prick skin test in the
general population: results
from the National Health
and Nutrition Examination
Survey 1988-1994 (NHANES
III). J Allergy Clin Immunol 2001;107:Suppl:S192.
abstract.
14.
Burks W, Sampson
HA, Bannon GA. Pea-
nut allergens. Allergy
1998;53:725-30.

15.
Bernhisel-Broadbent J,
Sampson HA. Cross-
allergenicity in the legume
botanical family in children
with food hypersensitiv-
ity. J Allergy Clin Immunol
1989;83:435-40.
16.
Sicherer SH, Burks AW,
Sampson HA. Clinical
features of acute allergic
reactions to peanut and tree
nuts in children. Pediatrics
1998;102:131. abstract.
17.
Sampson HA. Utility of
food-specific IgE con-
centrations in predicting
symptomatic food allergy.
J Allergy Clin Immunol
2001;107:891-6.
18.
Sicherer SH, Furlong TJ,
Munoz-Furlong A, Burks AW,
Sampson HA. A voluntary
registry for peanut and tree
nut allergy: characteristics
of the first 5149 registrants.
J Allergy Clin Immunol
2001;108:128-32.
19.
Skolnick HS,
Conover-Walker MK,
Koerner CB, Sampson HA,
Burks W, Wood RA. The
natural history of peanut
allergy. J Allergy Clin
Immunol 2001;107:367-74.
20.
Lin RY, Schwartz LB,
Curry A, et al. Histamine
and tryptase levels in
patients with acute allergic
reactions: an emergency
department-based study.
J Allergy Clin Immunol
2000;106:65-71.
21.
Sampson HA. Food allergy.
2. Diagnosis and manage-
ment. J Allergy Clin Immunol 1999;103:981-9.

22.
Hourihane JOB,
Bedwani SJ, Dean TP,
Warner JO. Randomised,
double-blind, cross-over
challenge study of allergenicity of peanut oils in subjects allergic to peanuts.
BMJ 1997;314:1084-8.
23.
Furlong TJ, DeSimone J,
Sicherer SH. Peanut and
tree nut allergic reactions
in restaurants and other
food establishments.
J Allergy Clin Immunol
2001;108:867-70.
24.
Sicherer SH, Furlong TJ,
DeSimone J, Sampson HA.
Self-reported allergic reactions to peanut on commercial airliners. J Allergy Clin
Immunol 1999;104:186-9.
25.
Simons FE, Gu X, Simons KJ.
Epinephrine absorption
in adults: intramuscular
versus subcutaneous injection. J Allergy Clin Immunol
2001;108:871-3.
26.
Strachan DP. Hay fever,
hygiene, and household size.
BMJ 1989;299:1259-60.
27.
Vadas P, Wai Y, Burks W,
Perelman B. Detection of
peanut allergens in breast
milk of lactating women.
JAMA 2001;285:1746-8.
28.
Frank L, Marian A, Visser M,
Weinberg E, Potter PC.
Exposure to peanuts in utero
and in infancy and the development of sensitization to
peanut allergens in young
children. Pediatr Allergy
Immunol 1999;10:27-32.

29.
Zeiger RS, Heller S, Mellon MH, et al. Effect of combined maternal and infant food-allergen avoidance on development of atopy in early infancy: a randomized study. J Allergy Clin Immunol 1989;84:72-89. [Erratum, J Allergy Clin Immunol 1989;84:677.]

30.
Sicherer SH, Furlong TJ, Maes HH, Desnick RJ, Sampson HA, Gelb BD. Genetics of peanut allergy: a twin study. J Allergy Clin Immunol 2000;106:53-6.

31.
Oppenheimer JJ, Nelson HS, Bock SA, Christensen F, Leung DYM. Treatment of peanut allergy with rush immunotherapy. J Allergy Clin Immunol 1992;90:256-62.

32.
Sampson HA. Immunological approaches to the treatment of food allergy. Pediatr Allergy Immunol 2001;12: Suppl 14:91-6.

33.
American Academy of Allergy, Asthma and Immunology. Anaphylaxis in schools and other childcare settings. J Allergy Clin Immunol 1998;102:173-6.

34.
Committee on Pediatric Emergency Medicine. Emergency preparedness for children with special health care needs. Pediatrics 1999;104:957. abstract.

35.
Sicherer SH, Furlong TJ, DeSimone J, Sampson HA. The US Peanut and Tree Nut Allergy Registry: characteristics of reactions in schools and day care. J Pediatr 2001;138:560-5.

36.
Committee on Toxicity of Chemicals in Food, Consumer Products, and the Environment. Peanut allergy. London: Department of Health, 1998:1-57.

37.
Altschul AS, Scherrer DL, Munoz-Furlong A, Sicherer SH. Manufacturing and labeling issues for commercial products: relevance to food allergy. J Allergy Clin Immunol 2001;108:468.

ADDENDUM

Since publication of this article, there has been further investigation of novel therapeutic agents for the treatment of peanut allergy.[1] One approach is to administer monthly injections of humanized recombinant anti-IgE antibodies, which may reduce mast-cell– and basophil-bound IgE sufficiently to prevent the activation of allergic responses, at least to small amounts of peanut protein. My colleagues and I conducted a a double-blind, randomized, dose-ranging trial of anti-IgE (TNX-901) administered subcutaneously on a monthly basis in patients with a history of immediate hypersensitivity to peanut.[2] Peanut allergy was confirmed, and the threshold dose of defatted peanut flour was established by a double-blind, placebo-controlled oral food challenge. We found that the highest monthly dose (450 mg) of TNX-901 significantly increased the threshold of sensitivity to peanut by oral challenge from a level of roughly half a peanut (178 mg) to almost nine peanuts (2805 mg) — an effect that should provide protection from most unintended ingestions. A decision was made not to go forward with TNX-901, but phase II trials have since been initiated with omalizumab (Xolair) to determine its efficacy in treating peanut-allergic patients.

1. Sampson HA. Immunolgical approaches to the treatment of food allergy. Pediatr Allergy Immunol 2001;12:Suppl 14:91-6.
2. Leung DY, Sampson HA, Yunginger JW, et al. Effect of anti-Ig E therapy in patients with peanut allergy. N Engl J Med 2003;348:986-93.

Carpal Tunnel Syndrome

JEFFREY N. KATZ, M.D., AND BARRY P. SIMMONS, M.D.

A 64-year-old, right-handed, retired woman presents with intermittent numbness, tingling, and burning pain in the three radial digits of both hands. She has had these symptoms for three months, and they awaken her several times each night. She has no atrophy of the thenar muscles. Sensation to light touch is intact. How should she be evaluated and treated?

THE CLINICAL PROBLEM

Hand, finger, or wrist symptoms account for 2.7 million office visits to physicians for new problems per year in the United States.[1] The differential diagnosis of discomfort of the hand and wrist includes entrapments of the nerves (such as carpal tunnel syndrome, entrapment of the ulnar nerve, and cervical radiculopathy), tendon disorders, overuse of muscles, nonspecific pain syndromes, and less common disorders. The prevalence of electrophysiologically confirmed, symptomatic carpal tunnel syndrome is about 3 percent among women and 2 percent among men, with peak prevalence in women older than 55 years of age.[2]

The carpal tunnel (Figure 1) is located at the base of the palm, just distal to the distal wrist crease. It is bounded on three sides by the carpal bones, which create an arch, and on the palmar side by the fibrous flexor retinaculum, or transverse carpal ligament. Nine flexor tendons (two extending to each finger and one to the thumb) traverse the carpal tunnel, along with the median nerve.

Carpal tunnel syndrome is caused by elevated pressure in the carpal tunnel[3]; this increased pressure produces ischemia of the median nerve, resulting in impaired nerve conduction and attendant paresthesia and pain. Early in the course, no morphologic changes are observable in the median nerve, neurologic findings are reversible, and symptoms are intermittent. Prolonged or frequent episodes of elevated pressure in the carpal tunnel may result in segmental demyelination and more constant and severe symptoms, occasionally with weakness. When there is prolonged ischemia, axonal injury ensues, and nerve dysfunction may be irreversible.[3,4]

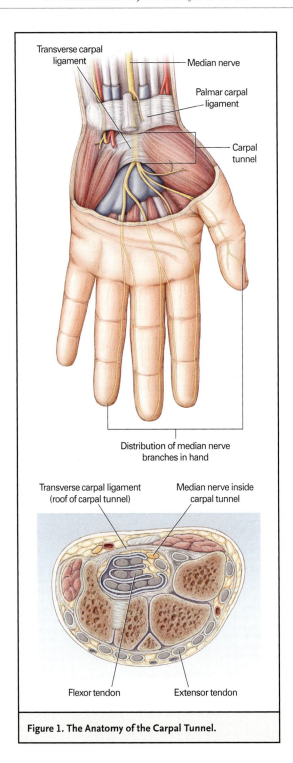

Transverse carpal
ligament

Median nerve

Palmar carpal
ligament

Carpal
tunnel

Distribution of median nerve
branches in hand

Transverse carpal ligament
(roof of carpal tunnel)

Median nerve inside
carpal tunnel

Flexor tendon

Extensor tendon

Figure 1. The Anatomy of the Carpal Tunnel.

A variety of conditions may be associated with carpal tunnel syndrome. These include pregnancy, inflammatory arthritis, Colles' fracture, amyloidosis, hypothyroidism, diabetes mellitus, acromegaly, and use of corticosteroids and estrogens.[5,6] Up to one third of cases of carpal tunnel syndrome occur in association with such medical conditions[7]; about 6 percent of patients have diabetes.[6] Carpal tunnel syndrome is also associated with repetitive activities of the hand and wrist, particularly with a combination of forceful and repetitive activities.[8-10] Occupations associated with a high incidence of carpal tunnel syndrome include food processing, manufacturing, logging, and construction work.[8,11]

The natural history of carpal tunnel syndrome is variable. One 11-year study of workers with carpal tunnel syndrome showed that, although abnormalities of nerve conduction tend to worsen over time, the prevalence of carpal-tunnel symptoms diminishes.[12]

STRATEGIES AND EVIDENCE

Diagnosis

A combination of electrodiagnostic studies (nerve-conduction studies and electromyography) and knowledge of the location and type of symptoms permits the most accurate diagnosis of carpal tunnel syndrome.[13] Symptoms consistent with carpal tunnel syndrome occur in up to 15 percent of the population,[2] and false negative[14] and false positive[15,16] results on electrodiagnostic testing have been well documented. Hence, both symptoms and electrodiagnostic studies must be interpreted carefully. Electrodiagnostic studies are most useful for confirming the diagnosis in suspected cases and ruling out neuropathy and other nerve entrapments.

History Carpal tunnel syndrome generally produces pain, tingling, burning, numbness, or some combination of these symptoms on the palmar aspect of the thumb, index finger, middle finger, and radial half of the ring finger. Patients often report only on detailed questioning that no such symptoms affect the fifth finger. A diagram of symptoms in the hand can help patients to localize symptoms. A diagram of symptoms rated as classic or probable carpal tunnel syndrome according to a standard rating system had a sensitivity of 61 percent and a specificity of 71 percent for the diagnosis of carpal tunnel syndrome in a clinic-based sample.[17] The sensitivity was lower and the specificity higher when the diagram was used to screen workers for carpal tunnel syndrome.[18] A history of nocturnal symptoms has moderate sensitivity (51 to 77 percent) and specificity (27 to 68 percent).[19] Often, patients report that they shake the symptomatic hand or hands when symptoms are at their worst. This response, the "flick sign," had both a sensitivity and a specificity that exceeded 90 percent in one study,[20] but it has not been evaluated further.

Physical Examination   Loss of two-point discrimination in the median-nerve distribution (inability to distinguish between one sharp point on the fingertip and two) as well as thenar atrophy occur late in the course of carpal tunnel syndrome. These signs have low sensitivity and high specificity.[17,19] Tests of the patient's ability to perceive varying degrees of vibratory stimulation[21] and direct pressure on the pulp of the finger[22] in the median-nerve distribution are technically demanding and have moderate sensitivity and specificity.

Several provocative tests may assist in the diagnosis. In Phalen's maneuver, the patient reports whether flexion of the wrist for 60 seconds elicits pain or paresthesia in the median-nerve distribution.[23] Studies of Phalen's maneuver report a wide range of values for sensitivity and specificity, from 40 to 80 percent.[17,19,21,22,24] Tinel's sign is judged to be present if tapping lightly over the volar surface of the wrist causes radiating paresthesia in the digits innervated by the median nerve.[22,23] The sensitivity of Tinel's sign ranges from 25 to 60 percent, although its specificity is higher (67 to 87 percent).[17,19,21,22,24] In the pressure provocation test,[25] the examiner's thumb is pressed over the carpal tunnel for 30 seconds. In the tourniquet test, a blood-pressure cuff is inflated around the arm to above systolic pressure for 60 seconds. Both tests are deemed positive if they elicit radiating paresthesia in the median-nerve distribution. Estimates of sensitivity and specificity for both of these tests vary widely.[20,26]

Since findings on physical examination and the history have limited diagnostic value, they are most useful when there is a reasonable clinical suspicion of carpal tunnel syndrome (as when a patient presents with hand symptoms). The history and physical examination have poor predictive value when the likelihood of carpal tunnel syndrome is low (as it is among participants in population-based or workplace screening programs).[17]

Treatment

Treating Associated Conditions   When carpal tunnel syndrome arises from rheumatoid arthritis or other types of inflammatory arthritis, treatment of the underlying condition generally relieves carpal-tunnel symptoms. Treatment of other associated conditions (such as hypothyroidism or diabetes mellitus) is also appropriate, although data are lacking on whether such treatment alleviates carpal tunnel syndrome. Similarly, it is not known whether stopping medications associated with carpal tunnel syndrome (such as corticosteroids or estrogen) leads to improvement, although taking such a step is also reasonable in the absence of contraindications.

Splinting   More than 80 percent of patients with carpal tunnel syndrome report that a wrist splint alleviates symptoms,[27] generally within days. Splinting also reduces sensory latency,[28] suggesting that the intervention may alter the underlying course of carpal tunnel syndrome. Splints are more effective if they maintain the wrist in neutral posture rather than in extension.[27] Commercially available splints are acceptable, provided that they maintain such a neutral position.

Medications Nonsteroidal antiinflammatory medications, diuretics, and pyridoxine (vitamin B_6) have each been studied in small, randomized trials, with no evidence of efficacy. One four-week randomized trial involving 91 patients had four treatment groups; one group received placebo, one received nonsteroidal antiinflammatory medication, one received a diuretic, and one received 20 mg of prednisolone daily for two weeks followed by 10 mg daily for another two weeks. The prednisolone group had a substantial reduction in symptoms, whereas the outcomes in the other medication groups did not differ from those in the placebo group.[29] In this small study, patients were not followed after the four-week course of treatment ended, nor did the study address the dose of corticosteroids needed to maintain a response. There were essentially no toxic effects of corticosteroids in this short-term trial, although risks including weight gain, hypertension, and hyperglycemia are recognized even with short-term treatment. Apart from this small, short-term study, there have been no other placebo-controlled trials of nonsteroidal antiinflammatory medications.

Local Corticosteroid Injection Patients who remain symptomatic after modification of their activities and splinting are candidates for injection of corticosteroids into the carpal tunnel. A 25-gauge needle may be used to inject 1 ml of 1 percent lidocaine just to the ulnar side of the palmaris longus tendon, proximal to the wrist crease. The needle is aimed toward the carpal tunnel at a 30-degree angle of entry. If there is no paresthesia on injection of a small amount of lidocaine, the rest of the lidocaine is injected followed by the depot corticosteroid.

Injection of corticosteroids is superior to injection of placebo,[30,31] improving symptoms in more than 75 percent of patients.[30,32-34] Local injection of corticosteroids is also associated with improvement in median-nerve conduction.[30,33,34] Symptoms generally recur within one year.[30,32] Risk factors for recurrence include severe abnormalities on electrodiagnostic testing, constant numbness, impaired sensibility, and weakness or thenar muscular atrophy.[30,32,34] The risks of infection and nerve damage resulting from corticosteroid injection are considered to be low but have not been formally studied. Many clinicians limit the number of injections into the carpal tunnel (as they would for other sites) to about three per year in order to minimize local complications (such as rupture of tendons and irritation of the nerves) and the possibility of systemic toxic effects (such as hyperglycemia or hypertension). The optimal number of injections per year has not been studied. Preliminary data suggest that iontophoresis with corticosteroid cream (a method that involves the use of an electrical current to deliver medication to deeper structures) may provide an alternative to corticosteroid injection.[35]

In general, conservative treatment is more successful in patients with mild nerve impairment. In one study,[32] 89 percent of patients with severe carpal tunnel syndrome (constant numbness with weakness, atrophy, or sensory loss) had recurrence of the syndrome within one year after a conservative program that included splinting and injection of corticosteroids into the carpal tunnel. Among patients with mild carpal tunnel syndrome (intermittent numbness and normal sensory and motor findings on physical examination), 60 percent had recurrence of symptoms after such conservative treatment.

Surgery   In general, the decision about whether to proceed with carpal-tunnel–release surgery should be driven by the preference of the patient. However, if a patient has symptoms and signs that are suggestive of axonal loss — constant numbness, symptoms for more than one year, loss of sensibility, and thenar muscular atrophy or weakness — surgery should be seriously considered.

There are several surgical approaches to carpal-tunnel release. In the traditional open procedure, the surgeon makes an incision 5 to 6 cm long, extending distally from the distal wrist crease, and releases the transverse carpal ligament under direct visualization. For endoscopic release, a device with either two portals[36] or one portal[37] is used to release the transverse carpal ligament. The endoscopic techniques carry a higher risk than open carpal-tunnel release of injury to the median nerve.[37-39] Relief of symptoms is similar with the open and the endoscopic procedures,[37,38] and many studies report that patients return to work earlier after the endoscopic surgery.[37-39]

In recent years, many surgeons have adopted a "mini"-open release that uses an incision of 2.0 to 2.5 cm to release the transverse carpal ligament under direct visualization. This approach is used in an attempt to achieve earlier recovery while avoiding the complications associated with the endoscopic approach.[40] The efficacies of the "mini"-open, endoscopic, and traditional open techniques have not been compared in an adequately powered randomized trial.

More than 70 percent of patients report being completely satisfied or very satisfied with the results of carpal-tunnel surgery (irrespective of whether they have undergone open or endoscopic surgery).[41] Similarly, 70 to 90 percent of subjects report being free of nocturnal pain after surgery.[38,41] There have been no randomized controlled trials comparing carpal-tunnel release with conservative therapy. After surgery, pain relief occurs within days, but hand strength does not reach preoperative levels for several months.[42] Tenderness of the surgical scar may also persist for up to a year after open release.[41] Patients with better general functional status and mental health have more favorable outcomes after carpal-tunnel release.[41,43]

Among workers undergoing carpal-tunnel release, involvement of an attorney (generally to dispute a decision about a workers' compensation claim) is associated with a worse surgical outcome.[43] Also, workers with less striking abnormalities on electrodiagnostic testing have worse outcomes.[44] This somewhat paradoxical finding may reflect the inclusion of cases in which symptoms arise from other disorders of the arm or hand, underscoring the importance of careful selection of patients for surgery.

Alternative Therapies   Acupuncture for carpal tunnel syndrome has not been evaluated in controlled studies. In a randomized trial, an intervention involving yoga-based stretching, strengthening, and relaxation in patients with carpal tunnel syndrome resulted in greater improvement in grip strength and reduction of pain than did splinting.[45] In one study, chiropractic therapy for carpal tunnel syndrome was as effective for pain as splints and medication,[46] but data are limited.

AREAS OF UNCERTAINTY

The benefit of modifying the patient's activities remains uncertain. It is reasonable to suggest that patients minimize forceful hand and wrist activities at home and work, since these activities increase carpal-tunnel pressure in patients with carpal tunnel syndrome,[47] and that patients minimize any activities that exacerbate their symptoms. The effects of ergonomically designed equipment and frequent rest breaks on the incidence and course of carpal tunnel syndrome have not been studied rigorously. Rigorous studies are also needed to define the effectiveness of various medications, acupuncture, dietary supplements, chiropractic, and yoga, as well as the optimal timing of carpal-tunnel surgery and the results of carpal-tunnel release with a "mini"-open incision.

GUIDELINES

The "Clinical Guideline on Wrist Pain" from the American Academy of Orthopedic Surgeons recommends that patients with suspected carpal tunnel syndrome modify their activities for two to six weeks while they are treated with wrist splints and nonsteroidal antiinflammatory medication. If these therapies are ineffective, or if the patient has thenar-muscle atrophy or weakness, the guidelines recommend referral to a specialist for consideration of injection or surgery.[48] The practice guidelines of the American College of Occupational and Environmental Medicine[49] suggest a similar approach and emphasize the importance of avoiding occupational activities that cause bothersome symptoms.

CONCLUSIONS AND RECOMMENDATIONS

Patients with discomfort of the hand and wrist, such as the woman described in the vignette, should be evaluated with a detailed history of symptoms (which can be facilitated with a diagram of hand pain) and a physical examination that includes tests of sensory and motor-nerve function and provocative maneuvers. Findings on such examination have limited diagnostic value, however, and will not establish the diagnosis with certainty. If carpal tunnel syndrome seems likely, conservative management with splinting should be initiated. If splinting causes discomfort during the performance of some hand-intensive tasks, it is advisable either to avoid the activity or to perform it without the splint. We suggest that patients reduce activities at home and work that exacerbate symptoms. Although the effects of nonsteroidal antiinflammatory medications on carpal tunnel syndrome have not been well studied, we generally suggest a trial of these agents if there are no contraindications. We do not recommend use of vitamin B_6 (because there is no evidence of efficacy) or oral corticosteroids (given the potential for toxic effects). We generally screen for and treat common underlying disorders — specifically, diabetes and hypothyroidism.

If the condition fails to improve, we recommend referral to a specialist with expertise in the diagnosis and management of carpal tunnel syndrome. If the diagnosis appears secure, the clinician should discuss the options of corticosteroid injection and surgical therapy with the patient. Injection is especially effective if there is no loss of sensibility or thenar-muscle atrophy and weakness and if symptoms are intermittent rather than constant. We perform electrodiagnostic studies if the diagnosis is uncertain, particularly if surgery is contemplated. For surgically treated patients, we favor the limited open incision for carpal-tunnel release.

Supported by grants (K24 AR 02123 and P60 AR 47782) from
the National Institutes of Health and by the Arthritis Foundation.

We are indebted to Drs. Peter Amadio, Alfred Franzblau, and David Rempel for their thoughtful reviews of an earlier version of the manuscript.

This article first appeared in the June 6, 2002, issue of the New England Journal of Medicine.

REFERENCES

1. Praemer A, Furner S, Rice DP. Musculoskeletal conditions in the United States. 2nd ed. Rosemont, Ill.: American Academy of Orthopaedic Surgeons, 1999.

2. Atroshi I, Gummesson C, Johnsson R, Ornstein E, Ranstam J, Rosen I. Prevalence of carpal tunnel syndrome in a general population. JAMA 1999;282:153-8.

3. Gelberman RH, Rydevik BL, Pess GM, Szabo RM, Lundborg G. Carpal tunnel syndrome: a scientific basis for clinical care. Orthop Clin North Am 1988;19:115-24.

4. Rempel D, Dahlin L, Lundborg G. Pathophysiology of nerve compression syndromes: response of peripheral nerves to loading. J Bone Joint Surg Am 1999;81:1600-10.

5. Solomon DH, Katz JN, Bahn R, Mogun H, Avorn J. Nonoccupational risk factors for carpal tunnel syndrome. J Gen Intern Med 1999;14:310-4.

6. Stevens JC, Beard CM, O'Fallon WM, Kurland LT. Conditions associated with carpal tunnel syndrome. Mayo Clin Proc 1992;67:541-8.

7. Atcheson SG, Ward JR, Lowe W. Concurrent medical disease in work-related carpal tunnel syndrome. Arch Intern Med 1998;158:1506-12.

8. Bernard BP, ed. Musculoskeletal disorders and workplace factors: a critical review of epidemiologic evidence for work-related musculoskeletal disorders of the neck, upper extremity, and low back. Cincinnati: National Institute for Occupational Safety and Health, July 1997. (DHHS (NIOSH) publication no. 97-141.)

9. Panel on Musculoskeletal Disorders and the Workplace, Commission on Behavioral and Social Sciences and Education, National Research Council and the Institute of Medicine. Musculoskeletal disorders and the workplace: low back and upper extremities. Washington, D.C.: National Academy Press, 2001.

10. Roquelaure Y, Mechali S, Dano C, et al. Occupational and personal risk factors for carpal tunnel syndrome in industrial workers. Scand J Work Environ Health 1997;23:364-9.

11. Silverstein B, Kalat J. Work related disorders of the back and upper extremity in Washington State, 1990-1997. SHARP technical report 40-2-1999. Olympia, Wash.: SHARP Program, 1999.

12. Nathan PA, Keniston RC, Myers LD, Meadows KD, Lockwood RS. Natural history of median nerve sensory conduction in industry: relationship to symptoms and carpal tunnel syndrome in 558 hands over 11 years. Muscle Nerve 1998;21:711-21.

13. Rempel D, Evanoff B, Amadio PC, et al. Consensus criteria for the classification of carpal tunnel syndrome in epidemiologic studies. Am J Public Health 1998;88:1447-51.

14. Hamanaka I, Okutsu I, Shimizu K, Takatori Y, Ninomiya S. Evaluation of carpal canal pressure in carpal tunnel syndrome. J Hand Surg [Am] 1995;20:848-54.

15. Homan MM, Franzblau A, Werner RA, Albers JW, Armstrong TJ, Bromberg MB. Agreement between symptom surveys, physical examination procedures and electrodiagnostic findings for carpal tunnel syndrome. Scand J Work Environ Health 1999;25:115-24.

16. Ferry S, Silman AJ, Pritchard T, Keenan J, Croft P. The association between different patterns of hand symptoms and objective evidence of median nerve compression: a community-based survey. Arthritis Rheum 1998;41:720-4.

17. Katz JN, Larson MG, Sabra A, et al. The carpal tunnel syndrome: diagnostic utility of the history and physical examination findings. Ann Intern Med 1990;112:321-7.

18. Franzblau A, Werner RA, Albers JW, Grant CL, Olinski R, Johnston E. Workplace surveillance for carpal tunnel syndrome using hand diagrams. J Occup Rehabil 1994;4:185-98.

19. D'Arcy CA, McGee S. The rational clinical examination: does this patient have carpal tunnel syndrome? JAMA 2000;283:3110-7. [Erratum, JAMA 2000;284:1384.]

20. Pryse-Phillips W. Validation of a diagnostic sign in carpal tunnel syndrome. J Neurol Neurosurg Psychiatry 1984;47:870-2.

21. Gerr F, Letz R, Harris-Abbott D, Hopkins LC. Sensitivity and specificity of vibrometry for detection of carpal tunnel syndrome. J Occup Environ Med 1995;37:1108-15.

22. Buch-Jaeger N, Foucher G. Correlation of clinical signs with nerve conduction tests in the diagnosis of carpal tunnel syndrome. J Hand Surg [Br] 1994;19:720-4.

23. Phalen GS. The carpal-tunnel syndrome: seventeen years' experience in diagnosis and treatment of six hundred fifty-four hands. J Bone Joint Surg Am 1966;48:211-28.

24. Golding DN, Rose DM, Selvarajah K. Clinical tests for carpal tunnel syndrome: an evaluation. Br J Rheumatol 1986;25:388-90.

25. Durkan JA. A new diagnostic test for carpal tunnel syndrome. J Bone Joint Surg Am 1991;73:535-8. [Erratum, J Bone Joint Surg Am 1992;74:311.]

26.
Kaul MP, Pagel KJ, Wheatley MJ, Dryden JD. Carpal compression test and pressure provocative test in veterans with median-distribution paresthesias. Muscle Nerve 2001;24:107-11.

27.
Burke DT, Burke MM, Steward GW, Cambre A. Splinting for carpal tunnel syndrome: in search of the optimal angle. Arch Phys Med Rehabil 1994;75:1241-4.

28.
Walker WC, Metzler M, Cifu DX, Swartz Z. Neutral wrist splinting in carpal tunnel syndrome: a comparison of night-only versus full-time wear instructions. Arch Phys Med Rehabil 2000;81:424-9.

29.
Chang M-H, Chiang H-T, Lee SS-J, Ger L-P, Lo Y-K. Oral drug of choice in carpal tunnel syndrome. Neurology 1998;51:390-3.

30.
Girlanda P, Dattola R, Venuto C, Mangiapane R, Nicolosi C, Messina C. Local steroid treatment in idiopathic carpal tunnel syndrome: short- and long-term efficacy. J Neurol 1993;240:187-90.

31.
Dammers JWHH, Veering MM, Vermeulen M. Injection with methylprednisolone proximal to the carpal tunnel: randomised double blind trial. BMJ 1999;319:884-6.

32.
Gelberman RH, Aronson D, Weisman MH. Carpal-tunnel syndrome: results of a prospective trial of steroid injection and splinting. J Bone Joint Surg Am 1980;62:1181-4.

33.
Giannini F, Passero S, Cioni R, et al. Electrophysiologic evaluation of local steroid injection in carpal tunnel syndrome. Arch Phys Med Rehabil 1991;72:738-42.

34.
Ayhan-Ardic FF, Erdem HR. Long-term clinical and electrophysiological results of local steroid injection in patients with carpal tunnel syndrome. Funct Neurol 2000;15:157-65.

35.
Banta CA. A prospective, nonrandomized study of iontophoresis, wrist splinting, and antiinflammatory medication in the treatment of early-mild carpal tunnel syndrome. J Occup Med 1994;36:166-8.

36.
Chow JCY. Endoscopic release of the carpal ligament for carpal tunnel syndrome: long-term results using the Chow technique. Arthroscopy 1999;15:417-21.

37.
Agee JM, McCarroll HR Jr, Tortosa RD, Berry DA, Szabo RM, Peimer CA. Endoscopic release of the carpal tunnel: a randomized prospective multicenter study. J Hand Surg [Am] 1992;17:987-95.

38.
Brown RA, Gelberman RH, Seiler JG III, et al. Carpal tunnel release: a prospective, randomized assessment of open and endoscopic methods. J Bone Joint Surg Am 1993;75:1265-75.

39.
Vasen AP, Kuntz KM, Simmons BP, Katz JN. Open versus endoscopic carpal tunnel release: a decision analysis. J Hand Surg 1999;24:1109-17.

40.
Hallock GG, Lutz DA. Prospective comparison of minimal incision "open" and two-portal endoscopic carpal tunnel release. Plast Reconstr Surg 1995;96:941-7.

41.
Katz JN, Keller RB, Simmons BP, et al. Maine Carpal Tunnel Study: outcomes of operative and nonoperative therapy for carpal tunnel syndrome in a community-based cohort. J Hand Surg [Am] 1998;23:697-710. [Erratum, J Hand Surg [Am] 1999;24:201.]

42.
Katz JN, Fossel KK, Simmons BP, Swartz RA, Fossel AH, Koris MJ. Symptoms, functional status, and neuromuscular impairment following carpal tunnel release. J Hand Surg [Am] 1995;20:549-55.

43.
Katz JN, Losina E, Amick BC III, Fossel AH, Bessette L, Keller RB. Predictors of outcomes of carpal tunnel release. Arthritis Rheum 2001;44:1184-93.

44.
Dennerlein JT, Soumekh FS, Fossel AH, Amick BC III, Keller RB, Katz JN. Longer distal motor latency predicts better outcomes of carpal tunnel release. J Occup Environ Med 2002;44:176-83.

45.
Garfinkel MS, Singhal A, Katz WA, Allan DA, Reshetar R, Schumacher HR Jr. Yoga-based intervention for carpal tunnel syndrome: a randomized trial. JAMA 1998;280:1601-3.

46.
Davis PT, Hulbert JR, Kassak KM, Meyer JJ. Comparative efficacy of conservative medical and chiropractic treatments for carpal tunnel syndrome: a randomized clinical trial. J Manipulative Physiol Ther 1998;21:317-26.

47.
Seradge H, Jia YC, Owens W. In vivo measurement of carpal tunnel pressure in the functioning hand. J Hand Surg [Am] 1995;20:855-9.

48.
American Academy of Orthopaedic Surgeons. Clinical guideline on wrist pain. National Guideline Clearinghouse, 1996. (Accessed January 31, 2006, at http://www.guideline.gov.)

49.
Harris JS, ed. Occupational medicine practice guidelines: evaluation and management of common health problems and functional recovery in workers. Beverly Farms, Mass.: OEM Press, 1998.

Postpartum Depression

KATHERINE L. WISNER, M.D., BARBARA L. PARRY, M.D., AND CATHERINE M. PIONTEK, M.D.

A woman visits the doctor for her six-week postpartum evaluation. She reports that she cannot sleep even if her baby sleeps. She cries daily and worries constantly. She does not feel hungry and is not eating regularly. Making decisions is overwhelming. She says she is not herself. How should this new mother be evaluated and treated?

THE CLINICAL PROBLEM

Postpartum depression, the most common complication of childbearing, occurs in 13 percent of women (one of every eight) after delivery.[1] Given that there are nearly 4 million births in the United States annually, a half-million women have this disorder every year.

STRATEGIES AND EVIDENCE

Definitions

Major depression is defined by the presence of five of the symptoms listed in Table 1, one of which must be either depressed mood or decreased interest or pleasure in activities. The symptoms reflect the physiologic dysregulation (disturbance of sleep, appetite, and cognition) that is characteristic of depression and must be present for most of the day nearly every day for two weeks or more. According to the *Diagnostic and Statistical Manual of Mental Disorders*, fourth edition (DSM-IV),[2] an episode of depression is considered to have postpartum onset if it begins within four weeks after delivery. However, onset within three months after delivery is the time frame commonly used by investigators on the basis of epidemiologic studies.[3] The patterns of symptoms in women with postpartum depression are similar to those in women who have episodes unrelated to childbirth.[4] Difficulties in the interactions between caretakers who are under stress and infants increase the risk of insecure attachment and cognitive and behavioral problems in children. The conse-

---

Table 1. Symptoms of Major Depression with Postpartum Onset.*

Major depression is defined by the presence of five of the following symptoms, one of which must be either depressed mood or decreased interest or pleasure†:

Depressed mood, often accompanied or overshadowed by severe anxiety

Markedly diminished interest or pleasure in activities

Appetite disturbance — usually loss of appetite with weight loss

Sleep disturbance — most often insomnia and fragmented sleep, even when the baby sleeps

Physical agitation (most commonly) or psychomotor slowing

Fatigue, decreased energy

Feelings of worthlessness or excessive or inappropriate guilt

Decreased concentration or ability to make decisions

Recurrent thoughts of death or suicidal ideation

---

* From the *Diagnostic and Statistical Manual of Mental Disorders,* fourth edition (DSM-IV).[2] Postpartum depression is defined in the DSM-IV as that which begins within four weeks after delivery.
† Symptoms must be present most of the day nearly every day for two weeks. A diagnosis of major depression also requires a decline from the woman's previous level of functioning and substantial impairment.

---

quences of parental mental illness, such as family discord, loss of income, and placement of children outside of the home, also affect child development.

Causes

The rapid decline in the levels of reproductive hormones that occurs after delivery is believed to contribute to the development of depression in susceptible women. In one study, such a decline after delivery was simulated in nonpregnant women with the use of leuprolide to induce a hypogonadal state, followed by treatment with supraphysiologic doses of estradiol and progesterone, and finally the withdrawal of both steroids under double-blind conditions.[5] Five of eight women with a history of postpartum depression, but none of eight women without previous depression, had mood changes. Women with a history of postpartum depression appear differentially sensitive to the effects on mood of the withdrawal of gonadal steroids.

Although it is tempting to attribute postpartum depression to hormonal decline, several other factors may predispose women to this condition. Stressful life events,[6] past episodes of depression (not necessarily related to childbearing), and a family history of mood disorders,[1,7] all recognized predictors of major depression in women,[6] are also predictors of postpartum depression. The likelihood of postpartum depression does not appear to be related to a woman's educational level, the sex of her infant, whether or not she breast-feeds, the mode of delivery, or whether or not the pregnancy was planned.[7]

Screening

The Edinburgh Postnatal Depression Scale (Supplementary Appendix 1, available with the full text of this article at http://www.nejm.org),[8] a 10-item questionnaire that is easy to administer, is an effective screening tool. One example of an item on the questionnaire is the following statement: "I have looked forward with enjoyment to things," to which responses are scored from 0, for "as much as I ever did," to 3, for "hardly at all." A cutoff score of 9 or 10 has been recommended in the United Kingdom for first-stage screening[9] and is a reliable indicator of the presence of postpartum depression in women in the United States as well.[10] If a woman has a total score on the Edinburgh Postnatal Depression Scale of 10 or higher or indicates that "the thought of harming myself has occurred to me" either "sometimes" (a score of 2) or "quite often" (a score of 3), a brief clinical interview to review symptoms and establish the diagnosis of depression is warranted.

An alternative to the Edinburgh Postnatal Depression Scale is to frame the required criterion for the diagnosis of depression as a screening question[2]: "Have you had depressed mood or decreased interest or pleasure in activities most of the day nearly every day for the past two weeks?" If the woman answers in the affirmative, the clinician can next determine whether at least five of the symptoms listed in Table 1 are present. The level of impairment and distress can be explored with the question "Has the depression made it hard for you to do your work, take care of things at home, or get along with people?"[2]

Evaluation and Differential Diagnosis

If the patient has considered a plan to act on suicidal thoughts or has thoughts about harming her infant, provisions for safety and urgent referral for psychiatric care are recommended. Women who have major functional impairment (as evidenced by the avoidance of family or friends, an inability to attend to hygiene, or an inability to care adequately for the infant) and those with coexisting substance abuse are also candidates for rapid referral. Women who report depressive symptoms without suicidal ideation or major functional impairment (or score between 5 and 9 on the Edinburgh Postnatal Depression Scale) should be evaluated again two to four weeks later in order to determine whether an episode of depression has evolved or whether symptoms have subsided.

A careful history taking and a physical examination are warranted in all women with postpartum depression. Thyroid function should be assessed, since both hypothyroidism and hyperthyroidism are more frequent during the postpartum period and may contribute to mood changes. However, in women with hyperthyroidism or hypothyroidism, treatment of both thyroid and depressive disorders is usually required.[7]

Postpartum depression must be distinguished from the "baby blues," which occur in the majority of new mothers. In this syndrome, symptoms such as weeping, sadness, irritability, anxiety, and confusion occur, peaking around the fourth day after delivery, and resolving by the tenth day. This transient mood disturbance does not consistently affect the woman's ability to function.

Postpartum psychosis represents a psychiatric emergency that requires immediate intervention because of the risk of infanticide and suicide. Onset usually occurs within the first two weeks after delivery. This disorder differs from other psychotic episodes because it usually involves extreme disorganization of thought, bizarre behavior, unusual hallucinations (which may be visual, olfactory, or tactile), and delusions, all of which suggest an organic cause.[4] Treatments for postpartum psychosis have been discussed in detail elsewhere.[11]

Postpartum psychosis is usually a manifestation of bipolar disorder.[12] A depressive episode (with or without psychotic features) can occur during the course of bipolar disorder. Therefore, all patients with postpartum depression should be screened with the following questions[2]: "Have you ever had four continuous days when you were feeling so good, high, excited, or 'hyper' that other people thought you were not your normal self or you got into trouble?" and "Have you experienced four continuous days when you were so irritable that you found yourself shouting at people or starting fights or arguments?" Positive responses to these questions necessitate psychiatric referral.

Antidepressant Treatment

For women who are given a diagnosis of major depression with postpartum onset, treatment with antidepressant drugs is appropriate. A selective serotonin-reuptake inhibitor should be tried initially because such agents are associated with a low risk of toxic effects in patients taking an overdose, as well as with ease of administration. However, if the patient has previously had a positive response to a specific drug from any class of antidepressants, that agent should be strongly considered.

The efficacy of antidepressant drugs for depression unrelated to childbearing supports their use for postpartum depression, and the available data confirm the assumption that they are effective against postpartum depression. Information about drugs used to treat depression[13-18] is presented in Table 2. However, only one placebo-controlled trial and three open trials that specifically addressed postpartum depression have been published. The selective serotonin-reuptake inhibitor fluoxetine was compared with psychotherapy,

Table 2. Pharmacotherapy for Postpartum Depression.

Drug	Recommended Range of Doses (mg/day)*	Side Effects	Implications for Use during Breast-Feeding
Selective serotonin-reuptake inhibitors			
Sertraline	50–200	Nausea, loose stools, tremors, insomnia, sexual dysfunction, possible drug interactions†	Drug and weakly active metabolite generally not detectable in infants; no reports of adverse events
Paroxetine	20–60	Nausea, drowsiness, fatigue, dizziness, sexual dysfunction, possible drug interactions†	No active metabolite; levels not detectable in infants; no reports of adverse events
Fluvoxamine	50–200	Nausea, drowsiness, anorexia, anxiety, sexual dysfunction, possible drug interactions†	No active metabolite; levels not detectable in infants; no reports of adverse events
Citalopram	20–40	Nausea, insomnia, dizziness, somnolence	One infant with a measurable level had colic; other infants had no problems and serum levels that were undetectable or just above the limit of detection
Fluoxetine	20–60	Nausea, drowsiness, anorexia, anxiety, sexual dysfunction, possible drug interactions†	Drug and active metabolite have comparatively long half-lives; serum levels similar to those in adults reported in some symptomatic infants; prenatal exposure adds to serum levels in breast-fed infants
Tricyclic antidepressants			
Nortriptyline	50–150	Sedation, weight gain, dry mouth, constipation, orthostatic hypotension, possible drug interactions†; base-line ECG recommended‡	Drug and metabolites generally below or slightly above limit of detectability; no reports of adverse events in infants
Desipramine	100–300	Sedation, weight gain, dry mouth, constipation, orthostatic hypotension, possible drug interactions†; base-line ECG recommended‡	Drug and metabolites below quantifiable level; no adverse effects
Serotonin–norepinephrine reuptake inhibitor			
Venlafaxine	75–300	Nausea, sweating, dry mouth, dizziness, insomnia, somnolence, sexual dysfunction	Undetectable or low serum levels of drug; metabolite usually measurable and levels similar to those in adults observed in some infants; drug level greater in breast milk than in maternal serum
Other			
Bupropion	300–450	Dizziness, headache, dry mouth, sweating, tremor, agitation, rare seizures, possible drug interactions†	Unknown
Nefazodone	300–600	Dry mouth, somnolence, nausea, dizziness, possible drug interactions†	No published data on serum levels in infants; sedation and poor feeding in a premature infant described
Mirtazapine	15–45	Somnolence, nausea, weight gain, dizziness	Unknown

* Treatment with any of these agents should be initiated at half of the lowest recommended therapeutic dose. Dosages are from the *Physicians' Desk Reference*, 55th ed.[13]

† Drug interactions are possible because of the drug's inhibition of the following cytochrome P450 (CYP) enzyme systems[17,18]: for sertraline, 2D6, 2C, and 3A4; for paroxetine, nortriptyline, desipramine, and bupropion, 2D6; for fluvoxamine, 1A2, 2C, and 3A4; for fluoxetine, 2D6, 2C, and 3A4; for nefazodone, 3A4.

‡ If the electrocardiogram (ECG) shows conduction defects, consider a non-tricyclic antidepressant.

and both treatments were similarly effective.[18] Fluoxetine was significantly more effective than placebo.[18] Sertraline,[19] venlafaxine,[20] and drugs grouped according to class (selective serotonin-reuptake inhibitors and tricyclic antidepressants[21]) were effective in open trials. Women with postpartum depression may be more likely to have a response to serotonergic agents, such as selective serotonin-reuptake inhibitors and venlafaxine, than to nonserotonergic tricyclic antidepressants.[19-21]

Because women who have recently given birth are often sensitive to the side effects of medications,[22] treatment should be initiated at half the recommended starting doses listed in Table 2 (e.g., 25 mg of sertraline per day or 10 mg of paroxetine per day) for four days, and doses should be increased by small increments (e.g., 25 mg of sertraline per week or 10 mg of paroxetine per week) as tolerated, until full remission is achieved. Slow increases in the dose are helpful in managing side effects. If the patient has a response to an initial trial of medication lasting six to eight weeks, the same dose should be continued for a minimum of six months after a full remission has been achieved, in order to prevent relapse.[23] If there is no improvement after six weeks of drug therapy, or if the patient has a response but then has a relapse, referral to a psychiatrist should be considered. The average duration of a postpartum episode of depression (without treatment) is seven months.[24] Fifty to 85 percent of patients with a single episode of major depression will have at least one more episode after the discontinuation of medication, and the risk increases with the number of previous episodes.[23] Therefore, long-term treatment for the prevention of recurrence should be considered for women who have had three or more episodes of severe depression.

Breast-Feeding

All antidepressants are excreted in breast milk. Optimal clinical management dictates the use of the lowest effective dose of antidepressants in a lactating mother. Observation of the infant's behavior before the mother is treated permits clinicians to avoid misinterpreting typical behavior as potentially drug-related.

The serum levels of antidepressants in infants of breast-feeding mothers have been evaluated in multiple studies.[25-41] The selective serotonin-reuptake inhibitor sertraline has been recommended as the first-line treatment for breast-feeding mothers on the basis of multiple case series by several investigators that suggest that this agent may be used with little risk.[42] Epperson and colleagues[27] evaluated the functional effects of very low levels of sertraline in breast-fed infants by assessing the platelet serotonin level. In humans, platelet and central neuronal serotonin transporters are identical. The expected marked decline in serotonin levels was observed in mothers after treatment, but there was minimal change in the infants who were exposed to small amounts of sertraline through breast milk. No reports of adverse effects in breast-fed infants whose mothers were treated with sertraline, paroxetine, or fluvoxamine have been published.

Colic has been reported in three infants who were breast-fed by mothers taking fluoxetine; when tested, the infants were shown to have serum levels of fluoxetine and norfluoxetine (the active metabolite of fluoxetine) that were in the therapeutic range for adults.[31,32] Chambers et al.[43] reported that breast-fed infants of fluoxetine-treated mothers gained significantly less weight after birth, although the mothers did not report unusual behavior in these infants. Unlike most antidepressants, fluoxetine has a highly active metabolite (norfluoxetine), and both agents have very long half-lives (84 and 146 hours, respectively).[41] Continuous exposure to fluoxetine through breast milk is more likely than exposure to other selective serotonin-reuptake inhibitors to lead to measurable serum levels of the antidepressant agent.[41] Prenatal exposure to fluoxetine may also contribute to measurable serum levels in infants of mothers who take this medication. In one report, "uneasy sleep" was described in an infant with a measurable serum level of citalopram, a selective serotonin-reuptake inhibitor with a shorter half-life[35]; however, this report is inconsistent with data on other selective serotonin-reuptake inhibitors that have similar half-lives. An unusually high level of sertraline was reported in one infant,[25] although the authors believed it to be a spurious finding. However, some infants may have particularly poor metabolism of antidepressants.[41]

Tricyclic antidepressants are not typically found in measurable amounts in nursing infants.[41] Since these agents are not first-line drugs for depression, only the representative drugs nortriptyline and desipramine (which have fewer side effects than others in the class) are listed in Table 2. Of the drugs in this class, nortriptyline has been studied the most as a treatment for breast-feeding women. The only adverse outcome reported with any tricyclic antidepressant, respiratory depression and sedation, occurred in an infant whose mother was taking doxepin.[41] Data are lacking on other classes of antidepressants.

Children who were exposed to tricyclic antidepressants through breast milk have been followed through preschool and compared with children who were not exposed to such drugs, and no developmental problems have been found.[44] However, there are no published long-term evaluations of infants exposed to selective serotonin-reuptake inhibitors through breast milk, and effects of antidepressants on developing neurotransmitter systems cannot be ruled out. Although substantial data have been published on antidepressant levels in infants exposed through breast milk, they reflect effects in full-term infants. Close clinical monitoring and measurement of serum levels are warranted for premature or sick newborns. In the cases of women who have a response only to drugs for which data are unavailable, decisions regarding treatment during breast-feeding must take into account this uncertainty. The importance of caretaking by capable parents, which is compromised by depression, and the benefits of breast-feeding should also be weighed in the decision-making process.

Prophylactic Treatment

Women who have a history of depression are justifiably concerned about recurrence after childbirth. After one postpartum episode, the risk of recurrence (defined as a return of symptoms that fulfill the DSM-IV criteria for major depression) is 25 percent.[10] Preventive therapy after delivery should be considered for women with any previous episode of depression.[10] The drug to which the patient previously had a response or a selective serotonin-reuptake inhibitor are reasonable choices; the tricyclic antidepressant nortriptyline did not confer protection, as compared with placebo.[10] At a minimum, postpartum management should include monitoring for recurrence, with a plan for rapid intervention if indicated.

Psychotherapy

In a study involving 120 women who had recently given birth, interpersonal psychotherapy, a 12-session treatment that focuses on changing roles and important relationships, was effective for the relief of depressive symptoms and improvement in psychosocial functioning in treated women as compared with controls who were on the waiting list for such therapy.[24] A group intervention based on interpersonal psychotherapy and delivered during pregnancy prevented postpartum depression in 35 economically disadvantaged women.[45] However, psychotherapy in addition to fluoxetine did not improve outcomes more than fluoxetine alone.[13]

Hormonal Therapy

Estradiol[46] has been evaluated as a treatment for postpartum depression. In a study comparing transdermal 17β-estradiol (200 μg per day) with placebo, the estradiol-treated group had a significant reduction in depression scores during the first month. However, nearly half the women also were treated with antidepressants, so the effect of estradiol alone remains uncertain. Prophylactic administration of a progestogen after delivery increased the risk of postpartum depression as compared with placebo.[47]

AREAS OF UNCERTAINTY

Antidepressants are effective for postpartum depression; however, it is not certain whether specific antidepressants or classes of antidepressants are more beneficial than others. The optimal approach to prophylaxis in high-risk patients is also unclear. The role of psychotherapy for patients with a partial response or no response to medication has not been explored. More data are needed on predictors of the response to therapy so that patients may be systematically matched with therapies. The role of gonadal steroids in causing postpartum depression remains unclear. In addition, data are needed about long-term physical and mental development in infants exposed to antidepressants through breast-feeding as well as prenatally.

GUIDELINES

To our knowledge, there are no treatment guidelines available that are specific to postpartum depression. Clinical-practice guidelines developed by the American Psychiatric Association for major depression in adults apply[23] (they are available at http://www.psych.org). The severity of symptoms, the preferences of the patient, and the response to treatment during previous episodes influence the recommendations for psychotherapy, antidepressants, or electroconvulsive therapy.

CONCLUSIONS AND RECOMMENDATIONS

Physicians must expect that one out of eight new mothers will have postpartum depression. In women with previous episodes of postpartum depression, the risk of recurrence is one in four. Since identification of postpartum depression is the first step, we recommend that women be screened after delivery with the Edinburgh Postnatal Depression Scale, which is brief, is highly acceptable to patients, and reliably detects the presence of postpartum depression (indicated by a score of 10 or higher).[8] Alternatively, women should be asked about depressed mood and other associated symptoms. Once depression has been identified, rapid implementation of treatment is advisable, because episodes may be long and the number and severity of sequelae increase with the duration of the episode. Depressed women should be asked about any intention to harm themselves or their children, which necessitates urgent referral for psychiatric care.

A selective serotonin-reuptake inhibitor should be the first-line drug because such agents carry a low risk of toxic effects in patients who take an overdose, are easy to administer, and have been used relatively frequently in breast-feeding women. Any drug should be initiated at half the usual starting dose. We administer medication for at least six months after full remission in order to prevent relapse,[23] and we consider long-term maintenance therapy for women with three or more episodes or episodes that featured serious disability. Women with postpartum depression may also respond to interpersonal psychotherapy. The goal of treatment is complete normalization of mood and physiologic and social functioning.

Women with this disorder need not feel alone in their suffering. They may find useful information in Marie Osmond's book *Behind the Smile: My Journey Out of Postpartum Depression*[48] and on the Web sites of the National Women's Health Information Center (http://www.4woman.gov) and groups such as Postpartum Support International (http://www.chss.iup.edu/postpartum) and Depression after Delivery (http://www.depressionafterdelivery.com).

Supported by grants (R01 57102 and R01 60335, to Dr. Wisner) from the National Institute of Mental Health.
An early draft of this paper was presented at the Summit on Women and Depression
sponsored by the American Psychological Association, Queenstown, Md., October 5–7, 2000.

This article first appeared in the July 18, 2002, issue of the New England Journal of Medicine.

REFERENCES

1.
O'Hara MW, Swain AM. Rates and risk of postpartum depression: a meta analysis. Int Rev Psychiatry 1996;8:37-54.

2.
The diagnostic and statistical manual of mental disorders, 4th ed.: DSM-IV. Washington, D.C.: American Psychiatric Association, 1994.

3.
Kendell RE, Chalmers JC, Platz C. Epidemiology of puerperal psychoses. Br J Psychiatry 1987;150:662-73. [Erratum, Br J Psychiatry 1987;151:135.]

4.
Wisner KL, Peindl KS, Hanusa BH. Symptomatology of affective and psychotic illnesses related to childbearing. J Affect Disord 1994;30:77-87.

5.
Bloch M, Schmidt PJ, Danaceau M, Murphy J, Nieman L, Rubinow DR. Effects of gonadal steroids in women with a history of postpartum depression. Am J Psychiatry 2000;157:924-30.

6.
Swendsen JD, Mazure CM. Life stress as a risk factor for postpartum depression: current research and methodological issues. Clin Psychol Sci Pract 2000;7:17-31.

7.
Wisner KL, Stowe ZN. Psychobiology of postpartum mood disorders. Semin Reprod Endocrinol 1997;15:77-89.

8.
Cox JL, Holden JM, Sagovsky R. Detection of postnatal depression: development of the 10-item Edinburgh Postnatal Depression Scale. Br J Psychiatry 1987;150:782-6.

9.
Cox J. Origins and development of the 10-item Edinburgh Postnatal Depression Scale. In: Cox J, Holden J, eds. Perinatal psychiatry, use and misuse of the Edinburgh Postnatal Depression Scale. London: Gaskell, 1994:115-23.

10.
Wisner KL, Perel JM, Peindl KS, Hanusa BH, Findling RL, Rapport D. Prevention of recurrent postpartum depression: a randomized clinical trial. J Clin Psychiatry 2001;62:82-6.

11.
Parry BL, Hamilton J. Postpartum psychiatric syndromes. In: Risch SC, Janowsky DS, eds. The art of psychopharmacology. New York: Guilford Press, 1992.

12.
Wisner KL, Peindl KS, Hanusa BH. Psychiatric episodes in women with young children. J Affect Disord 1995;34:1-11.

13.
Physicians' desk reference. 55th ed. Montvale, N.J.: Medical Economics, 2001.

14.
Preskorn SH. Clinical pharmacology of selective serotonin reuptake inhibitors. Caddo, Okla.: Professional Communications, 1996:75-105.

15.
Richelson E. Pharmacology of antidepressants — characteristics of the ideal drug. Mayo Clin Proc 1994;69:1069-81.

16.
Nemeroff CB, DeVane CL, Pollack BG. Newer antidepressants and the cytochrome P_{450} system. Am J Psychiatry 1996;153:311-20.

17.
Brosen K. Differences in interactions of SSRIs. Int Clin Psychopharmacol 1998;13:Suppl 5:S45-S47.

18.
Appleby L, Warner R, Whitton A, Faragher B. A controlled study of fluoxetine and cognitive-behavioural counselling in the treatment of postnatal depression. BMJ 1997;314:932-6.

19.
Stowe ZN, Casarella J, Landry J, Nemeroff CB. Sertraline in the treatment of women with postpartum major depression. Depression 1995;3:49-55.

20.
Cohen LS, Viguera AC, Bouffard SM, et al. Venlafaxine in the treatment of postpartum depression. J Clin Psychiatry 2001;62:592-6.

21.
Wisner KL, Peindl KS, Gigliotti TV. Tricyclics vs SSRIs for postpartum depression. Arch Womens Mental Health 1999;1:189-91.

22.
Wisner KL, Perel JM, Peindl KS, Findling RL, Hanusa BH. Effects of the postpartum period on nortriptyline pharmacokinetics. Psychopharmacol Bull 1997;33:243-8.

23.
American Psychiatric Association. Guidelines for the treatment of patients with major depressive disorder (revision). Am J Psychiatry 2000;157:Suppl:1-45.

24.
O'Hara MW, Stuart S, Gorman LL, Wenzel A. Efficacy of interpersonal psychotherapy for postpartum depression. Arch Gen Psychiatry 2000;57:1039-45.

25.
Wisner KL, Perel JM, Blumer J. Serum sertraline and N-desmethylsertraline levels in breast-feeding mother-infant pairs. Am J Psychiatry 1998;155:690-2.

26.
Stowe ZN, Owens MJ, Landry JC, et al. Sertraline and desmethylsertraline in human breast milk and nursing infants. Am J Psychiatry 1997;154:1255-60.

27.
Epperson N, Czarkowski KA, Ward-O'Brien D, et al. Maternal sertraline treatment and serotonin transport in breast-feeding mother-infant pairs. Am J Psychiatry 2001;158:1631-7.

28.
Hendrick V, Fukuchi A, Altshuler L, Widawski M, Wertheimer A, Brunhuber MV. Use of sertraline, paroxetine and fluvoxamine by nursing women. Br J Psychiatry 2001;179:163-6.

29.
Stowe ZN, Cohen LS, Hostetter A, Ritchie JC, Owens MJ, Nemeroff CB. Paroxetine in human breast milk and nursing infants. Am J Psychiatry 2000;157:185-9.

30.
Misri S, Kim J, Riggs KW, Kostaras X. Paroxetine levels in postpartum depressed women, breast milk, and infant serum. J Clin Psychiatry 2000;61:828-32.

31.
Lester BM, Cucca J, Andreozzi L, Flanagan P, Oh W. Possible association between fluoxetine hydrochloride and colic in an infant. J Am Acad Child Adolesc Psychiatry 1993;32:1253-5.

32.
Kristensen JH, Ilett KF, Hackett LP, Yapp P, Paech M, Begg EJ. Distribution and excretion of fluoxetine and norfluoxetine in human milk. Br J Clin Pharmacol 1999;48:521-7.

33.
Piontek CM, Wisner KL, Perel JM, Peindl KS. Serum fluvoxamine levels in breast-fed infants. J Clin Psychiatry 2001;62:111-3.

34.
Jenson PN, Olesen OV, Bertelsen A, Linnet K. Citalopram and desmethyl-citalopram concentrations in breast milk and in serum of mother and infant. Ther Drug Monit 1997;19:236-9.

35.
Schmidt K, Olesen OV, Jensen PN. Citalopram and breast-feeding: serum concentration and side effects in the infant. Biol Psychiatry 2000;47:164-5.

36.
Hendrick V, Altshuler L, Wertheimer A, Dunn WA. Venlafaxine and breast-feeding. Am J Psychiatry 2001;158:2089-90.

37.
Ilett KF, Hackett LP, Dusci LJ, et al. Distribution and excretion of venlafaxine and O-desmethylvenlafaxine in human milk. Br J Clin Pharmacol 1998;45:459-62.

38.
Ilett KF, Kristensen JH, Hackett LP, Paech MJ, Rampono J. Distribution of venlafaxine and its O-desmethyl metabolite in human milk and their effects in breastfed infants. Br J Clin Pharmacol 2002;53:17-22.

39.
Rampono J, Kirstensen JH, Hackett LP, Paech M, Kohan R, Ilett KF. Citalopram and desmethylcitalopram in human milk: distribution, excretion and effects in breast fed infants. Br J Clin Pharmacol 2000;50:263-8.

40.
Yapp P, Ilett KF, Kristensen JH, Hackett LP, Paech MJ, Rampono J. Drowsiness and poor feeding in a breast-fed infant: association with nefazodone and its metabolites. Ann Pharmacother 2000;34:1269-72.

41.
Wisner KL, Perel JM, Findling RL. Antidepressant treatment during breast-feeding. Am J Psychiatry 1996;153:1132-7.

42.
Altshuler LL, Cohen LS, Moline ML, Kahn DA, Carpenter D, Docherty JP. The Expert Consensus Guideline Series: treatment of depression in women. Postgrad Med 2001; (Special Number):1-107.

43.
Chambers CD, Anderson PO, Thomas RG, et al. Weight gain in infants breast-fed by mothers who take fluoxetine. Pediatrics 1999;104:1120-1. abstract.

44.
Yoshida K, Smith B, Craggs M, Kumar RC. Investigation of pharmacokinetics and of possible adverse effects in infants exposed to tricyclic antidepressants in breast-milk. J Affect Disord 1997;43:225-37.

45.
Zlotnick C, Johnson SL, Miller IW, Pearlstein T, Howard M. Postpartum depression in women receiving public assistance: pilot study of an interpersonal-therapy-oriented group intervention. Am J Psychiatry 2001;158:638-40.

46.
Gregoire AJP, Kumar R, Everitt B, Henderson AF, Studd JWW. Transdermal oestrogen for treatment of severe postnatal depression. Lancet 1996;347:930-3.

47.
Lawrie TA, Hofmeyr GJ, De Jager M, Berk M, Paiker J, Viljoen E. A double-blind randomised placebo controlled trial of postnatal norethisterone enanthate: the effect on postnatal depression and serum hormones. Br J Obstet Gynaecol 1998;105:1082-90.

48.
Osmond M. Behind the smile: my journey out of postpartum depression. New York: Warner Books, 2001.

ADDENDUM

Since the publication of this article, authors of a meta-analysis have identified the incidence of postpartum depression to be 14.5 percent (one in seven new mothers) in the first three postpartum months.[1] A pooled analysis of studies of antidepressant levels in lactating mothers, breast milk, and nursing infants[2] indicated that maternal treatment with nortriptyline, paroxetine, and sertraline usually results in nonquantifiable serum levels in breast-fed infants, and it concluded that these are drugs of choice for the breast-feeding woman; however, established efficacy of another drug in a given patient must be considered in the decision-making process.

A small placebo-controlled randomized trial of non-depressed women with a history of postpartum depression suggested that sertraline might prevent recurrence. As compared with the placebo group, women randomized to a six-month course of sertraline immediately postpartum were significantly less likely to experience a postpartum major depression.[3]

1. Gaynes BN, Gavin N, Meltzer-Brody S, et al. Perinatal depression: prevalence, screening accuracy, and screening outcomes. (Accessed January 31, 2006, at http://www.ahrq.gov/clinic/epcsums/peridepsum.htm.)

2. Weissman AM, Levy BT, Hartz AJ, et al. Pooled analysis of antidepressant levels in lactating mothers, breast milk, and nursing infants. Am J Psychiatry 2004;161:1066-78.

3. Wisner KL, Perel JM, Peindl KS, Hanusa BH, Piontek CM, Findling RL. Prevention of postpartum depression: a pilot randomized clinical trial. Am J Psychiatry 2004;161:1290-2.

Preventing Falls in Elderly Persons

MARY E. TINETTI, M.D.

A 79-year-old woman with a history of congestive heart failure, arthritis, depression, and difficulty sleeping presents for a follow-up visit. She takes several prescription medications, including an antidepressant, a diuretic, an angiotensin-converting–enzyme inhibitor, and a beta-blocker, as well as over-the-counter sleep and allergy medications. Her chronic conditions appear to be stable. Her daughter reports that the patient has fallen twice during the past six months. What can be done to prevent future falls?

THE CLINICAL PROBLEM

More than one third of persons 65 years of age or older fall each year, and in half of such cases the falls are recurrent.[1,2] Approximately 1 in 10 falls results in a serious injury, such as hip fracture, other fracture, subdural hematoma, other serious soft-tissue injury, or head injury.[3-5] Falls account for approximately 10 percent of visits to the emergency department and 6 percent of urgent hospitalizations among elderly persons.[4,6] Independently of other health conditions, falls are associated with restricted mobility; a decline in the ability to carry out activities such as dressing, bathing, shopping, or housekeeping; and an increased risk of placement in a nursing home.[7-9]

Although a few falls have a single cause, the majority result from interactions between long-term or short-term predisposing factors and short-term precipitating factors in a person's environment.[1-5] Each of the following conditions has been shown to increase the subsequent risk of falling in two or more observational studies: arthritis; depressive symptoms; orthostasis; impairment in cognition, vision, balance, gait, or muscle strength; and the use of four or more prescription medications. Furthermore, the risk of falling consistently increases as the number of these risk factors increases.[1,2] The risk of falling increased in a cohort of elderly persons living in the community, for example, from 8 percent among those with no risk factors to 78 percent among those with four or more risk factors.[1]

Although there is a clear relation between falling and the use of a higher number of medications, the risks associated with individual classes of drugs have been more variable.[10,11] To date, serotonin-reuptake inhibitors, tricyclic antidepressants, neuroleptic agents, benzodiazapines, anticonvulsants, and class IA antiarrhythmic medications have been shown to have the strongest link to an increased risk of falling.[10-12]

During the month after hospital discharge, the risk of falling is high, particularly among elderly persons frail enough to require home health care.[13] Other periods of high risk include those in which there are episodes of acute illness or exacerbations of chronic illness.

As discussed in the next section of this article, several single and multifactorial, health care–based strategies have proved effective in reducing the rate of falling in clinical trials.[14-21] However, implementation of these approaches for the prevention of falling may be complicated, for at least two reasons. First, clinicians are more experienced at managing discrete diseases than at managing multifactorial conditions, such as falling. Second, although many components of an effective fall-prevention strategy are relatively straightforward, others require tradeoffs and the weighing of risks and benefits. Perhaps the most complicated component of a strategy to prevent falls involves reduction in the use of medications. Medications may be appropriately recommended for the treatment of a disease, but they also have adverse effects; falling is one of the most common adverse events related to drugs.[22-24] Many elderly patients have several chronic conditions for which multiple medications are prescribed, further increasing the associated risks, including falling.

STRATEGIES AND EVIDENCE

Assessment and Intervention

Because falls result from various combinations of factors, an effective and efficient clinical strategy for risk assessment and management must address many predisposing and precipitating factors. However, a clinically sensible strategy can be extrapolated from the available clinical-trial data, augmented by observational data from well-designed studies.[1-5,10-21]

A rational approach to the prevention of falls is presented in Figure 1. Because elderly persons may not volunteer the information, physicians should, on at least a yearly basis, ask their elderly patients about any falls and ask about and look for any difficulties with balance or gait. Brief screens such as the "Get-Up and Go" test, which involves looking for unsteadiness as the patient gets up from a chair without using his or her arms, walks a few meters, and returns, is easily incorporated into short clinical encounters.[25,26] Other assessments provide more specific information about balance and gait abnormalities.[27]

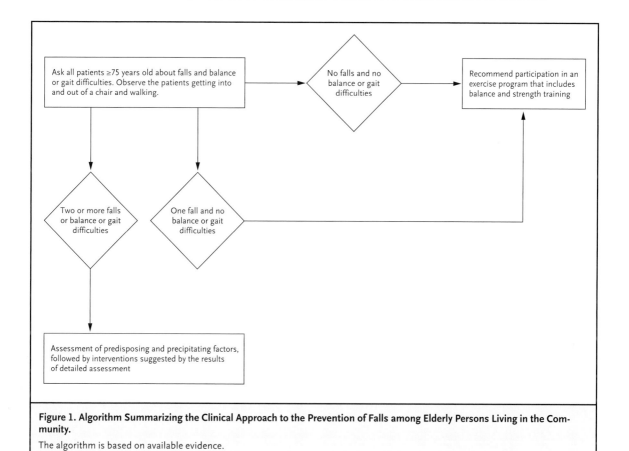

Figure 1. Algorithm Summarizing the Clinical Approach to the Prevention of Falls among Elderly Persons Living in the Community.

The algorithm is based on available evidence.

Although there is no consensus about the optimal time to initiate screening, the rate of falling and the prevalence of risk factors for falling increase steeply after the age of 70 years.[1-4]

Single-intervention strategies that have proved effective among elderly persons deemed at risk for falling, either because of the presence of a known risk factor or because of a history of falls, include professionally supervised balance and gait training and muscle-strengthening exercise; gradual discontinuation of psychotropic medications; and modification of hazards in the home after hospital discharge (Table 1).[14-21] In one study, tapering and discontinuation of psychotropic medications, including benzodiazepines, other sleep medications, neuroleptic agents, and antidepressants, over a 14-week period were associated with a 39 percent reduction in the rate of falling.[17] Although nonspecific advice about modification of home hazards directed at untargeted groups of elderly persons has not proved effective, standardized assessment of home hazards by an occupational thera-

Table 1. Strategies Shown in Randomized Clinical Trials to Be Effective in Reducing the Occurrence of Falls among Elderly Persons Living in the Community.*

Strategy	Estimated Risk Reduction	No. of Trials with Positive Results†
	%	
Health care–based strategy‡		
Balance and gait training and strengthening exercise	14–27	2 of 3
Reduction in home hazards after hospitalization	19	1 of 1
Discontinuation of psychotropic medication	39	1 of 1
Multifactorial risk assessment with targeted management§	25–39	3 of 3
Community-based strategy¶		
Specific balance or strength exercise programs	29–49	2 of 2

* The trials are those reported in the Cochrane review[14] that included at least six months of follow-up and involved persons living in the community. Among the strategies that have not been shown to be effective are multifactorial risk assessment without targeted management (none of three trials with positive results[28-30]), low-intensity general exercise programs (none of seven trials with positive results[31-37]), and cognitive–behavioral, educational, and self-management programs (one of six trials with positive results[38-43]).

† Positive results were defined as relative risks with 95 percent confidence intervals that did not include 1.[15,16,19-21]

‡ Participants were recruited from clinical settings, and interventions were carried out by health care professionals. Participants had reported previous falls or balance or gait difficulties or had one or more risk factors for falling.

§ The specific assessments and interventions varied among the trials. The trial personnel directed or carried out specific interventions on the basis of the results of the assessments.

¶ Participants were recruited from community sites, and interventions were not carried out by health care professionals. Participants were not recruited on the basis of previous falls, balance or gait difficulties, or risk factors.[44,45]

pist, along with specific recommendations and follow-up after hospital discharge, was associated with a 20 percent reduction in the risk of falling.[14,18] The most commonly recommended modifications in that study were the removal of rugs, a change to safer footwear, the use of nonslip bathmats, the use of lighting at night, and the addition of stair rails. Adherence to the recommended interventions ranged from 19 percent for the installation of stair rails to 75 percent for the use of bathmats.[18]

Whereas multifactorial assessments not linked to targeted interventions have been ineffective in preventing falls,[14,28-30] the most consistently successful approach to prevention has been multifactorial assessment, followed by interventions targeting the identified risk factors.[19-21] Such targeted assessment and management strategies have been shown to reduce the occurrence of falling by 25 to 39 percent (Table 1). Successful components of these interventions include review and possible reduction of medications; balance

Table 2. Recommended Components of Clinical Assessment and Management for Older Persons Living in the Community Who Are at Risk for Falling.

Assessment and Risk Factor	Management
Circumstances of previous falls*	Changes in environment and activity to reduce the likelihood of recurrent falls
Medication use High-risk medications (e.g., benzodiazepines, other sleeping medications, neuroleptics, antidepressants, anticonvulsants, or class IA antiarrhythmics)*†‡ Four or more medications‡	Review and reduction of medications
Vision* Acuity <20/60 Decreased depth perception Decreased contrast sensitivity Cataracts	Ample lighting without glare; avoidance of multifocal glasses while walking; referral to an ophthalmologist
Postural blood pressure (after ≥5 min in a supine position, immediately after standing, and 2 min after standing)‡ ≥20 mm Hg (or ≥20%) drop in systolic pressure, with or without symptoms, either immediately or after 2 min of standing	Diagnosis and treatment of underlying cause, if possible; review and reduction of medications; modification of salt restriction; adequate hydration[46]; compensatory strategies (e.g., elevation of head of bed, rising slowly, or dorsiflexion exercises); pressure stockings; pharmacologic therapy if the above strategies fail
Balance and gait†‡ Patient's report or observation of unsteadiness Impairment on brief assessment (e.g., the Get-Up and Go test[25,26] or performance-oriented assessment of mobility[27])	Diagnosis and treatment of underlying cause, if possible; reduction of medications that impair balance; environmental interventions; referral to physical therapist for assistive devices and for gait and progressive balance training
Targeted neurologic examination Impaired proprioception* Impaired cognition* Decreased muscle strength†‡	Diagnosis and treatment of underlying cause, if possible; increase in proprioceptive input (with an assistive device or appropriate footwear that encases the foot and has a low heel and thin sole); reduction of medications that impede cognition; awareness on the part of caregivers of cognitive deficits; reduction of environmental risk factors; referral to physical therapist for gait, balance, and strength training
Targeted musculoskeletal examination: examination of legs (joints and range of motion) and examination of feet*	Diagnosis and treatment of the underlying cause, if possible; referral to physical therapist for strength, range-of-motion, and gait and balance training and for assistive devices; use of appropriate footwear; referral to podiatrist
Targeted cardiovascular examination† Syncope Arrhythmia (if there is known cardiac disease, an abnormal electrocardiogram, and syncope)	Referral to cardiologist; carotid-sinus massage (in the case of syncope)
Home-hazard evaluation after hospital discharge†‡	Removal of loose rugs and use of nightlights, nonslip bathmats, and stair rails; other interventions as necessary

* Recommendation of this assessment is based on observational data that the finding is associated with an increased risk of falling.
† Recommendation of this assessment is based on one or more randomized controlled trials of a single intervention.
‡ Recommendation of this assessment is based on one or more randomized controlled trials of a multifactorial intervention strategy that included this component.

and gait training, muscle-strengthening exercise; evaluation of postural blood pressure, followed by strategies to reduce any decreases in postural blood pressure; home-hazard modifications; and targeted medical and cardiovascular assessments and treatments. Ascertainment of the circumstances surrounding previous falls may reveal precipitating factors, such as environmental hazards, risks associated with the activity at the time of the fall, and acute host factors, such as acute illness or immediate effects of medication, that may be amenable to intervention.

Specific recommendations for assessment and intervention are summarized in Table 2. The assessments can be performed either by the patient's usual physician or by a geriatric specialist. All medications, including over-the-counter medications, should be thoroughly reviewed and considered for possible elimination or dose reduction; the goal should be to maximize the overall health and functional benefits of the medications while minimizing their adverse effects, such as falls. Psychotropic medications warrant particular attention, since there is very strong evidence that use of these medications is linked to the occurrence of falls.[10,11,17] Reducing the total number of medications to four or fewer, if feasible, has also been demonstrated to reduce the risk of falling.[47]

When assessed appropriately, clinically significant postural hypotension is detected in up to 30 percent of elderly persons.[46,48] Moreover, some elderly persons with postural hypotension do not report symptoms, such as dizziness or lightheadedness.[46] Evidence from trials of single and multifactorial interventions suggests that all elderly persons who have any abnormalities on balance and gait testing should be referred to physical therapy for a comprehensive evaluation as well as rehabilitation.[15,16,19-21]

In addition to direct observation of the elderly person while he or she stands from a sitting position and walks, a targeted neurologic examination may reveal potentially treatable causes of balance or gait impairment. Proprioceptive impairment due to a neuropathy, for example, is a common cause of balance impairment in elderly persons. A decreased sensation of vibration, a frequent but abnormal finding in this population, is a more sensitive marker of neuropathy than a decrease in the sensation of position. A gait that worsens when the eyes are closed and improves when minor support is given by the examiner is a further clue to proprioceptive problems.

Persons who have fallen should be asked about loss of consciousness. Given recent evidence that some elderly persons are unaware of episodes of loss of consciousness, syncope should also be considered in those who report "just going down."[49]

Laboratory Tests and Imaging

The role of laboratory and ancillary testing in the prevention of falls has not been well studied. Laboratory tests that might reasonably be performed in all persons at risk for falling include a complete blood count; measurement of serum electrolytes, blood urea nitrogen, creatinine, glucose, and vitamin B_{12}; and assessment of thyroid function. These tests are relatively inexpensive, and abnormal results, which are likely to be prevalent, suggest the presence of a treatable entity. Other tests should be reserved for persons in whom the presence of an abnormality is suggested by the history and results of physical examination. Neuroimaging is indicated only if there is a head injury or new, focal neurologic findings on the physical examination or if a central nervous system process is suspected on the basis of the history or examination results. Electroencephalography is rarely helpful and is indicated only if there is a high degree of clinical suspicion of seizure. Similarly, ambulatory cardiac monitoring is helpful only rarely; in elderly persons, this technique is associated with frequent false positives and false negatives.[50] An evaluation for arrhythmia is warranted only if there is clinical evidence of this diagnosis, such as a known history of cardiac events or an abnormal electrocardiogram.

Education and Other Measures

Though repeatedly shown to be ineffective as a sole intervention,[38-43] education is an important component of strategies to manage the risk of falling. The person at risk and his or her family members should be educated about the multifactorial nature of most falls, about the specific risk factors for falling that are present, and about recommended interventions. Persons at risk for falling who live alone or who spend large amounts of time alone should be taught what to do if they fall and cannot get up, and they should have a personal emergency-response system or a telephone that is accessible from the floor.

For healthy elderly persons who have not fallen and who do not report or show balance or gait difficulties, the available evidence suggests that community-based exercise programs not supervised by health care professionals that include progressive balance-training and strengthening components may reduce the likelihood of a fall (Table 1).[14,44,45] Nonspecific, general exercise programs,[31-37] self-management and cognitive–behavioral approaches,[38-43] and home-hazard modifications for older persons without a history of falling or recent hospitalization have not proved effective.[14,38,51]

Low bone density increases the risk of hip and other fractures and should be identified and treated. The guidelines of the National Osteoporosis Foundation recommend that all women 65 years of age or older and women less than 65 years of age who are postmenopausal and who have additional risk factors for osteoporotic fractures (such as a lean habitus, a history of fractures, or a history of cigarette smoking) should undergo bone mineral density measurement to assess the risk of fractures and to ascertain whether pharmacologic or nonpharmacologic treatment would be appropriate.[52] A discussion of the prevention and treatment of osteoporosis is beyond the scope of this article, but information is available from the National Osteoporosis Foundation (http://www.nof.org/physguide).[52] In addition to other therapies, hip protectors appear to reduce the risk of hip fracture among persons at high risk.[53]

AREAS OF UNCERTAINTY

It remains to be determined whether the strategies that have proved effective in reducing the occurrence of falls are equally effective in reducing the most serious injuries that occur as a result of falling, such as fractures and head injuries. Observational data suggest that the risk factors for falls and for serious injuries due to falls are similar[3-5]; trials of fall-prevention strategies to date, however, have not had sufficient power to detect whether they have an effect on the incidence of serious injury.[14]

The exercise programs found to be effective have been short term, usually lasting one year or less. Since most of the benefits of exercise are maintained only as long as the exercise regimen is maintained, methods for enhancing long-term adherence are needed. The optimal intensity, frequency, and type of exercise needed to minimize the risk of falling and of incurring injury while maximizing mobility remain to be determined.

Studies suggest that the number of medications prescribed can be reduced safely and effectively.[14,47,54] However, practical methods are needed to balance the benefits of medications for the treatment of specific diseases with the risk of adverse events, including falls, in elderly persons.

There may be an overlap between falling and the presence of syncope: preliminary data suggest that patients who have had recurrent, unexplained falls and who have bradycardia in response to carotid-sinus stimulation have fewer falls with cardiac pacing.[49] Until these findings are confirmed in clinical trials, however, pacemaker therapy for the prevention of unexplained falls cannot be recommended.

GUIDELINES

The U.S. Preventive Services Task Force recommends that all persons 75 years of age or older, as well as those 70 to 74 years of age who have a known risk factor, be counseled about specific measures to prevent falls.[55] It also recommends that elderly persons at high risk for falling receive individualized, multifactorial interventions in settings where adequate resources to deliver such services are available.

The American Geriatrics Society, the British Geriatrics Society, and the American Academy of Orthopaedic Surgeons have released joint, evidence-based guidelines for the prevention of falls.[56] They recommend that all elderly patients be asked about any falls that have occurred during the previous year and that they undergo a quick test of gait and balance. The age at which screening should begin is not stipulated in the guidelines. A more comprehensive assessment, followed by a multifactorial intervention strategy, is recommended for patients who report recurrent falls, who present after a fall, or who have difficulties with balance or gait.

CONCLUSIONS AND RECOMMENDATIONS

All patients 75 years of age or older (or 70 years of age or older, if they are known to be at increased risk for falling) should be asked whether they have a history of falls and, if they do, should be carefully questioned about the circumstances of the falls and examined for potential risk factors. Strategies involving multifactorial assessment and intervention effectively reduce the rate of falling.

In the case of the patient described in the vignette, a review of the circumstances of her previous falls may identify high-risk activities that should be discontinued, such as carrying laundry up and down stairs. Her depressive symptoms should be reviewed to assess the tradeoff between the amelioration of depression and the risk of falling associated with her use of antidepressant medication. Efforts should be made to encourage the patient to eliminate over-the-counter sleep and allergy medications, both of which have anticholinergic effects and thus probably contribute to her risk of falling. Because her congestive heart failure is stable, it may be possible to reduce the dose of her diuretic or her cardiac medications. Any evidence of postural hypotension would further support an attempt to reduce the dose of her cardiac medications. Adequate hydration should be ensured, while avoiding fluid overload or serious hyponatremia.[57] If, as is likely, she has any balance or gait problems, she should be referred to a physical therapist who will train her in the use of an appropriate assistive device, such as a cane or walker, and who will prescribe a progressive program of balance and gait training and muscle strengthening. If her bone mineral density is low, I would advise her to wear hip protectors and to take calcium and vitamin D supplements, along with a bisphosphonate. These interventions will reduce by one third her risk of falling and of sustaining a hip fracture.

Additional information on the prevention of falls, including educational material for patients, can be obtained from the National Institute on Aging (http://www.nia.nih.gov), the Centers for Disease Control and Prevention (http://www.cdc.gov), and the American Geriatrics Society (http://www.americangeriatrics.org/education/forum).

This article first appeared in the January 2, 2003, issue of the New England Journal of Medicine.

REFERENCES

1.
Tinetti ME, Speechley M, Ginter SF. Risk factors for falls among elderly persons living in the community. N Engl J Med 1988; 319:1701-7.

2.
Nevitt MC, Cummings SR, Kidd S, Black D. Risk factors for recurrent nonsyncopal falls: a prospective study. JAMA 1989;261:2663-8.

3.
Nevitt MC, Cummings SR, Hudes ES. Risk factors for injurious falls: a prospective study. J Gerontol 1991;46: M164-M170.

4.
Sattin RW. Falls among older persons: a public health perspective. Annu Rev Public Health 1992;13:489-508.

5.
Tinetti ME, Doucette J, Claus E, Marottoli RA. Risk-factors for serious injury during falls by older persons in the community. J Am Geriatr Soc 1995;43:1214-21.

6.
Runge JW. The cost of injury. Emerg Med Clin North Am 1993;11:241-53.

7.
Kosorok MR, Omenn GS, Diehr P, et al. Restricted activity days among older adults. Am J Public Health 1992;82:1263-7.

8.
Tinetti ME, Williams CS. The effect of falls and fall injuries on functioning in community-dwelling older persons. J Gerontol A Biol Sci Med Sci 1998;53:M112-M119.

9.
Tinetti ME, Williams CS. Falls, injuries due to falls, and the risk of admission to a nursing home. N Engl J Med 1997;337:1279-84.

10.
Leipzig RM, Cumming RG, Tinetti ME. Drugs and falls in older people: a systematic review and meta-analysis. I. Psychotropic drugs. J Am Geriatr Soc 1999;47:30-9.

11.
Leipzig RM, Cumming RG, Tinetti ME. Drugs and falls in older people: a systematic review and meta-analysis. II. Cardiac and analgesic drugs. J Am Geriatr Soc 1999;47:40-50.

12.
Thapa PB, Gideon P, Cost TW, Milam AB, Ray WA. Antidepressants and the risk of falls among nursing home residents. N Engl J Med 1998;339:875-82.

13.
Mahoney J, Sager M, Dunham NC, Johnson J. Risk of falls after hospital discharge. J Am Geriatr Soc 1994;42:269-74.

14.
Gillespie LD, Gillespie WJ, Robertson MC, Lamb SE, Cumming RG, Rowe BH. Interventions for preventing falls in elderly people. Cochrane Database Syst Rev 2001;3:CD000340.

15.
Campbell AJ, Robertson MC, Gardner MM, Norton RN, Tilyard MW, Buchner DM. Randomised controlled trial of a general practice programme of home based exercises to prevent falls in elderly women. BMJ 1997;315:1065-9.

16.
Robertson MC, Devlin N, Gardner MM, Campbell AJ. Effectiveness and economic evaluation of a nurse delivered home exercise programme to prevent falls. 1. Randomised controlled trial. BMJ 2001;322:697-701.

17.
Campbell AJ, Robertson MC, Gardner MM, Norton RN, Buchner DM. Psychotropic medication withdrawal and a home-based exercise program to prevent falls: a randomized, controlled trial. J Am Geriatr Soc 1999;47:850-3.

18.
Cumming RG, Thomas M, Szonyi G, et al. Home visits by an occupational therapist for assessment and modification of environmental hazards: a randomized trial of falls prevention. J Am Geriatr Soc 1999;47:1397-402.

19.
Close J, Ellis M, Hooper R, Glucksman E, Jackson S, Swift C. Prevention of falls in the elderly trial (PROFET): a randomised controlled trial. Lancet 1999;353:93-7.

20.
Wagner EH, LaCroix AZ, Grothaus L, et al. Preventing disability and falls in older adults: a population-based randomized trial. Am J Public Health 1994;84:1800-6.

21.
Tinetti ME, Baker DI, McAvay G, et al. A multifactorial intervention to reduce the risk of falling among elderly people living in the community. N Engl J Med 1994;331:821-7.

22.
Gray SL, Mahoney JE, Blough DK. Adverse drug events in elderly patients receiving home health services following hospital discharge. Ann Pharmacother 1999;33:1147-53.

23.
Field TS, Gurwitz JH, Avorn J, et al. Risk factors for adverse drug events among nursing home residents. Arch Intern Med 2001;161:1629-34.

24.
Hanlon JT, Schmader KE, Koronkowski MJ, et al. Adverse drug events in high risk older outpatients. J Am Geriatr Soc 1997;45:945-8.

25.
Mathias S, Nayak US, Isaacs B. Balance in elderly patients: the "get-up and go" test. Arch Phys Med Rehabil 1986;67:387-9.

26.
Podsiadlo D, Richardson S. The timed "Up & Go": a test of basic functional mobility for frail elderly persons. J Am Geriatr Soc 1991;39:142-8.

27.
Tinetti ME. Performance-oriented assessment of mobility problems in elderly patients. J Am Geriatr Soc 1986;34:119-26.

28.
Vetter NJ, Lewis PA, Ford D. Can health visitors prevent fractures in elderly people? BMJ 1992;304:888-90.

29.
van Haastregt JC, Diederiks JP, van Rossum E, de Witte LP, Voorhoeve PM, Crebolder HF. Effects of a programme of multifactorial home visits on falls and mobility impairments in elderly people at risk: randomised controlled trial. BMJ 2000;321:994-8.

30.
Coleman EA, Grothaus LC, Sandhu N, Wagner EH. Chronic care clinics: a randomized controlled trial of a new model of primary care for frail older adults. J Am Geriatr Soc 1999;47:775-83.

31.
Lord SR, Ward JA, Williams P, Strudwick M. The effect of a 12-month exercise trial on balance, strength, and falls in older women: a randomized controlled trial. J Am Geriatr Soc 1995;43:1198-206.

32.
MacRae PG, Feltner ME, Reinsch S. A 1-year exercise program for older women: effects on falls, injuries, and physical performance. J Aging Physical Activity 1994;2:127-42.

33.
Steinberg M, Cartwright C, Peel N, Williams G. A sustainable programme to prevent falls and near falls in community dwelling older people: results of a randomised trial. J Epidemiol Community Health 2000;54:227-32.

34.
McMurdo ME, Mole PA, Paterson CR. Controlled trial of weight bearing exercise in older women in relation to bone density and falls. BMJ 1997;314:569.

35.
Means KM, Rodell DE, O'Sullivan PS, Cranford LA. Rehabilitation of elderly fallers: pilot study of a low to moderate intensity exercise program. Arch Phys Med Rehabil 1996;77:1030-6.

36.
Ebrahim S, Thompson PW, Baskaran V, Evans K. Randomized placebo-controlled trial of brisk walking in prevention of postmenopausal osteoporosis. Age Ageing 1997;26:253-60.

37.
Reinsch S, MacRae P, Lachenbruch PA, Tobis JS. Attempts to prevent falls and injury: a prospective community study. Gerontologist 1992;32:450-6.

38.
Hornbrook MC, Stevens VJ, Wingfield DJ, Hollis JF, Greenlick MR, Ory MG. Preventing falls among community-dwelling older persons: results from a randomized trial. Gerontologist 1994;34:16-23.

39.
Fabacher D, Josephson K, Pietruszka F, Linderborn K, Morley JE, Rubenstein LZ. An in-home preventive assessment program for independent older adults: a randomized controlled trial. J Am Geriatr Soc 1994;42:630-8.

40.
Carpenter GI, Demopoulos GR. Screening the elderly in the community: controlled trial of dependency surveillance using a questionnaire administered by volunteers. BMJ 1990;300:1253-6.

41.
van Rossum E, Frederiks CM, Philipsen H, Portengen K, Wiskerke J, Knipschild P. Effects of preventive home visits to elderly people. BMJ 1993;307:27-32.

42.
Gallagher EM, Brunt H. Head over heels: impact of a health promotion program to reduce falls in the elderly. Can J Aging 1996;15:84-96.

43.
Jitapunkul S. A randomised controlled trial of regular surveillance in Thai elderly using a simple questionnaire administered by nonprofessional personnel. J Med Assoc Thai 1998;81:352-6.

44.
Wolf SL, Barnhart HX, Kutner NG, McNeely E, Coogler C, Xu T. Reducing frailty and falls in older persons: an investigation of Tai Chi and computerized balance training. J Am Geriatr Soc 1996;44:489-97.

45.
Buchner DM, Cress ME, de Lateur BJ, et al. The effect of strength and endurance training on gait, balance, fall risk, and health services use in community-living older adults. J Gerontol A Biol Sci Med Sci 1997;52:M218-M224.

46.
Tilvis RS, Hakala SM, Valvanne J, Erkinjuntti T. Postural hypotension and dizziness in a general aged population: a four-year follow-up of the Helsinki Aging Study. J Am Geriatr Soc 1996;44:809-14.

47.
Tinetti ME, McAvay G, Claus E. Does multiple risk factor reduction explain the reduction in fall rate in the Yale FICSIT trial? Am J Epidemiol 1996;144:389-99.

48.
Luukinen H, Koski K, Laippala P, Kivela SL. Prognosis of diastolic and systolic orthostatic hypotension in older persons. Arch Intern Med 1999;159:273-80.

49.
McIntosh S, Da Costa D, Kenny RA. Outcome of an integrated approach to the investigation of dizziness, falls and syncope in elderly patients referred to a "syncope" clinic. Age Ageing 1993;22:53-8.

50.
Adams ME, Antczak-Bouckoms A, Frazier HS, Lau J, Chalmers TC, Mosteller F. Assessing the effectiveness of ambulatory cardiac monitoring for specific clinical indicators: introduction. Int J Technol Assess Health Care 1993;9:97-101.

51.
Stevens M, D'Arcy J, Holman C, Bennett N. Preventing falls in older people: impact of an intervention to reduce environmental hazards in the home. J Am Geriatr Soc 2001;49:1442-7.

52.
Osteoporosis clinical practice guidelines. Washington, D.C.: National Osteoporosis Foundation, 2002. (Accessed January 31, 2006, at http://www.nof.org/professionals/clinical/clinical.htm.)

53.
Parker MJ, Gillespie LD, Gillespie WJ. Hip protectors for preventing hip fractures in the elderly. Cochrane Database Syst Rev 2001;2:CD001255.

54.
Muir AJ, Sanders LL, Wilkinson WE, Schmader K. Reducing medication regimen complexity: a controlled trial. J Gen Intern Med 2001;16:77-82.

55.
Preventive Services Task Force. Guide to clinical preventive services: report of the U.S. Preventive Services Task Force. 2nd ed. Baltimore: Williams & Wilkins, 1996:659-85.

56.
American Geriatrics Society, British Geriatrics Society, American Academy of Orthopaedic Surgeons Panel on Falls Prevention. Guideline for the prevention of falls in older persons. J Am Geriatr Soc 2001;49:664-72.

57.
Shannon JR, Diedrich A, Biaggioni I, et al. Water drinking as a treatment for orthostatic syndromes. Am J Med 2002;112:355-60.

Suspected Appendicitis

ERIK K. PAULSON, M.D., MATTHEW F. KALADY, M.D.,
AND THEODORE N. PAPPAS, M.D.

An otherwise healthy 22-year-old woman comes to the emergency department with acute abdominal pain of 18 hours' duration in the right lower quadrant. On physical examination, she is afebrile, with tenderness on deep palpation in the right lower quadrant, and has no peritoneal signs. Pelvic examination reveals tenderness in the right adnexa without a mass. How should this patient be further evaluated?

THE CLINICAL PROBLEM

Approximately 3.4 million patients with abdominal pain seek medical care at emergency departments in the United States annually.[1] The various underlying causes of the pain range from benign processes to acute life-threatening disorders. Timely diagnosis and treatment of conditions for which a delay in care may have grave consequences remain a challenge.

More than 250,000 appendectomies are performed in the United States each year, making it the most common abdominal operation performed on an emergency basis.[2] Although the diagnosis of appendicitis in young men who have abdominal pain is usually straightforward,[3] the diagnostic considerations are broader for premenopausal women with the same clinical presentation. In addition, abdominal pain in patients at the extremes of age often presents a diagnostic challenge because of delays in seeking medical care or difficulty obtaining a history and performing an accurate physical examination. Since delayed diagnosis and treatment of appendicitis are associated with an increased rate of perforation, with resulting increases in morbidity and mortality rates,[4-6] timely intervention is crucial.

To minimize the risk of appendiceal perforation while patients await treatment, surgeons have traditionally favored early laparotomy, even in the absence of a definitive diagnosis. In approximately 20 percent of patients who undergo exploratory laparotomy because of suspected appendicitis, the appendix is normal. When advanced age or female sex confounds the usual signs and symptoms of appendicitis, the error rate in managing pain in the right lower quadrant can approach 40 percent.[7] In an effort to improve

Table 1. Sensitivity and Specificity of Clinical Findings for the Diagnosis of Acute Appendicitis.

Finding	Sensitivity	Specificity	Study
		percent	
Signs			
Fever	67	69	Wagner et al.[8]
Guarding	39–74	57–84	Wagner et al.,[8] Jahn et al.[9]
Rebound tenderness	63	69	Wagner et al.[8]
Indirect tenderness (Rovsing's sign)	68	58	Jahn et al.[9]
Psoas sign	16	95	Wagner et al.[8]
Symptoms			
Right-lower-quadrant pain	84	90	Wagner et al.[8]
Nausea	58–68	37–40	Wagner et al.,[8] Jahn et al.[9]
Vomiting	49–51	45–69	Wagner et al.,[8] Jahn et al.[9]
Onset of pain before vomiting	100	64	Wagner et al.[8]
Anorexia	68	36	Wagner et al.[8]

diagnostic accuracy, observation of the patient, laparoscopy, and diagnostic imaging have been used when the clinical presentation is equivocal.

STRATEGIES AND EVIDENCE

History and Physical Examination

The history taking and physical examination remain the diagnostic cornerstone in evaluating pain in the right lower quadrant. Although no single aspect of the clinical presentation accurately predicts the presence of the disease, a combination of various signs and symptoms may support the diagnosis. The specificity and sensitivity of common signs and symptoms of appendicitis are presented in Table 1. The three signs and symptoms that are most predictive of acute appendicitis are pain in the right lower quadrant, abdominal rigidity, and migration of pain from the periumbilical region to the right lower quadrant.[8] The duration of pain, defined as the time from the onset of symptoms to presentation, has also been shown to be an important predictor, since patients with appendicitis have a significantly shorter duration of pain than do patients with other disorders.[10]

For women with appendicitis, the most common misdiagnoses include pelvic inflammatory disease, gastroenteritis, abdominal pain of unknown origin, urinary tract infection, ruptured ovarian follicle, and ectopic pregnancy.[11] In a retrospective study of signs and symptoms that differentiated appendicitis from pelvic inflammatory disease in women with abdominal pain who were seen in the emergency department,[12] the findings that were most predictive of pelvic inflammatory disease included a history of the disorder, a history of vaginal discharge, vaginal discharge on examination, urinary symptoms, abnormalities on urinalysis, tenderness outside the right lower quadrant, and cervical-motion tenderness. A history of anorexia was not helpful in differentiating appendicitis from pelvic inflammatory disease.[12]

Laboratory Testing

Laboratory tests are performed as part of the initial evaluation of right-lower-quadrant pain in order to rule out or confirm specific disorders. In all women of reproductive age who present with acute abdominal pain, the serum β-human chorionic gonadotropin level should be measured to rule out uterine or ectopic pregnancy. Although approximately 70 to 90 percent of patients with acute appendicitis have an elevated leukocyte count, leukocytosis is also characteristic of several other acute abdominal and pelvic diseases and thus has poor specificity for the diagnosis of acute appendicitis.[13-17] Use of the leukocyte count alone to make management decisions in cases of suspected appendicitis may result in missed diagnoses or unnecessary surgery.

Approximately 10 percent of patients with abdominal pain who are seen in the emergency department have urinary tract disease.[18] A urinalysis may confirm or rule out urologic causes of abdominal pain. Although the inflammatory process of acute appendicitis may cause pyuria, hematuria, or bacteriuria in as many as 40 percent of patients,[19] urinary erythrocyte counts exceeding 30 cells per high-power field or leukocyte counts exceeding 20 cells per high-power field suggest a urinary tract disorder.

Observation and Laparoscopy

When the history and findings on physical examination are consistent with the diagnosis of appendicitis, appendectomy is often performed without further evaluation. If the initial clinical presentation does not suggest the need for immediate surgery, the patient may be observed for 6 to 10 hours in order to clarify the diagnosis.[20,21] This practice may reduce the rate of unnecessary laparotomy without increasing the rate of appendiceal perforation.[22-24] However, with the improved diagnostic accuracy of computed tomography (CT), early use of CT may result in lower overall costs and use of hospital resources[25] than the observation strategy.

Diagnostic laparoscopy has been advocated to clarify the diagnosis in equivocal cases and has been shown to reduce the rate of unnecessary appendectomy.[26] It is most effective for female patients, since a gynecologic cause of pain is identified in approximately 10 to

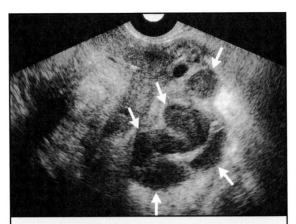

Figure 1. Endovaginal Ultrasonogram in a 46-Year-Old Premenopausal Woman with Right-Lower-Quadrant Pain, Adnexal Tenderness, and an Elevated White-Cell Count.

A carefully performed ultrasonographic examination of the right lower quadrant failed to show the appendix or the cause of pain. Endovaginal ultrasonographic examination of the right adnexa shows a fluid-filled, dilated, tubular structure (arrows), which is consistent with the presence of a hydrosalpinx or pyosalpinx. The patient underwent exploratory laparotomy, and a pyosalpinx was identified. Salpingo-oophorectomy was performed, and the patient had an uneventful recovery.

20 percent of such patients.[27,28] However, diagnostic laparoscopy is an invasive procedure with approximately a 5 percent rate of complications, which in most cases are associated with the use of a general anesthetic.[27]

Conventional Radiography

Abdominal radiography has low sensitivity and specificity for the diagnosis of acute appendicitis.[29,30] Similarly, contrast-enema examination has a low accuracy. In the era of cross-sectional imaging, neither test has a role in the diagnosis of acute appendicitis.[29-31]

Ultrasonography

A carefully performed ultrasonographic study has a sensitivity of 75 to 90 percent, a specificity of 86 to 100 percent, and a positive predictive value of 89 to 93 percent for the diagnosis of acute appendicitis,[32-37] with an overall accuracy of 90 to 94 percent.[9] In addition, ultrasonography may identify alternative diagnoses, such as pyosalpinx or ovarian torsion, in as many as 33 percent of female patients with suspected appendicitis[38,39] (Figure 1). Although appendicitis may be ruled out if the appearance of the appendix is normal on ultrasonography, a normal appendix is seen in less than 5 percent of patients.[33,35,40]

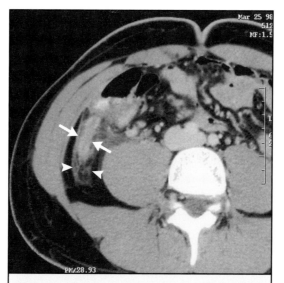

Figure 2. CT Scan in an 18-Year-Old Man with Abdominal Pain and Nausea.

CT examination of the right lower quadrant after the administration of intravenous and enteric contrast material shows a dilated, fluid-filled appendix with a thickened wall (arrows). There are inflammatory changes in the adjacent fat tissue (arrowheads). Laparotomy confirmed the diagnosis of acute appendicitis, and an appendectomy was performed. The patient had an uneventful recovery.

Most physicians hesitate to make clinical decisions about appendicitis when the appendix itself is not seen on imaging studies. Therefore, the failure to see the appendix, whether it is diseased or normal, fundamentally limits the usefulness of ultrasonography for the diagnosis of appendicitis.

Computed Tomography

With improvements in CT, including multislice spiral CT, the entire abdomen can be scanned at high resolution in thin slices during a single period of breath-holding. Such scanning virtually eliminates motion and misregistration artifacts and routinely results in high-quality, high-resolution images of the appendix and periappendiceal tissue. For patients with suspected appendicitis, spiral CT has a sensitivity of 90 to 100 percent, a specificity of 91 to 99 percent, a positive predictive value of 95 to 97 percent, and an accuracy of 94 to 100 percent.[33,41-49] In a retrospective review of 650 consecutive adults with clinical findings suggestive of acute appendicitis, CT had a sensitivity of 97 percent, a specificity of 98 percent, and an accuracy of 98 percent; alternative disorders were diagnosed in 66 percent of patients.[50]

CT has also proved to be accurate in patients in whom the diagnosis is uncertain. In one study, 107 consecutive patients in the emergency department who had pain in the right lower quadrant but equivocal clinical or physical findings were evaluated by means of contrast-enhanced CT.[45] All the patients underwent appendectomy, and the histologic diagnosis was compared with the CT diagnosis. CT had a sensitivity of 92 percent, a specificity of 85 percent, a positive predictive value of 75 percent, a negative predictive value of 95 percent, and an overall accuracy of 90 percent.

CT findings that are diagnostic of appendicitis, such as a distended appendix, a thickened appendiceal wall, and periappendiceal inflammation, are shown in Figure 2. Since CT provides a view of the entire abdomen and pelvis, alternative diagnoses may be readily identified.[38,39] Alternative diagnoses include, but are not limited to, colitis, diverticulitis, small-bowel obstruction, inflammatory bowel disease, adnexal cysts, acute cholecystitis, acute pancreatitis, and ureteral obstruction.[50]

Computed Tomography versus Ultrasonography

Two prospective studies directly comparing the efficacy of CT with that of ultrasonography in adults have shown the superiority of CT in diagnosing appendicitis.[38,39] In one study, 100 consecutive patients with suspected appendicitis underwent imaging, regardless of the degree of diagnostic certainty on the basis of the history and physical examination.[38] As compared with ultrasonography, CT had greater sensitivity (96 percent vs. 76 percent), greater accuracy (94 percent vs. 83 percent), and a higher negative predictive value (95 percent vs. 76 percent). There were smaller differences in specificity (89 percent for CT and 91 percent for ultrasonography) and the positive predictive value (96 percent and 95 percent, respectively). Among patients who did not have appendicitis, an alternative diagnosis was detected more frequently with CT than with ultrasonography. In cases in which there were conflicting interpretations of the CT and ultrasonographic findings, the CT findings were more frequently correct. Abscesses and phlegmons were also more likely to be detected by CT.[38]

Similar findings were reported in a prospective trial of 120 patients with an equivocal clinical presentation of appendicitis.[39] CT and ultrasonography had a sensitivity of 95 percent and 87 percent, specificity of 89 percent and 74 percent, positive predictive value of 97 percent and 92 percent, and negative predictive value of 83 percent and 63 percent, respectively. Among patients who did not have acute appendicitis, the correct alternative diagnosis was based on CT studies more frequently than on ultrasonographic studies. CT detected an abscess in 15 percent of patients, whereas ultrasonography detected an abscess in 9 percent of patients. There was no difference in diagnostic accuracy between men and women with the use of either CT or ultrasonography.[39]

Effect of Imaging on Outcome

Although CT has been shown to be sensitive and specific for the diagnosis of acute appendicitis, retrospective studies of its effects on management decisions and rates of unnecessary appendectomy have had conflicting results.[51,52] However, prospective studies have directly addressed these questions.[24,53] One study prospectively evaluated CT in 100 consecutive patients with suspected appendicitis for whom the initial management plan was either immediate surgery or admission for observation.[25] The initial plan was compared with the actual care received after CT studies had been performed. The accuracy of CT in diagnosing appendicitis was 98 percent, and it led to a change in management in 59 patients, including avoidance of an unnecessary appendectomy, avoidance of admission for observation (on the basis of normal CT findings), prompt surgery (on the basis of CT evidence of appendicitis), and identification of an alternative disease process. Taking into account the costs of an unnecessary appendectomy, one day of inpatient observation, and the CT scan, the use of CT resulted in an average cost savings of $447 per patient.[25]

Another study included 99 patients for whom a surgical consultation was obtained because of suspected appendicitis.[53] After the initial management plan had been established, all patients underwent CT and ultrasonographic studies of the right lower quadrant. Approximately two hours later, each patient was reevaluated clinically, and the treating physicians were informed of the imaging results. The surgical team then developed a final plan, using all the available information. Forty-four patients were initially scheduled for appendectomy, 49 were to be admitted for observation, and 6 were to be discharged. Among the 44 patients originally scheduled for surgery, CT combined with repeated clinical examination led to cancellation of the planned surgery for 6 patients, none of whom were found to have appendicitis; all 6 were women. Overall, of the 18 women initially assigned to surgery, 9 (50 percent) had appendicitis. Six of the 9 women who did not have appendicitis were spared unnecessary surgery by the use of CT, with the rate of unnecessary appendectomy reduced from 50 percent (9 of 18) to 17 percent (3 of 18), a difference that was statistically significant. The fact that only 50 percent of the women initially designated to have surgery actually had appendicitis emphasizes the difficulty of establishing the correct diagnosis in women.

In contrast, of the 26 men initially assigned to surgery, 24 (92 percent) had appendicitis and 2 (8 percent) did not. The addition of CT did not influence the decision to operate in any of these men. There were no men or women in whom the use of ultrasonography alone led to the cancellation of a planned surgery.

Among the 49 patients for whom observation was planned, the CT findings, combined with repeated clinical examination, led to the discharge of 13 patients from the hospital and immediate appendectomy in 10 patients. Given the costs of observation in the hospital, CT, and appendectomy (both in patients who had appendicitis and in those who did not), the authors calculated that this approach resulted in an average cost savings of $206 per patient.

AREAS OF UNCERTAINTY

Whether CT should be performed with the use of intravenous iodinated contrast material or enteric contrast material is a controversial matter.[33,41,42,47] Recent work indicates that intravenous contrast material improves the delineation of a thickened appendiceal wall, as well as the detection of inflammation within and surrounding the appendix, leading to improved diagnostic accuracy.[49] The primary purpose of using enteric contrast material is to permit definitive identification of the terminal ileum and cecum, since terminal ileitis can mimic appendicitis both clinically and radiographically.[33] The enteric contrast material can be delivered orally or rectally. Some suggest scanning solely in the region of the appendix[48]; others suggest scanning the entire abdomen and pelvis.[44,49,50] The spiral CT technique with slice thicknesses of no more than 5 mm is critical for accurate imaging of acute appendicitis.[32,33,46] In addition to the scanning technique, the skill and experience of the radiologist influence the usefulness of the examination.

GUIDELINES

To our knowledge, no major medical organization has proposed specific guidelines for the evaluation of patients with acute pain in the right lower quadrant.

CONCLUSIONS AND RECOMMENDATIONS

The evaluation of acute pain in the right lower quadrant is a common clinical problem. The diagnosis relies heavily on an accurate history and physical examination. Figure 3 shows our proposed approach. A patient, male or female, who presents with acute abdominal pain that has migrated from the umbilicus to the right lower quadrant and that is associated with tenderness in the right lower quadrant should be taken directly to the operating room for an appendectomy. The expected diagnostic accuracy in these circumstances approaches 95 percent and is probably not improved by imaging. If the clinical presentation is equivocal or if there is the suspicion of a mass or perforation with abscess formation, we advocate CT imaging to help establish the diagnosis, as in the patient described in the clinical vignette. CT has demonstrated superiority over transabdominal ultrasonography for identifying appendicitis, associated abscess, and alternative diagnoses. We reserve the use of ultrasonography for the evaluation of women who are pregnant and women in whom there is a high degree of suspicion of gynecologic disease.

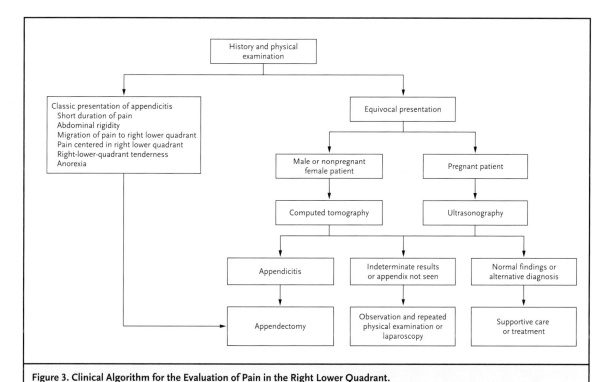

Figure 3. Clinical Algorithm for the Evaluation of Pain in the Right Lower Quadrant.

The algorithm is for suspected cases of acute appendicitis. If gynecologic disease is suspected, a pelvic and endovaginal ultrasonographic examination should be considered.

The results of imaging can be broadly classified as positive for appendicitis, indeterminate, or negative for appendicitis. If imaging suggests the presence of appendicitis, we recommend that an appendectomy be performed without further delay. If the appendix is not seen or if the results of imaging are otherwise indeterminate, we suggest further clinical observation and repeated physical examination or laparoscopy, with appropriate intervention. Finally, if CT studies show the presence of another disorder or an absence of abnormalities, there is no need for appendectomy, and supportive care or appropriate alternative treatment can be provided. This strategy can reduce the cost of observation, since a normal CT scan rules out appendicitis with a high degree of accuracy. We believe that adherence to these guidelines will increase diagnostic accuracy, leading to timely intervention, while reducing the rate of unnecessary appendectomy, and largely eliminating the costs of unnecessary imaging or observation.

We are indebted to David L. Simel, M.D., for his thoughtful comments on the manuscript.

This article first appeared in the January 16, 2003, issue of the New England Journal of Medicine.

REFERENCES

1.
McCraig LF, Burt CW. National Hospital Ambulatory Medical Care Survey: 1999 emergency department summary. Advance data from vital and health statistics. No. 320. Hyattsville, Md.: National Center for Health Statistics, 2001:24. (DHHS publication no. (PHS) 2001-1250 01-0357.)

2.
Owings MF, Kozak LJ. Ambulatory and inpatient procedures in the United States, 1996. Vital and health statistics. Series 13. No. 139. Hyattsville, Md.: National Center for Health Statistics, November 1998:26. (DHHS publication no. (PHS) 99-1710.)

3.
Mutter D, Vix M, Bui A, et al. Laparoscopy not recommended for routine appendectomy in men: results of a prospective randomized study. Surgery 1996;120:71-4.

4.
Von Titte SN, McCabe CJ, Ottinger LW. Delayed appendectomy for appendicitis: causes and consequences. Am J Emerg Med 1996;14:620-2.

5.
Rusnak RA, Borer JM, Fastow JS. Misdiagnosis of acute appendicitis: common features discovered in cases after litigation. Am J Emerg Med 1994;12:397-402.

6.
Graff L, Russell J, Seashore J, et al. False-negative and false-positive errors in abdominal pain evaluation: failure to diagnose acute appendicitis and unnecessary surgery. Acad Emerg Med 2000;7:1244-55.

7.
Andersson RE, Hugander A, Thulin AJ. Diagnostic accuracy and perforation rate in appendicitis: association with age and sex of the patient and with appendectomy rate. Eur J Surg 1992;158:37-41.

8.
Wagner JM, McKinney WP, Carpenter JL. Does this patient have appendicitis? JAMA 1996;276:1589-94.

9.
Jahn H, Mathiesen FK, Neckelmann K, Hovendal CP, Bellstrom T, Gottrup F. Comparison of clinical judgment and diagnostic ultrasonography in the diagnosis of acute appendicitis: experience with a score-aided diagnosis. Eur J Surg 1997;163:433-43.

10.
John H, Neff U, Kelemen M. Appendicitis diagnosis today: clinical and ultrasonic deductions. World J Surg 1993;17:243-9.

11.
Rothrock SG, Green SM, Dobson M, Colucciello SA, Simmons CM. Misdiagnosis of appendicitis in non-pregnant women of childbearing age. J Emerg Med 1995;13:1-8.

12.
Webster DP, Schneider CN, Cheche S, Daar AA, Miller G. Differentiating acute appendicitis from pelvic inflammatory disease in women of childbearing age. Am J Emerg Med 1993;11:569-72.

13.
Hale DA, Molloy M, Pearl RH, Schutt DC, Jaques DP. Appendectomy: a contemporary appraisal. Ann Surg 1997;225:252-61.

14.
Lewis FR, Holcroft JW, Boey J, Dunphy JE. Appendicitis: a critical review of diagnosis and treatment in 1,000 cases. Arch Surg 1975;110:677-84.

15.
Eriksson S, Granstrom L, Carlstrom A. The diagnostic value of repetitive preoperative analyses of C-reactive protein and total leucocyte count in patients with suspected acute appendicitis. Scand J Gastroenterol 1994;29:1145-9.

16.
Dueholm S, Bagi P, Bud M. Laboratory aid in the diagnosis of acute appendicitis: a blinded, prospective trial concerning diagnostic value of leukocyte count, neutrophil differential count, and C-reactive protein. Dis Colon Rectum 1989;32:855-9.

17.
Thompson MM, Underwood MJ, Dookeran KA, Lloyd DM, Bell PR. Role of sequential leucocyte counts and C-reactive protein measurements in acute appendicitis. Br J Surg 1992;79:822-4.

18.
Powers RD, Guertler AT. Abdominal pain in the ED: stability and change over 20 years. Am J Emerg Med 1995;13:301-3.

19.
Puskar D, Bedalov G, Fridrih S, Vuckovic I, Banek T, Pasini J. Urinalysis, ultrasound analysis, and renal dynamic scintigraphy in acute appendicitis. Urology 1995;45:108-12.

20.
Andersson RE, Hugander A, Ravn H, et al. Repeated clinical and laboratory examinations in patients with an equivocal diagnosis of appendicitis. World J Surg 2000;24:479-85.

21.
Kirby CP, Sparnon AL. Active observation of children with possible appendicitis does not increase morbidity. ANZ J Surg 2001;71:412-3.

22.
Jones PF. Suspected acute appendicitis: trends in management over 30 years. Br J Surg 2001;88:1570-7.

23.
Graff L, Radford MJ, Werne C. Probability of appendicitis before and after observation. Ann Emerg Med 1991;20:503-7.

24.
Colson M, Skinner KA, Dunnington G. High negative appendectomy rates are no longer acceptable. Am J Surg 1997;174:723-7.

25.
Rao PM, Rhea JT, Novelline RA, Mostafavi AA, McCabe CJ. Effect of computed tomography of the appendix on treatment of patients and use of hospital resources. N Engl J Med 1998;338:141-6.

26.
Sauerland S, Lefering R, Neugebauer EAM. Laparoscopic versus open surgery for suspected appendicitis. Cochrane Database Syst Rev 2002;1:CD001546.

27.
Moberg AC, Ahlberg G, Leijonmarck CE, et al. Diagnostic laparoscopy in 1043 patients with suspected acute appendicitis. Eur J Surg 1998;164:833-41.

28.
Thorell A, Grondal S, Schedvins K, Wallin G. Value of diagnostic laparoscopy in fertile women with suspected appendicitis. Eur J Surg 1999;165:751-4.

29.
Uses, limitations, and technical considerations. In: Baker SR, Cho KC. The abdominal plain film with correlative imaging. 2nd ed. Stamford, Conn.: Appleton & Lange, 1999:1-13.

30.
Rao PM, Rhea JT, Rao JA, Conn AK. Plain abdominal radiography in clinically suspected appendicitis: diagnostic yield, resource use, and comparison with CT. Am J Emerg Med 1999;17:325-8.

31.
Balthazar EJ. Diseases of the appendix. In: Gore RM, Levine MS, eds. Textbook of gastrointestinal radiology. 2nd ed. Vol. 1. Philadelphia: W.B. Saunders, 2000:1123-50.

32.
Birnbaum BA, Jeffrey RB Jr. CT and sonographic evaluation of acute right lower quadrant abdominal pain. AJR Am J Roentgenol 1998;170:361-71.

33.
Birnbaum BA, Wilson SR. Appendicitis at the millennium. Radiology 2000;215:337-48.

34.
Jeffrey RB Jr, Laing FC, Lewis RF. Acute appendicitis: high-resolution real-time US findings. Radiology 1987;163:11-4.

35.
Jeffrey RB Jr, Laing FC, Townsend RR. Acute appendicitis: sonographic criteria based on 250 cases. Radiology 1988;167:327-9.

36.
Abu-Yousef MM, Bleicher J, Maher JJ, Urdaneta LF, Franken EA Jr, Metcalf AM. High-resolution sonography of acute appendicitis. AJR Am J Roentgenol 1987;149:53-8.

37.
Puylaert JB. Acute appendicitis: US evaluation using graded compression. Radiology 1986;158:355-60.

38.
Balthazar EJ, Birnbaum BA, Yee J, Megibow AJ, Roshkow J, Gray C. Acute appendicitis: CT and US correlation in 100 patients. Radiology 1994;190:31-5.

39.
Pickuth D, Heywang-Kobrunner SH, Spielmann RP. Suspected acute appendicitis: is ultrasonography or computed tomography the preferred imaging technique? Eur J Surg 2000;166:315-9.

40.
Puylaert JBCM, Rutgers PH, Lalisang RI, et al. A prospective study of ultrasonography in the diagnosis of appendicitis. N Engl J Med 1987;317:666-9.

41.
Lane MJ, Katz DS, Ross BA, Clautice-Engle TL, Mindelzun RE, Jeffrey RB Jr. Unenhanced helical CT for suspected acute appendicitis. AJR Am J Roentgenol 1997;168:405-9.

42.
Lane MJ, Liu DM, Huynh MD, Jeffrey RB Jr, Mindelzun RE, Katz DS. Suspected acute appendicitis: nonenhanced helical CT in 300 consecutive patients. Radiology 1999;213:341-6.

43.
Lane M, Mindelzun R. Appendicitis and its mimickers. Semin Ultrasound CT MR 1999;20:77-85.

44.
Kamel IR, Goldberg SN, Keogan MT, Rosen MP, Raptopoulos V. Right lower quadrant pain and suspected appendicitis: nonfocused appendiceal CT — review of 100 cases. Radiology 2000;217:159-63.

45.
Stroman DL, Bayouth CV, Kuhn JA, et al. The role of computed tomography in the diagnosis of acute appendicitis. Am J Surg 1999;178:485-9.

46.
Weltman DI, Yu J, Krumenacker J Jr, Huang S, Moh P. Diagnosis of acute appendicitis: comparison of 5- and 10-mm CT sections in the same patient. Radiology 2000;216:172-7.

47.
Walker S, Haun W, Clark J, McMillin K, Zeren F, Gilliland T. The value of limited computed tomography with rectal contrast in the diagnosis of acute appendicitis. Am J Surg 2000;180:450-5.

48.
Rao P, Rhea J, Novelline R, et al. Helical CT technique for the diagnosis of appendicitis: prospective evaluation of a focused appendix CT examination. Radiology 1997;202:139-44.

49.
Jacobs JE, Birnbaum BA, Macari M, et al. Acute appendicitis: comparison of helical CT diagnosis focused technique with oral contrast material versus nonfocused technique with oral and intravenous contrast material. Radiology 2001;220:683-90.

50.
Raman SS, Lu DS, Kadell BM, Vodopich DJ, Sayre J, Cryer H. Accuracy of nonfocused helical CT for the diagnosis of acute appendicitis: a 5-year review. AJR Am J Roentgenol 2002;178:1319-25.

51.
Lee SL, Walsh AJ, Ho HS. Computed tomography and ultrasonography do not improve and may delay the diagnosis and treatment of acute appendicitis. Arch Surg 2001;136:556-62.

52.
Rao PM, Rhea JT, Rattner DW, Venus LG, Novelline RA. Introduction of appendiceal CT: impact on negative appendectomy and appendiceal perforation rates. Ann Surg 1999;229:344-9.

53.
Wilson EB, Cole JC, Nipper ML, Cooney DR, Smith RW. Computed tomography and ultrasonography in the diagnosis of appendicitis: when are they indicated? Arch Surg 2001;136:670-5.

Mammographic Screening for Breast Cancer

SUZANNE W. FLETCHER, M.D., AND JOANN G. ELMORE, M.D., M.P.H.

A 44-year-old woman who is a new patient has no known current health problems and no family history of breast or ovarian cancer. Eighteen months ago, she had a normal screening mammogram. She recently read that mammograms may not help to prevent death from breast cancer and that "the patient should decide." But she does not think she knows enough. She worries that there is a breast-cancer epidemic. What should her physician advise?

THE CLINICAL PROBLEM

In 1990, for the first time in 25 years, mortality from breast cancer in the United States began dropping; by 1999, the age-adjusted mortality rate was at its lowest level (27.0 per 100,000 population) since 1973.[1] Meanwhile, by 1997, 71 percent of women in the United States who were 40 years of age or older reported having undergone mammography during the previous two years — an increase from 54 percent in 1989.[2] Ironically, just as screening (or better treatment or both) seemed to be lowering mortality from breast cancer nationally, questions were raised about the validity of the studies that had led to widespread screening. For more than two decades, expert groups uniformly agreed that screening mammography reduces mortality from breast cancer among women in their 50s and 60s, even though they disagreed about other age groups.[3] However, questions were raised in 2000, when two Danish investigators concluded that only three of eight randomized trials were of sufficient quality to determine the effectiveness of mammography and that the combined results of these three trials showed no benefit. This report led to confusion about the usefulness of screening mammography.

STRATEGIES, EVIDENCE, AND AREAS OF UNCERTAINTY

Women are interested in knowing about breast cancer and want information from their doctors.[4,5] When women and their physicians are making decisions about screening, they need information about the underlying risk of the condition being screened for, the

Table 1. Chances of the Development of and Death from Breast Cancer within the Next 10 Years.*

Age	Cases of Invasive Breast Cancer	Death from Breast Cancer	Death from Any Cause
	no./1000 women		
40 Yr	15	2	21
50 Yr	28	5	55
60 Yr	37	7	126
70 Yr	43	9	309
80 Yr	35	11	670

* Rates for breast cancer and death from breast cancer were calculated on the basis of data from Feuer and Wun[6]; rates of death from any cause were calculated on the basis of data from Anderson and DeTurk.[7]

effectiveness of the procedure in preventing an untoward outcome such as death, and the potential ill effects of screening, such as false positive tests. (For policymakers and payers, cost-effectiveness is an important factor in decisions about the allocation of finite resources.) Clinical information about each of these issues with regard to breast cancer and mammography is summarized below.

The Risk of Development of and Death from Breast Cancer

The average 10-year risk of the development of and death from breast cancer is shown in Table 1, along with the 10-year risk of death from any cause (in order to provide context).[6,7] A computerized tool for calculating an individual woman's risk of breast cancer, the Breast Cancer Risk Assessment Tool (available at http://bcra.nci.nih.gov/brc/), can be used to calculate the five-year risk and the lifetime risk. The tool uses the woman's age, history of first-degree relatives with breast cancer (up to two relatives), number of previous breast biopsies (and whether any revealed atypical hyperplasia), age at menarche, and age at first delivery. It assumes regular screening and no history of breast cancer and does not include several known risk factors and several known protective factors (see Supplementary Appendix 1, available with the full text of this article at http://www.nejm.org).[8] Overall, the tool has been found to predict breast cancer well, but its ability to discriminate at the individual level was not much better than that of predictions that would have occurred by chance,[9] so its usefulness is similar to that of Table 1. For women with a strong family history of breast cancer, ovarian cancer, or both, a program that can be used to estimate the risk of genetic mutations in the *BRCA1* and *BRCA2* genes is available at http://astor.som.jhmi.edu/brcapro/. The program has been found to be effective in predicting risk on an individual level.[10]

Mammography and Mortality from Breast Cancer

There have been eight randomized trials of the effectiveness of mammography: four trials in Sweden comparing mammography with no screening; one in Edinburgh, Scotland, one in New York, and one in Canada comparing the combination of mammography and clinical breast examination with no screening; and one in Canada evaluating the effect of the addition of mammography to a standardized, 10-to-15-minute clinical breast examination. The studies differed with respect to the years in which they were conducted, the type of mammography used, the interval between mammographic examinations, the method of assigning women to the screened and unscreened groups, the number of screening visits, the age of the women who were included, and the methods of analysis.[3,11] For women between 50 and 69 years of age, all reports of studies comparing screening with no screening showed protective effects of screening, and meta-analyses that included all trials demonstrated statistically significant 20 to 35 percent reductions in mortality from breast cancer.

A widely cited meta-analysis published in 2000[12] (updated in 2001[13]) by Gotzsche and Olsen raised questions about the efficacy of mammography. The authors concluded that the methods used in five of the eight studies were so flawed that they had to be excluded from the meta-analysis. Appropriate randomization should lead to very similar groups, but for five of the studies (and part of a sixth, the Malmö II Trial), there were significant differences between the screened group and the control group in some of the characteristics; Gotzsche and Olsen suggested that these differences might bias the trial results. Also, numbers varied among different reports on the same trials. Finally, according to a combined analysis of the four Swedish studies, mortality from breast cancer, but not overall mortality, decreased in the screened group, raising the possibility of bias in determining the cause of death, as well as the possibility that treatments resulting from findings on screening could be dangerous. A meta-analysis of the remaining three studies showed no protective effect of mammography.

The investigators defended their trials. Several trials included some subjects who were later determined to be ineligible, and reports sometimes used the woman's age instead of the date of birth, accounting for differing numbers. The cluster randomization that was used in several trials probably led to small, unimportant base-line differences between groups.[14,15] In an updated analysis of the four Swedish studies published after the critique, unadjusted overall mortality was lower in the screened group (relative risk, 0.98 [95 percent confidence interval, 0.96 to 1.00]).[16] (Detailed responses to the criticisms of Gotzsche and Olsen are reviewed in Supplementary Appendix 2, available with the full text of this article at http://www.nejm.org.) In addition, Gotzsche and Olsen were criticized for not considering other methodologic aspects, such as the age of participants (one of the trials included only women in their 40s); the number, type, and quality of screenings and the intervals between them; compliance with the assigned strategy; and contamination (the degree to which women in control groups underwent screening mammography).[14,15,17,18] Finally, they included a study that compared two methods of screening[19] and had no unscreened control group.

In summary, criticisms of all but one of the trials excluded from the meta-analysis have been answered. In-depth independent reviews of the criticisms concluded that they do not negate the effectiveness of mammography, especially for women older than 50 years of age.[3,18,20]

Women in Their 40s

For many years, there has been controversy over the use of screening mammography for women in their 40s.[21] In general, the effect of screening younger women has been slower to appear and less dramatic than the effect among women older than 50 years of age. These differences may result from mammographically denser breasts in younger women (leading to reduced sensitivity of mammography), faster spread of some cancers in younger women, or both. Meta-analyses show that screening in this age group decreased 15-year mortality from breast cancer by about 20 percent.[3,22]

Because trial results are presented according to women's ages at the time of entry into the studies, some women who entered in their late 40s received a diagnosis of breast cancer in their 50s; therefore, some of the benefit ascribed to the screening of women in their 40s would have occurred if the women had waited until 50 years of age to be screened.[23,24] Also, although analyses are usually presented according to the decade of life, it is likely that a gradual change occurs as a woman ages. The latest analysis of the four Swedish trials — the first to examine screening effects according to five-year age increments — found that screening was most effective after 55 years of age.[16]

Mammography in Women Older than 70 Years of Age

Too few women older than 70 years of age participated in randomized trials to permit conclusions to be drawn about the effects of mammographic screening in this age group. One case–control study in the Netherlands found that screening women between 65 and

74 years of age led to a 55 percent decrease in mortality from breast cancer (relative risk of death from breast cancer, 0.45 [95 percent confidence interval, 0.20 to 1.02]).[25]

Risks Associated with Mammography

False Positive Mammograms   Because most women do not have breast cancer at the time of screening, there is potential to do harm with false positive results that necessitate further investigation before a woman can be declared to be free of disease. Nationally, an average of 11 percent of screening mammograms are read as abnormal and necessitate further diagnostic evaluation[26]; breast cancer is found in about 3 percent of women with an abnormal mammogram (representing 0.3 percent of all mammograms). Therefore, on average, a woman has about a 10.7 percent chance of a false positive result with each mammogram. Because women are screened repeatedly, a woman's risk of having a false positive mammogram increases over time. One study estimated that after 10 mammograms, about half of women (49 percent [95 percent confidence interval, 40 to 64]) will have had a false positive result, which will have led to a needle biopsy or an open biopsy in 19 percent (95 percent confidence interval, 10 to 41).[27]

False positive mammograms increase patients' anxiety; the degree of anxiety is related to the intensity of the additional diagnostic procedures and the recency of the screening mammogram.[20] One study found that in the 12 months after a false positive mammogram, women initiated more health care visits for both breast-related and non–breast-related problems.[28] However, false positive mammograms increase women's adherence to further screening.[29-31]

The risk of a false positive mammogram varies according to characteristics of the woman and radiologic factors: a younger age, an increasing number of breast biopsies, a positive family history of breast cancer, estrogen use, an increasing interval between screenings, the lack of comparison with previous mammograms, and a tendency by the radiologist to consider mammograms abnormal (as determined by the percentage of mammograms read as abnormal) were independent risk factors for a false positive result in one study.[32] Having mammographically dense breasts also increases the risk of false positive (or false negative) mammograms.[33-35] Many characteristics of patients are immutable, but obtaining mammograms during the luteal phase of the menstrual cycle may decrease mammographic sensitivity.[36] Also, a preliminary investigation found that stopping hormone-replacement therapy 10 to 30 days before a repeated mammogram eliminated or reduced mammographic abnormalities.[37]

Lowering the recall rate (the percentage of mammograms that result in recommendations for further tests) is likely to reduce the risk of false positive mammograms. Because of the trade-off between sensitivity and specificity, it is important not to lower the radiographic threshold for recall so much that cancers are missed. The Agency for Health Care Policy and Research recommends that the false positive rate be no more than 10 percent.[38] The malpractice climate in this country may work against the lowering of the threshold, since failure to diagnose breast cancer is the leading reason for malpractice suits.[39] Comparison of current and previous mammograms decreases the false positive rate, as does the use of screening intervals of 18 months or less.

Possible Overdiagnosis — Ductal Carcinoma in Situ   Ductal carcinoma in situ was a relatively rare diagnosis before the introduction of mammography. In 1973, the incidence in the United States was 2.4 cases per 100,000 women; by 1998, it was 30.7 per 100,000 women, accounting for approximately 14 percent of all breast cancers diagnosed.[1] With treatment, the prognosis is excellent. In one study, women given a diagnosis of ductal carcinoma in situ had a 9-year survival rate that was the same as or better than that in the general population,[40] and in another study, the risk of death from breast cancer within 10 years after the diagnosis of ductal carcinoma in situ was 1.9 percent.[41]

Such an excellent prognosis could be attributable to the detection of lesions before they become invasive cancers, which could save lives. However, if ductal carcinoma in situ were the usual precursor to early invasive cancer, the incidence of early-stage invasive breast cancer should decrease as the incidence of in situ cancer increases, but the opposite is happening. Also, autopsy studies in women who died from causes unrelated to breast cancer have shown a substantial "reservoir" of ductal carcinoma in situ in such women.[42] Therefore, detection of ductal carcinoma in situ may be an example of overdiagnosis — finding early neoplasms, many of which will never become invasive breast cancer.

Unfortunately, ductal carcinoma in situ can progress to invasive cancer. The eight-year rate of recurrence in one study of treatment with only surgical excision was 27 percent, and half the recurrences were invasive cancers.[43] It is not clear who is at risk for recurrence and whether survival results would be the same if surgery were undertaken only after early invasive cancer had been diagnosed. In sum, women who undergo screening mammography are more likely than other women to be given a diagnosis of ductal carcinoma in situ. Whether finding it saves lives or merely increases the number of women who receive a diagnosis of breast cancer is not yet clear.

Other Risks   Many women have pain during mammography, but few report that pain deters them from obtaining subsequent mammograms.[44-48] The risks associated with radiation are small. It has been estimated that 10 years' worth of annual mammographic

Table 2. North American Recommendations for Routine Mammographic Screening in Women at Average Risk Who Are 40 Years of Age or Older.*

Group (Date)	Frequency of Screening	Initiation of Screening		
		40–49 Yr of Age	50–69 Yr of Age	≥70 Yr of Age
	yr			
Government-sponsored and private groups				
U.S. Preventive Services Task Force (2002)†	1–2	Yes	Yes	Yes‡
Canadian Task Force on Preventive Health Care (1998, 1999, 2001)	1–2	No	Yes	No
National Institutes of Health consensus conference (1997)		No§	—	—
American Cancer Society (1997)	1	Yes	Yes	Yes
National Cancer Institute (2002)	1–2	Yes	Yes	Yes
Medical societies				
American College of Obstetricians and Gynecologists (2000)	1–2 if 40–49 yr old 1 yr if ≥50 yr old	Yes	Yes	Yes
American Medical Association (1999)	1	Yes	Yes	Yes
American College of Radiology (1998)	1	Yes	Yes	Yes
American College of Preventive Medicine (1996)	1–2	No¶	Yes	Yes
American Academy of Family Physicians (2001)	1–2	No§¶	Yes	No
American Geriatrics Society (1999)	1–2	—	—	Yes‡
Advocacy groups				
National Breast Cancer Coalition (2000)		No	—§	No
National Alliance of Breast Cancer Organizations (2002)	1	Yes	Yes	Yes
Susan B. Komen Foundation (2002)	1	Yes	Yes	Yes

* Adapted from the U.S. Preventive Services Task Force.[3] A "no" recommendation may be a statement that there is insufficient evidence for a positive recommendation.
† Recommendations are for mammography with or without clinical breast examination.
‡ There is an explicit recommendation to screen women older than 70 years of age.
§ Recommendations note that women should be counseled about the risks and benefits of mammography.
¶ Recommendations note that women at high risk should be screened beginning at 40 years of age.

screenings in 10,000 women will cause one additional breast cancer.[49] False negative interpretations are possible and are more common in younger women and in those with dense breasts.[50-52]

Recommendations from several leading groups regarding mammographic screening are summarized in Table 2.[3] After the analysis by Gotzsche and Olsen, some, but not all, reconsidered and changed their recommendations. For example, the editorial board of the Physician Data Query data base of the National Cancer Institute (which does not issue recommendations, as such) backed away from concluding that mammography is effective; instead, the board now concludes that mammography "may" decrease mortality.[23] The U.S. Preventive Services Task Force moved in the opposite direction and extended its recommendations for the use of screening to include women ranging from 40 years of age to more than 70 years of age.[3]

Recommendations from expert groups with regard to screening women in their 40s have long varied, but over time, more groups have moved toward endorsing the same approach for this age group as for older women. Most groups have not issued explicit recommendations for women older than 70 years and merely recommend that screening begin at a certain age. More groups have begun calling for shared decision making about breast-cancer screening, but the information to be shared has not been specified.

CONCLUSIONS AND RECOMMENDATIONS

General Conclusions

Breast cancer is common, but when viewed over a 10-year period, the risk for the average woman is relatively small. During the past few years, scientific controversy about the benefits of screening mammography has increased. As with most screening tests, there are hazards — primarily, risks of false positive mammograms, with associated anxiety and unnecessary biopsies, and perhaps a risk of overdiagnosis.

When the benefits of medical interventions are controversial and when hazards exist, shared decision making is needed, with the clinician providing facts and the patient assessing her situation from the vantage point of her personal values. In addition, the climate in the United States with regard to malpractice makes discussions between clinician and patient about breast-cancer screening essential for all women beginning at 40 years of age. To save time, information can be provided by handouts and an office practice that is organized to address the concerns of patients.

Women vary in terms of how much they want to participate in decisions about screening. In one survey of women younger than 50 years of age, 49 percent wanted to share in decision making, 44 percent wanted to make the decision themselves, and 7 percent wanted the physician to decide.[5] However, 79 percent wanted information from the doctor. Because of varying

Table 3. Recommendations Regarding Breast-Cancer Screening in Women.

Age	Recommendations
Any	Ask about family history of breast cancer, ovarian cancer, or both on both maternal and paternal sides. Consider referral or counseling for possible genetic testing if risk of a *BRCA1* or *BRCA2* gene mutation is at least 10 percent (to calculate risk, see http:// astor. som.jhmi.edu/brcapro/) or the patient has one of the following: a first-degree relative with a known deleterious mutation for breast cancer; ≥2 relatives given a diagnosis of breast cancer before 50 yr of age, ≥1 of them a first-degree relative; ≥3 relatives given a diagnosis of breast cancer, ≥1 of them before 50 yr of age; ≥2 relatives given a diagnosis of ovarian cancer; ≥1 relative given a diagnosis of breast cancer and ≥1 relative given a diagnosis of ovarian cancer.
40–70 Yr	Begin discussions about breast-cancer screening at 40 yr of age. Recommend screening mammography every 1–2 yr between 50 and 69 yr of age. Use information on the chances of development of or death from breast cancer within the next 5 yr (as given in the National Cancer Institute Breast Cancer Assessment Tool) or 10 yr.* Also give information on benefits and hazards of mammography.† Emphasize the increasing risk of breast cancer, increasing benefit of screening, and decreased harms associated with screening with increasing age. Record decision about screening in the medical record.
>70 Yr	For women with life expectancy of ≥10 yr, consider screening as above, making clear that risks of breast cancer are known but less is known about the benefits and harms of screening. Record decision about screening in the medical record.

* This information is presented in Table 1.
† This information is shown in Figures 1 and 2.

individual values, and because women have a good deal of fear about breast cancer,[53] physicians should be prepared for a decision different from the one they would recommend.

A woman needs some knowledge of her risk of breast cancer and the benefits and hazards of screening — specifically, her risks of the development of and death from breast cancer and her chances of successful treatment with screening and without screening, of having a false positive mammogram or an invasive breast procedure, and of having ductal carcinoma in situ diagnosed. Numerical risks may be best explained with the use of pictures or graphs, with discussion of absolute as well as relative risks (occurring over meaningful periods), and through comparisons with other risks.[54]

Specific Recommendations

All women, regardless of age, should be asked whether they have a family history of breast cancer, ovarian cancer, or both (Table 3).[55,56] For women without strong family histories, discussions about breast-cancer screening should begin at 40 years of age and continue

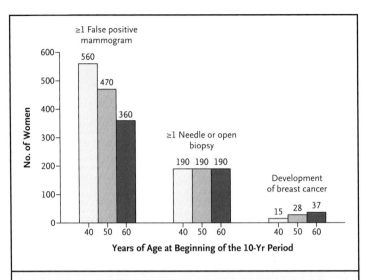

Figure 1. Chances of False Positive Mammograms, Need for Biopsies, and Development of Breast Cancer among 1000 Women Who Undergo Annual Mammography for 10 Years.

All numbers are rounded. The numbers for 10-year rates of false positive mammograms and breast biopsies come from a single study in which, overall, the rate of false positive mammograms was 6.5 percent,[27] and the rate may be different in other settings. Data on the development of breast cancer are broken down further in Figure 2.

until life expectancy is less than 10 years. Evidence supporting the usefulness of mammographic screening is strongest for women between 50 and 69 years of age, and screening should be routinely recommended for women in this age group. For women 40 to 49 years of age (such as the patient described in the vignette), shared decision making is especially important, because the absolute benefit of screening is smaller and the risks associated with it are greater. Screening should be routinely discussed, and the patient and clinician should decide together according to the woman's values.

For women who want more information, Table 1, the Breast Cancer Risk Assessment Tool, or both can be used to estimate the individual risk of breast cancer. Women should be reminded that the risk of breast cancer increases with age and that the one-in-eight risk is a lifetime risk for a newborn who lives for 90 years.

The chances of being helped or harmed by screening mammography are summarized in Figure 1 and Figure 2, which contain information that may be useful to patients. These figures show the chances that yearly screening mammography in women of different ages will result in a false positive mammogram, an invasive breast procedure, or a diagnosis of

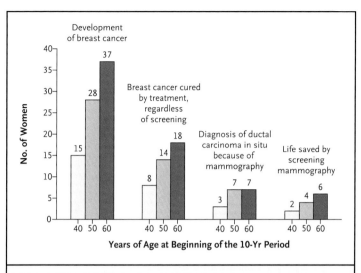

Figure 2. Chances of Breast-Cancer–Related Outcomes among 1000 Women Who Undergo Annual Mammography for 10 Years.

All numbers are rounded. The numbers for the incidence of invasive breast cancer and ductal carcinoma in situ, as well as the number of women whose lives are saved by treatment (those surviving at least 20 years after the first diagnosis of breast cancer) regardless of screening, were calculated on the basis of data from the Surveillance, Epidemiology, and End Results program.[1,57] The numbers of women whose lives are saved because of screening (those surviving at least 15 years after diagnosis) were calculated on the assumption of a reduction of 20 percent in mortality from breast cancer among women 40 to 49 years of age and a reduction of 30 percent among women 50 to 69 years of age; these numbers are approximate.

ductal carcinoma in situ or invasive breast cancer. Women should be made aware that at least half the patients given a diagnosis of breast cancer survive regardless of the use or nonuse of screening — a fact that many women do not understand.[57,58] Recently, survival rates have been improving, but how much of this improvement is attributable to treatment itself and how much to earlier diagnosis due to screening are difficult to determine. The number of women "saved" is calculated according to the estimates that screening of women in their 40s reduces mortality from breast cancer by about 20 percent and screening of women in their 50s or 60s reduces it by about 30 percent. It should be emphasized that these numbers may vary, depending on the efficacy of mammography in reducing mortality. Individual women will interpret these numbers differently depending on their own values.

To decrease the risk of false positive results, patients should be referred to experienced mammographers with recall rates of no more than 10 percent. They should be encouraged to obtain previous mammograms for comparison and should undergo screening more frequently than every 18 months.

Women often are unaware of the difference between screening and diagnostic examinations to evaluate a breast symptom or abnormal finding. In one study, cancer was diagnosed in about 10 percent of women older than 40 years of age who reported a breast mass and in almost 5 percent of those with any breast-related problem.[59] Clinicians and women should not be falsely reassured by a previously normal screening mammogram in the case of a new breast-related problem.

This article first appeared in the April 24, 2003, issue of the New England Journal of Medicine.

REFERENCES

1.
Ries LAG, Eisner MP, Kosary CL, et al., eds. SEER cancer statistics review, 1973-1999. Bethesda, Md.: National Cancer Institute, 2002. (Accessed August 29, 2005, at http://seer.cancer.gov/csr/1973_1999/.)

2.
Blackman DK, Bennett EM, Miller DS. Trends in self-reported use of mammograms (1989–1997) and Papanicolaou tests (1991–1997) — behavioral risk factor surveillance system. MMWR CDC Surveill Summ 1999;48(SS-6):1-22.

3.
Preventive Services Task Force. Screening for breast cancer: recommendations and rationale. Ann Intern Med 2002;137:344-6.

4.
Johnson JD, Meishcke H. Differences in evaluations of communication channels for cancer-related information. J Behav Med 1992;15:429-45.

5.
Kinsinger L, Harris R, Karnitschnig J. Interest in decision-making about breast cancer screening in younger women. J Gen Intern Med 1998;13: Suppl:98. abstract.

6.
Feuer EJ, Wun LM. DevCan: probability of developing or dying of cancer. 4.1. Bethesda, Md.: National Cancer Institute, 1999.

7.
Anderson RN, DeTurk PB. United States life tables, 1999. National vital statistics reports. Vol. 50. No. 6. Hyattsville, Md.: National Center for Health Statistics, 2002. (DHHS publication no. (PHS) 2002-1120 02-0141.)

8.
Clemons M, Goss P. Estrogen and the risk of breast cancer. N Engl J Med 2001;344:276-85. [Erratum, N Engl J Med 2001;344:1804.]

9.
Rockhill B, Spiegelman D, Byrne C, Hunter DJ, Colditz GA. Validation of the Gail et al. model of breast cancer risk prediction and implications for chemoprevention. J Natl Cancer Inst 2001;93:358-66.

10.
Berry DA, Iversen ES Jr, Gudbjartsson DF, et al. BRCAPRO validation, sensitivity of genetic testing of BRCA1/BRCA2, and prevalence of other breast cancer susceptibility genes. J Clin Oncol 2002;20:2701-12.

11.
Fletcher SW, Black W, Harris R, Rimer BK, Shapiro S. Report of the International Workshop on Screening for Breast Cancer. J Natl Cancer Inst 1993;85:1644-56.

12.
Gotzsche PC, Olsen O. Is screening for breast cancer with mammography justifiable? Lancet 2000;355:129-34.

13.
Olsen O, Gotzsche PC. Cochrane review on screening for breast cancer with mammography. Lancet 2001;358:1340-2.

14.
Screening mammography re-evaluated. Lancet 2000;355:747-8, 752.

15.
Screening for breast cancer with mammography. Lancet 2001;358:2164-8.

16.
Nystrom L, Andersson I, Bjurstam N, Frisell J, Nordenskjold B, Rutqvist LE. Long-term effects of mammography screening: updated overview of the Swedish randomised trials. Lancet 2002;359:909-19. [Erratum, Lancet 2002;360:724.]

17.
Basinski A. Commentary on "Review: High-quality studies do not show reductions in breast cancer mortality for women screened with mammography." ACP J Club 2000;133:67. [Comment on: Gotzsche PC, Olsen O. Is screening for breast cancer with mammography justifiable? Lancet 2000;355:129-34.]

18.
The benefit of population screening for breast cancer with mammography. The Hague, the Netherlands: Health Council of the Netherlands, 2002. (Publication no. 2002/03E.)

19.
Miller AB, Baines CJ, To T, Wall C. Canadian National Breast Screening Study. 2. Breast cancer detection and death rates among women 50 to 59 years. CMAJ 1992;147:1477-88. [Erratum, CMAJ 1993;148:718.]

20.
Vainio H, Bianchini F. Breast cancer screening. Lyons, France: IARC Press, 2002.

21.
Breast cancer screening for women ages 40-49. Vol. 15. No. 1. Bethesda, Md.: National Institutes of Health Consensus Development Program, 1997. (Accessed August 29, 2005, at http://consensus.nih.gov/cons/103/103_intro.htm.)

22.
Berry DA. Benefits and risks of screening mammography for women in their forties: a statistical appraisal. J Natl Cancer Inst 1998;90:1431-9.

23.
Breast Cancer (PDQ): screening. Bethesda, Md.: National Cancer Institute, 2003. (Accessed August 29, 2005, at http://www.cancer.gov/cancerinfo/pdq/screening/breast/.)

24.
Fletcher SW. Breast cancer screening among women in their forties: an overview of the issues. In: National Institutes of Health Consensus Conference on breast cancer screening for women ages 40–49. Journal of the National Cancer Institute Monographs. No. 22. Bethesda, Md.: National Cancer Institute, 1997;22:5-9.

25.
van Dijck JA, Verbeek AL, Beex L, et al. Mammographic screening after the age of 65 years: evidence for a reduction in breast cancer mortality. Int J Cancer 1996;66:727-31.

26.
Brown ML, Houn F, Sickles EA, Kessler LG. Screening mammography in community practice: positive predictive value of abnormal findings and yield of follow-up diagnostic procedures. AJR Am J Roentgenol 1995;165:1373-7.

27.
Elmore JG, Barton MB, Moceri VM, Polk S, Arena PJ, Fletcher SW. Ten-year risk of false positive screening mammograms and clinical breast examinations. N Engl J Med 1998;338:1089-96.

28.
Barton MB, Moore SM, Polk S, Shtatland E, Elmore JG, Fletcher SW. Increased patient concern after false-positive mammograms: clinician documentation and subsequent ambulatory visits. J Gen Intern Med 2001;16:150-6.

29.
Burman ML, Taplin SH, Herta DF, Elmore JG. Effect of false-positive mammograms on interval breast cancer screening in a health maintenance organization. Ann Intern Med 1999;131:1-6.

30.
Pisano ED, Earp JA, Schell M, Vokaty K, Denham A. Screening behavior of women after a false-positive mammogram. Radiology 1998;208:245-9.

31.
Lerman C, Trock B, Rimer BK, Boyce A, Jepson C, Engstrom PF. Psychological and behavioral implications of abnormal mammograms. Ann Intern Med 1991;114:657-61.

32.
Christiansen CL, Wang F, Barton MB, et al. Predicting the cumulative risk of false-positive mammograms. J Natl Cancer Inst 2000;92:1657-66.

33.
Fajardo LL, Hillman BJ, Frey C. Correlation between breast parenchymal patterns and mammographers' certainty of diagnosis. Invest Radiol 1988;23:505-8.

34.
Laya MB, Gallagher JC, Schreiman JS, Larson EB, Watson P, Weinstein L. Effect of postmenopausal hormonal replacement therapy on mammographic density and parenchymal pattern. Radiology 1995;196:433-7.

35.
Laya MB, Larson EB, Taplin SH, White E. Effect of estrogen replacement therapy on the specificity and sensitivity of screening mammography. J Natl Cancer Inst 1996;88:643-9.

36.
White E, Velentgas P, Mandelson MT, et al. Variation in mammographic breast density by time in menstrual cycle among women aged 40-49 years. J Natl Cancer Inst 1998;90:906-10.

37.
Harvey JA, Pinkerton JV, Herman CR. Short-term cessation of hormone replacement therapy and improvement of mammographic specificity. J Natl Cancer Inst 1997;89:1623-5.

38.
Bassett LW, Hendrick RE, Bassford TL, et al. Quality determinants of mammography. Clinical practice guideline. No. 13. Rockville, Md.: Agency for Health Care Policy and Research, October 1994. (AHCPR publication no. 95-0632.)

39.
Breast cancer study. Washington, D.C.: Physician Insurers Association of America, June 1995.

40.
Ernster VL, Barclay J, Kerlikowske K, Grady D, Henderson C. Incidence of and treatment for ductal carcinoma in situ of the breast. JAMA 1996;275:913-8.

41.
Ernster VL, Barclay J, Kerlikowske K, Wilkie H, Ballard-Barbash R. Mortality among women with ductal carcinoma in situ of the breast in the population-based Surveillance, Epidemiology and End Results program. Arch Intern Med 2000;160:953-8.

42.
Welch HG, Black WC. Using autopsy series to estimate the disease "reservoir" for ductal carcinoma in situ of the breast: how much more breast cancer can we find? Ann Intern Med 1997;127:1023-8.

43.
Fisher B, Costantino J, Redmond C, et al. Lumpectomy compared with lumpectomy and radiation therapy for the treatment of intraductal breast cancer. N Engl J Med 1993;328:1581-6.

44.
Andrews FJ. Pain during mammography: implications for breast screening programmes. Australas Radiol 2001;45:113-7.

45.
Kemmers-Gels ME, Groenendijk RP, van den Heuvel JH, Boetes C, Peer PG, Wobbes TH. Pain experienced by women attending breast cancer screening. Breast Cancer Res Treat 2000;60:235-40.

46.
Dullum JR, Lewis EC, Mayer JA. Rates and correlates of discomfort associated with mammography. Radiology 2000;214:547-52.

47.
Kornguth PJ, Keefe FJ, Conaway MR. Pain during mammography: characteristics and relationship to demographic and medical variables. Pain 1996;66:187-94.

48.
Rutter DR, Calnan M, Vaile MS, Field S, Wade KA. Discomfort and pain during mammography: description, prediction, and prevention. BMJ 1992;305:443-5.

49.
Feig SA. Assessment of radiation risk from screening mammography. Cancer 1996;77:818-22.

50.
Ma L, Fishell EK, Wright B, Hanna W, Allan S, Boyd NF. Case-control study of factors associated with failure to detect breast cancer by mammography. J Natl Cancer Inst 1992;84:781-5.

51.
Holland R, Hendriks JH, Mravunac M. Mammographically occult breast cancer: a pathologic and radiologic study. Cancer 1983;52:1810-9.

52.
Kerlikowske K, Grady D, Barclay J, Sickles EA, Ernster V. Effect of age, breast density, and family history on the sensitivity of first screening mammography. JAMA 1996;276:33-8.

53.
Black WC, Nease RF Jr, Tosteson ANA. Perceptions of breast cancer risk and screening effectiveness in women younger than 50 years of age. J Natl Cancer Inst 1995;87:720-31.

54.
Edwards A, Elwyn G, Mulley A. Explaining risks: turning numerical data into meaningful pictures. BMJ 2002;324:827-30.

55.
Statement of the American Society of Clinical Oncology: genetic testing for cancer susceptibility, adopted on February 20, 1996. J Clin Oncol 1996;14:1730-6.

56.
BRCA1 genetic screening. Guideline NGC-0461. Rockville, Md.: Kaiser Permanente, 1998.

57.
Ries LAG, Kosary CL, Hankey BF, Miller BA, Harras A, Edwards BK, eds. SEER cancer statistics review, 1973-1994. Bethesda, Md.: National Cancer Institute, 1997. (NIH publication no. 97-2789.)

58.
Silverman E, Woloshin S, Schwartz LM, Byram SJ, Welch HG, Fischhoff B. Women's views on breast cancer risk and screening mammography: a qualitative interview study. Med Decis Making 2001;21:231-40.

59.
Barton MB, Elmore JG, Fletcher SW. Breast symptoms among women enrolled in a health maintenance organization: frequency, evaluation, and outcome. Ann Intern Med 1999;130:651-7.

Emergency Contraception

CAROLYN WESTHOFF, M.D.

A healthy 19-year-old woman comes in for a routine appointment. She is sexually active in a monogamous relationship. Pregnancy is not currently desired. Her partner uses condoms most of the time. She is uncertain of the date of her last menstrual period but has had sexual intercourse several times since her last menses, including unprotected intercourse four days earlier. A high-sensitivity urine test for pregnancy is negative. Should emergency contraception be prescribed?

THE CLINICAL PROBLEM

About 3 million unintended pregnancies occur each year in the United States.[1] Most of these result from the nonuse of contraception or from a noticeable contraceptive failure, such as a broken condom,[2] and could be prevented with the use of emergency contraception.

A fertile couple has a 25 percent chance of pregnancy with repeated unprotected intercourse during a single menstrual cycle. In a large, prospective study of couples seeking pregnancy, a single act of unprotected intercourse occurring about one to two days before ovulation was associated with a 24 percent probability that conception would lead to successful pregnancy.[3,4] However, among women 19 to 26 years of age (the age group in which fertility is greatest), the chance of pregnancy may be as high as 50 percent when unprotected intercourse occurs during this interval.[5]

Because sperm can survive in the female genital tract for five to six days, fertilization may occur days after sexual activity. Even the most sensitive pregnancy test will not be positive until after the implantation of a fertilized egg in the uterus, an event that occurs about seven days after fertilization.[6]

STRATEGIES AND EVIDENCE

Immediate use of an emergency contraceptive will reduce a woman's risk of pregnancy to 1 to 2 percent. The effectiveness depends on the regimen used and on the time between

Table 1. Types of Emergency Contraception.		
Class	**Dose**	**Brands Available in the United States**
Combined oral contraceptives	100 µg of ethinyl estradiol and 0.5 mg of levonorgestrel twice 12 hr apart	Preven (Gynétics) Ovral (Wyeth)*
Progestin-only oral contraceptives	1.5 mg of levonorgestrel once or 0.75 mg twice 12 hr apart	Plan B (Women's Capital Corporation)
Copper T intrauterine device	—	ParaGard T 380A (Ortho-McNeil)
Antiprogestins	10 mg of mifepristone	None at this dose

* Other hormonal contraceptives that are effective for emergency contraception, along with the doses and instructions for use, are listed at http://www.not-2-late.com.

unprotected intercourse and treatment. Table 1 lists the main types of emergency contraception.

The Yuzpe Regimen

An approach first studied in the 1970s by Yuzpe et al. is the use of two doses of a combination oral contraceptive containing 100 µg of ethinyl estradiol and 1.0 mg of the progestin norgestrel.[7] This treatment has been approved by the Food and Drug Administration (FDA) and is available by prescription (Preven, Gynétics); two tablets are given twice, 12 hours apart (a total of four tablets).[8] A similar approach with the same efficacy is to use pills from a package of combination birth-control pills that contain the progestin norgestrel; each dose must contain 1.0 mg of norgestrel or 0.5 mg of its active isomer levonorgestrel, along with 100 µg of ethinyl estradiol. Depending on the brand of pill, two to five pills are required per dose. This treatment reduces the risk of pregnancy to about 2 percent, as compared with about 8 percent in the absence of treatment.[9] The main side effects are nausea (in at least 50 percent of women) and vomiting (in about 20 percent), which can be minimized or prevented by prior or concomitant treatment with an antiemetic (e.g., 10 mg of metoclopramide).[10] The next menses after treatment will usually occur within one week before or after the expected date; if menses do not occur within three to four weeks after treatment, then a pregnancy test is indicated.

Progestin-Only Regimen

A newer, more effective approach to emergency contraception is the use of progestin-only contraceptive tablets. An FDA-approved product (Plan B, Women's Capital Corporation) is available in the United States and consists of 0.75-mg tablets of levonorgestrel, to be taken within 72 hours after unprotected intercourse in two doses separated by 12 hours.[11]

Clinical trials directly comparing a progestin-only regimen with a combined estrogen–progestin regimen indicate that the progestin-only approach is more effective, reducing the risk of pregnancy to 1 percent and the incidence of nausea and vomiting to 22 percent and 8 percent, respectively.[12] Recent data indicate that the levonorgestrel-only treatment can be given once in a single dose, rather than twice in a divided dose, with the same efficacy.[13] In contrast, a single dose of combination hormonal contraceptive pills (including 200 μg of ethinyl estradiol) cannot be recommended, given the lack of data regarding its effectiveness and the likelihood of more severe side effects.

Timing of Use

Both the combination and the progestin-only regimens of emergency contraception were originally studied for use up to three days after a single unprotected act of intercourse. Data from a large, randomized clinical trial demonstrated that pregnancy rates were lowest when emergency contraception was initiated within 12 hours after unprotected intercourse, with a monotonic decrement in effectiveness as the interval between unprotected intercourse and treatment increased. The pregnancy rate was less than 1 percent when treatment was given within 12 hours, as compared with over 3 percent when treatment was given 61 to 72 hours after intercourse.[13,14] Other studies, however, have not shown a strong relation between the timing of therapy and efficacy.[15] Two observational studies indicate that treatment 72 to 120 hours after intercourse results in pregnancy rates similar to those in studies of earlier treatment.[16,17] Emergency contraception should thus be offered for any act of unprotected intercourse that has occurred in the preceding five days, even if the patient has had other unprotected acts earlier in the same menstrual cycle. Because the length of the menstrual cycle varies and the day of ovulation is generally unknown even in women who report having regular cycles,[18] treatment is indicated regardless of the cycle day on which unprotected intercourse occurred.

Other Approaches

Other strategies for postcoital contraception are either less well studied or less available than progestin-only or combination regimens. Combination oral contraceptives that contain other progestins may be similar in effectiveness to pills containing levonorgestrel. In a randomized clinical trial that included nearly 1200 women, the pregnancy rate after two doses of a norethindrone-containing oral contraceptive (2.0 mg per dose) did not differ significantly from the rate after two doses of a levonorgestrel-containing pill (the Yuzpe regimen) (2.7 percent and 2.0 percent, respectively).[19]

Insertion of a copper-containing intrauterine device (IUD) up to five days after unprotected intercourse also reduces the risk of pregnancy. This approach is supported by published case series that included 879 insertions of an IUD after intercourse, with only one pregnancy.[20] A randomized clinical trial compared the use of two different copper-bearing IUDs among 192 women requesting emergency contraception, most of whom were nulliparous. Follow-up data were available for 98 percent of the women at six weeks; there were no pregnancies and no cases of pelvic inflammatory disease.[21] However, the number of pregnancies that would have been expected without treatment was not clear.

An important benefit of IUD insertion is that it provides continued contraception; 80 percent of the trial participants continued using the IUD after completion of the study.[21] In other studies of hormonal emergency contraception, pregnancies occurred in women who had additional acts of unprotected intercourse later in the same cycle,[19] indicating the importance of providing ongoing contraception immediately. An IUD is more expensive than hormonal emergency contraception but is cost effective for women who choose to use it long-term.[22] The copper IUD is approved by the FDA for use for up to 10 years, and clinical data indicate that its effectiveness lasts for at least 12 years.

Mifepristone, a progesterone-receptor antagonist used for medical abortion, is another alternative. Randomized clinical trials show that a single 10-mg dose of mifepristone is as effective as the levonorgestrel-containing regimens,[13] with an even lower incidence of nausea and vomiting. However, the 10-mg dose is not commercially available in the United States. The 200-mg tablet that is used for medical abortion is available in the United States only to physicians who establish an account with the distributor, severely limiting access. In addition, mifepristone is more expensive than other hormonal therapies. New antiprogestins are being studied for this indication and may have similar effectiveness.[23]

Safety of Emergency Contraception

A theoretical concern is that the use of combined oral contraceptives for emergency contraception might increase the risk of thrombotic events, such as venous thromboembolism or stroke, that are associated with long-term use of these products.[24,25] Such adverse events did not occur in the clinical trials evaluating these agents; however, the studies lacked power to detect rare events. A Medline search for reports of thrombotic events that occurred in association with hormonal emergency contraception yielded four case reports of cerebrovascular complications[26-29] — all of which followed the use of combination hormonal therapy. No case reports of cerebrovascular events were identified in association with the use of progestin-only emergency contraceptives, nor were there reports of deep-vein thrombosis or pulmonary embolism after either type of hormonal contraception.

Population-based or case–control studies of cerebral thrombosis after emergency contraception have not been performed. A population-based retrospective cohort study[30] assessed the risk of venous thromboembolism among users of combination hormonal emergency contraception, on the basis of data from the General Practice Research Database in the United Kingdom. The analysis included 73,302 women who received 100,615 prescriptions for postcoital contraception between 1989 and 1996; of these women, 19 had a deep-vein thrombosis or a pulmonary embolus during follow-up. There were no venous thromboembolic events during the 45 days after the receipt of any prescription for emergency contraception. In contrast, the risk of venous thromboembolism was increased during pregnancy and with ongoing use of oral contraceptives — observations that support the validity of the analysis.

There are no absolute contraindications to the use of hormonal emergency contraception. Even for women who have contraindications to the long-term use of combination hormonal contraception (such as liver disease or a history of thromboembolism),[31] the balance of risks and benefits may favor the brief hormonal exposure resulting from emergency contraception over the possibility of a high-risk pregnancy. Progestin-only emergency contraception or the insertion of an IUD should be considered first in women with these or other medical contraindications to combination oral contraceptives, especially given the effectiveness of these approaches and the low rate of side effects. Insertion of an IUD for emergency contraception should be performed according to the regular guidelines for IUD use.[32] This approach should be avoided, for instance, in women with active, recent, or recurrent pelvic infections.

Outcomes of Pregnancy after Emergency Contraception

Pregnancies can be established, but not diagnosed, at the time of emergency contraceptive use or can be associated with the failure of the emergency contraceptive. Although case reports have described ectopic pregnancy after the use of emergency contraception, there is no good evidence of an increased risk of this outcome.[33,34] In a large World Health Organization trial, only 42 pregnancies were identified after nearly 2000 treatments,[12] and none were ectopic. Five of these pregnancies were continued, with normal outcomes. No studies have been large enough to quantify the teratogenic risk among the very small number of pregnancies that follow the use of emergency contraception. However, observations that there is no increase in birth defects among pregnancies exposed to daily use of combined oral contraceptives are reassuring.[35]

Patients who had a recent menstrual period at the usual time and with the usual flow do not need a pregnancy test before using emergency contraception.[36] If the patient's menstrual history is either vague or unusual, then a pretreatment pregnancy test may allow earlier diagnosis of a pregnancy that is already established, facilitating earlier prenatal care,[37] or an earlier abortion. A physical examination is unnecessary before treatment.[38]

Advance Prescribing

Emergency contraception is currently available by prescription only; therefore, there may be a substantial delay between the time women identify the need for treatment and the time they receive it.[39] Clinicians can help prevent this problem by providing emergency contraception in advance of need. Several clinical trials, three of them randomized, have compared the effects of advance provision of emergency contraception with the effects of education alone.[40-44] All these trials found that advance provision increased the use of emergency contraception, that the use was appropriate, that women did not abandon or decrease the use of their regular contraceptives, and that advance provision led to a reduction in the number of unintended pregnancies. These studies were too small, however, to identify a significant difference in the pregnancy rate. No serious adverse events were observed.

Possible Over-the-Counter Status

The FDA is currently evaluating an application for a switch to over-the-counter status for the levonorgestrel-only formulation of emergency contraceptive. Hormonal emergency contraception is highly suitable for such a switch. The dose is the same for everyone, there are no contraindications to its use, adverse events are rare, and there is no potential for addiction.[45] Repeated use is safe and reasonably effective but is unlikely to replace long-term contraception, owing to the expense and side effects such as menstrual changes.[46]

AREAS OF UNCERTAINTY

The mechanism of action of emergency contraception is incompletely understood. It does not interfere with an established, postimplantation pregnancy. The use of emergency contraception can delay ovulation and decrease the probability of fertilization after ovulation[47]; at least some of its effect appears to occur after ovulation.[48]

Immediate initiation of long-term contraception is desirable to reduce the risk of pregnancy after treatment. A small, nonrandomized study in which the use of oral contraceptives was initiated on the same day as a levonorgestrel-only emergency contraceptive found that this approach was highly acceptable to patients[49] and was associated with higher rates of continuation of the oral contraceptive than was waiting to start long-term contraception. Whether immediate initiation of oral contraceptives influences the effectiveness of therapy or increases the rate of side effects has not been studied.

GUIDELINES

Both the American Medical Association and the American College of Obstetricians and Gynecologists (ACOG) encourage physicians and other professionals to discuss emergency contraception as part of routine family planning and contraceptive counseling and promote efforts to expand access to such treatment, including making it available in physicians' offices.[50,51] ACOG recommends both combination and progestin-only hormonal methods but advises that the progestin-only approach be considered first. ACOG also specifically supports efforts to make emergency oral contraception available to women over the counter in a designated product.[52]

CONCLUSIONS AND RECOMMENDATIONS

The patient described in the clinical vignette, who had had unprotected intercourse four days earlier, should receive emergency contraception as soon as possible. The preferred regimen is the levonorgestrel-only product at a dose of 1.5 mg, since this is highly effective and generally well tolerated. If supplies are not available in the physician's office, the physician should be able to identify a local pharmacy that stocks this product. In addition, the physician should provide refills of this prescription or provide a separate prescription that the patient can use in case she has unprotected intercourse again. Having emergency contraception readily available does not lead to the abandonment of other forms of contraception.

The use of regular contraception should also be emphasized, along with condom use to reduce the transmission of sexually transmitted diseases. If hormonal contraception is chosen, it should be initiated immediately, rather than waiting for the patient's next menstrual period. Some pregnancies in clinical trials resulted from additional acts of unprotected intercourse later in the same menstrual cycle. Ample refills should be provided, since running out of pills is a major reason for unintended pregnancy among users of oral contraceptives.[2] A need for emergency contraception should prompt consideration of screening for sexually transmitted diseases, such as chlamydia.[53] A follow-up pregnancy test is indicated if the patient does not have withdrawal bleeding after finishing her first pack of oral contraceptives or, for those who do not immediately begin taking oral contraceptives, if menses do not occur within three to four weeks after treatment.

Until a dedicated product is widely available over the counter, emergency contraception should routinely be provided in advance of need. Eligible women should include those who are not currently sexually active, since they are unlikely to have an ongoing method of contraception and are at risk if they become sexually active.

Dr. Westhoff reports having received research grants from Berlex Laboratories and honorariums for consulting from Barr Laboratories.

This article first appeared in the November 6, 2003, issue of the New England Journal of Medicine.

REFERENCES

1.
Henshaw SK. Unintended pregnancy in the United States. Fam Plann Perspect 1998;30:24-9, 46.

2.
Jones RK, Darroch JE, Henshaw SK. Contraceptive use among U.S. women having abortions in 2000-2001. Perspect Sex Reprod Health 2002;34:294-303.

3.
Wilcox A, Weinberg C, Baird D. Timing of sexual intercourse in relation to ovulation. N Engl J Med 1995;333:1517-21.

4.
Baird D, Weinberg C, Zhou H, et al. Preimplantation urinary hormone profiles and the probability of conception in healthy women. Fertil Steril 1999;71:40-9.

5.
Dunson DB, Colombo B, Baird DD. Changes with age in the level and duration of fertility in the menstrual cycle. Hum Reprod 2002;17:1399-403.

6.
Norwitz E, Schust D, Fisher SJ. Implantation and the survival of early pregnancy. N Engl J Med 2001; 345:1400-8.

7.
Yuzpe AA, Smith RP, Rademaker AW. A multicenter clinical investigation employing ethinyl estradiol combined with dl-norgestrel as postcoital contraceptive agent. Fertil Steril 1982;37:508-13.

8.
Preven emergency contraceptive. Somerville, N.J.: Gynetics, Inc., 2000 (package insert).

9.
Trussell J, Rodriguez G, Ellertson C. Updated estimates of the effectiveness of the Yuzpe regimen of emergency contraception. Contraception 1999;59:147-51.

10.
Raymond EG, Creinin MD, Barnhart KT, Lovvorn AE, Rountree RW, Trussell J. Meclizine for prevention of nausea associated with the use of emergency contraceptive pills: a randomized trial. Obstet Gynecol 2000;95:271-7.

11.
Plan B. Washington, D.C.: Women's Capital Corporation, 2003 (package insert).

12.
Task Force on Postovulatory Methods of Fertility Regulation. Randomised controlled trial of levonorgestrel versus the Yuzpe regimen of combined oral contraceptives for emergency contraception. Lancet 1998;353:428-32.

13.
von Hertzen H, Piaggio G, Ding J, et al. Low dose mifepristone and two regimens of levonorgestrel for emergency contraception. Lancet 2002;360:1803-10.

14.
Piaggio G, von Hertzen H, Grimes D, Van Look PFA. Timing of emergency contraception with levonorgestrel or the Yuzpe regimen. Lancet 1999;353:721.

15.
Trussell J, Ellertson C, Rodriguez G. The Yuzpe regimen of emergency contraception. Obstet Gynecol 1996;88:150-4.

16.
Ellertson C, Evans M, Ferden S, et al. Extending the time limit for starting the Yuzpe regimen of emergency contraception to 120 hours. Obstet Gynecol 2003;101:1168-71.

17.
Rodrigues I, Grou F, Joly J. Effectiveness of emergency contraceptive pills between 72 and 120 hours after unprotected sexual intercourse. Am J Obstet Gynecol 2001;184:531-7.

18.
Wilcox AJ, Dunson D, Baird DD. The timing of the "fertile window" in the menstrual cycle. BMJ 2000;321:1259-62.

19.
Ellertson C, Webb A, Blanchard K, et al. Modifying the Yuzpe regimen of emergency contraception. Obstet Gynecol 2003;101:1160-6.

20.
Fasoli M, Parazzini F, Cecchetti G, La Vecchia C. Post-coital contraception. Contraception 1989;39:459-68.

21.
D'Souza RE, Masters T, Bounds W, Guillebaud J. Randomised controlled trial assessing the acceptability of GyneFix versus Gyne-T380S for emergency contraception. J Fam Plann Reprod Health Care 2003;29:23-9.

22.
Trussell J, Koenig J, Ellertson C, Stewart F. Preventing unintended pregnancy. Am J Public Health 1997;87:932-7.

23.
Stratton P, Hartog B, Hajizadeh N, et al. A single mid-follicular dose of CDB-2914, a new antiprogestin, inhibits folliculogenesis and endometrial differentiation in normally cycling women. Hum Reprod 2000;15:1092-9.

24.
Effect of different progestagens in low oestrogen oral contraceptives on venous thromboembolic disease. Lancet 1995;346:1582-8.

25.
Schwartz SM, Petitti DB, Siscovick DS, et al. Stroke and use of low-dose oral contraceptives in young women. Stroke 1998;29:2277-84.

26.
Sanchez-Ojanguren J, Escudero D, Zapata A. Occlusion of the right common carotid artery due to oral estrogen overdose. Rev Neurol 1998;27:604-6.

27.
Lake SR, Vernon S. Emergency contraception and retinal vein thrombosis. Br J Ophthalmol 1999;83:630-1.

28.
Sanchez-Guerra M, Valle N, Blanco L, Combarros O, Pascual J. Brain infarction after postcoital contraception in a migraine patient. J Neurol 2003;249:774.

29.
Hamandi K, Scolding J. Emergency contraception and stoke. J Neurol 2003;250:615-6.

30.
Vasilakis C, Jick SS, Jick H. The risk of venous thromboembolism in users of postcoital contraceptive pills. Contraception 1999;59:79-83.

31.
Improving access to quality care in family planning. 2nd ed. Geneva: World Health Organization, 2000.

32.
Speroff L, Darney PD. A clinical guide for contraception. 3rd ed. Baltimore: Williams & Wilkins, 2001.

33.
Nielsen C, Miller L. Ectopic gestation following emergency contraceptive pill administration. Contraception 2000;62:275-6.

34.
Sheffer-Mimouni G, Pauzner D, Maslovitch S, Lessing JB, Gamzu R. Ectopic pregnancies following emergency levonorgestrel contraception. Contraception 2003;67:267-9.

35.
Bracken MB. Oral contraception and congenital malformations in offspring. Obstet Gynecol 1990;76:552-7.

36.
Grimes DA, Raymond EG. Bundling a pregnancy test with the Yupze regimen of emergency contraception. Obstet Gynecol 1999;94:471-3.

37.
Arab L, Carriquiry A, Steck-Scott S, Gaudet MM. Ethnic differences in the nutrient intake adequacy of premenopausal US women. J Am Diet Assoc 2003;103:1008-14.

38.
Stewart FH, Harper CC, Ellertson CE, Grimes DA, Sawaya GF, Trussell J. Clinical breast and pelvic examination requirements for hormonal contraception. JAMA 2001;285:2232-9.

39.
Trussell J, Duran V, Shochet T, Moore K. Access to emergency contraception. Obstet Gynecol 2000;95:267-70.

40.
Glasier A, Baird D. The effects of self-administering emergency contraception. N Engl J Med 1998;339:1-4.

41.
Raine T, Harper C, Leon K, Darney P. Emergency contraception. Obstet Gynecol 2000;96:1-7.

42.
Jackson R, Bimla Schwarz E, Freedman L, Darney P. Advance supply of emergency contraception: effect on use and usual contraception — a randomized trial. Obstet Gynecol 2003;102:8-16.

43.
Ellertson C, Ambardekar S, Hedley A, Coyaji K, Trussell J, Blanchard K. Emergency contraception. Obstet Gynecol 2001;98:570-5.

44.
Ng E, Damus K, Bruck L, MacIsaac L. Advance provision of levonorgestrel-only emergency contraception versus prescription. Obstet Gynecol 2003;101: Suppl:13S. abstract.

45.
Grimes DA. Switching emergency contraception to over-the-counter status. N Engl J Med 2002;347:846-9.

46.
Efficacy and side effects of immediate postcoital levonorgestrel used repeatedly for contraception. Contraception 2000;61:303-8.

47.
Croxatto H. Emergency contraception pills: how do they work? IPPF Med Bull 2002;36:1-2.

48.
Trussell J, Raymond EG. Statistical evidence about the mechanism of action of the Yuzpe regimen of emergency contraception. Obstet Gynecol 1999;93:872-6.

49.
Westhoff C, Kerns J, Morroni C, Cushman LF, Tiezzi L, Murphy PA. Quick start. Contraception 2002;66:141-5.

50.
American Medical Association. Policy Statement H-75.985: access to emergency contraception. Chicago: American Medical Association.

51.
ACOG Practice Bulletin. Gynecology: emergency oral contraception. ACOG Pract Bull 2001;25:1-14.

52.
Statement of the American College of Obstetricians and Gynecologists supporting the availability of over-the-counter emergency contraception. Washington, D.C.: American College of Obstetricians and Gynecologists, February 2001.

53.
Berg AO, Allan JD, Frame PS, et al. Screening for chlamydia infection: recommendations and rationale. Am J Nurs 2002;102:87-92.

ADDENDUM

Since publication of this article in 2003, the FDA reveiwed an application for a switch to over-the-counter status for emergency contraception (Plan B). There was scientific agreement among, and strong guidance from, the FDA advisory panel favoring the switch.

The FDA continues to defer action on the matter; thus, emergency contraception remains available only by prescription. The prolonged FDA inaction on this application lacks scientific or clinical justification.[1,2]

1. Wood AJJ, Drazen JM, Greene MF. A sad day for science at the FDA. N Engl J Med 2005;353:1197-9.
2. Wood SF. Women's health and the FDA. N Engl J Med 2005;353:1650-1.

Preven, one manufacturer's formulation of combined oral contraceptives mentioned in Table 1, is no longer available.

Dysplastic Nevi

JEAN MARIE NAEYAERT, M.D., PH.D.,

AND LIEVE BROCHEZ, M.D., PH.D.

A 26-year-old man comes to establish primary care. Physical examination reveals multiple moles on his body, which he describes as "funny-looking." There is no family history of melanoma. He thinks that one of his two brothers (15 years of age) and his father have the same kind of moles. How should this case be managed?

THE CLINICAL PROBLEM

Various names are used in the literature for dysplastic nevi, including BK moles (after the initials of the first two patients in whom these lesions were described),[1] Clark's nevi, and atypical moles or nevi. All these terms refer to lesions with specific clinicopathological characteristics associated with an increased risk of melanoma.

A dysplastic nevus is typically a macular lesion that is 5 mm or more in diameter, usually with irregular, fuzzy borders (Figure 1).[2] Under oblique or lateral illumination, most lesions are slightly elevated and have a smooth or pebbled surface. Some have a central papule surrounded by a macular pigmented rim, creating a "fried-egg" appearance. Their pigmentation is variegated shades of tan and brown. Some lesions have a characteristic reddish hue and blanch with pressure under a glass microscope slide. Dysplastic nevi may be present anywhere on the skin, including the so-called doubly protected areas (breasts and buttocks) and the scalp, but they are most common on the trunk, especially on the upper back.[3] In preadolescent children who are members of a family with dysplastic nevus–melanoma syndrome, dysplastic nevi may first appear on the scalp.[4]

Dysplastic nevi usually become clinically apparent at puberty or adolescence, but true dysplastic nevi have been described in prepubertal children.[1,4] The dysplastic nevi continue to appear throughout life. Their number may vary greatly, from one to hundreds. In patients with multiple lesions, there is marked heterogeneity among lesions, resulting in a highly characteristic clinical phenotype (Figure 2). Counts of dysplastic nevi are highly correlated with total nevus counts (increasing as the total count increases), independent of a personal or family history of melanoma.[5]

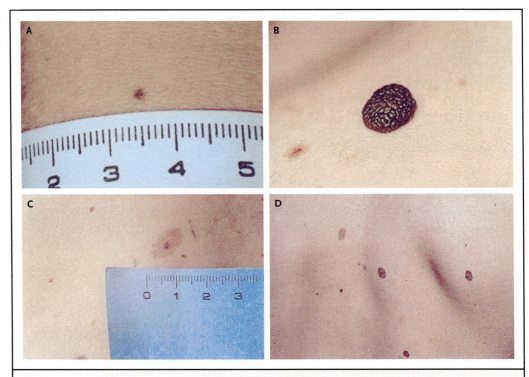

Figure 1. Clinical Characteristics of Atypical Nevi as Compared with Common Nevi.

Common nevi (Panels A and B) are macular or papular, symmetric lesions that have a regular, well-defined border, are homogeneous in color, and are usually less than 5 mm in diameter. Atypical nevi (Panels C and D) are macular or maculopapular lesions that are slightly asymmetric, with an irregular, ill-defined border; they vary in color (from shades of tan to pink or red) and are usually 5 mm or more in diameter. The scale markers in Panels A and C show centimeters.

The term "dysplastic nevus syndrome" is used arbitrarily. Some clinicians use it to describe patients with only one atypical nevus,[6] although the "classic" dysplastic nevus syndrome refers to patients who have the triad of 100 or more nevi, at least 1 nevus 8 mm or larger in diameter, and at least 1 nevus with clinically atypical features.[7] The syndrome can occur sporadically or in a familial setting. To diagnose sporadic dysplastic nevus syndrome with certainty, clinical examination of first-degree relatives is necessary.[8] Although there has been concern that nonspecialists might not reliably recognize the clinical phenotype, a recent study showed that identification of the phenotype with the use of a specific scoring system was a skill that could be easily learned by health care professionals who are not specialists.[9]

Pathological Diagnosis of Dysplastic Nevi

The pathological diagnosis of a dysplastic nevus requires the identification of both specific cytologic and architectural abnormalities (Figure 3). Interobserver agreement in the

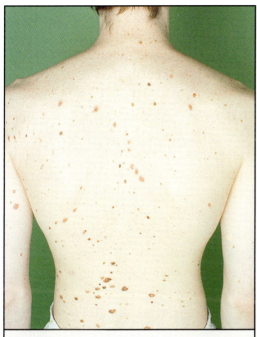

Figure 2. A 26-Year-Old Man with Atypical Nevi.

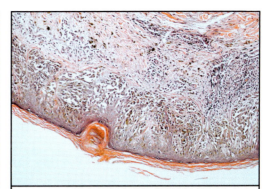

Figure 3. Pathological Appearance of a Dysplastic Nevus.

The pathological diagnosis is based on the presence of two major criteria and at least two minor criteria. The major criteria are basilar proliferation of atypical nevomelanocytes, extending three rete ridges beyond a dermal melanocytic component (if present), and intraepidermal melanocytic proliferation (lentiginous or epithelioid). The minor criteria are concentric eosinophilic fibrosis enveloping the rete ridges or lamellar fibroplasia beneath the tips of the rete ridges, neovascularization, a dermal inflammatory response, and fusion of the rete ridges due to the confluence of adjacent melanocytic nests. In the lesion shown, all the criteria are met.

pathological diagnosis of melanocytic dysplasia is hampered by the lack of universally accepted diagnostic criteria. In studies that use preset criteria for diagnosis, interobserver agreement is moderate to good.[10-12] Reproducibility in grading atypia remains poor to moderate because of the nonuniform criteria used.[11-13]

Clinicopathological Correlations

The presence or absence of atypical clinical features correlates, imperfectly, with the presence or absence of histologic dysplasia. In a study involving 101 patients with a history of sporadic melanoma in whom the most clinically atypical nevus was removed, the likelihood of histologic dysplasia ranged from 7 percent among lesions with no or only one clinically atypical feature (a diameter of 5 mm or more, an ill-defined or irregular border, or color variation) to 23 percent in cases with two atypical features and 62 percent in cases with three atypical features.[14] Among nevi without histologic dysplasia, only 4 percent had all three clinically atypical features.[14] In another study, roughly 30 percent of common (nondysplastic) nevi met the histologic criteria for dysplasia (architectural atypia, cytologic atypia, and a dermal host response), albeit minimally.[15]

In a population-based study, histologic findings of melanocytic dysplasia were associated with higher total nevus counts. Among subjects from whom biopsy specimens were obtained from the two most clinically atypical nevi, the histologic concordance between the biopsy results was higher than would be expected on the basis of chance alone, suggesting that melanocytic dysplasia is not randomly distributed but, rather, that some persons appear to have a predisposition to melanocytic dysplasia.[16]

Epidemiologic Characteristics

The estimated prevalence of clinically atypical nevi ranges from 7 percent to 18 percent in population-based samples,[17,18] and the prevalence of histologic melanocytic dysplasia is approximately 10 percent.[19,20] The reported frequency of clinically atypical nevi among patients with a history of melanoma is higher, ranging from 34 percent to 59 percent.[18,21-24] The variations in the estimates of prevalence probably reflect, at least in part, the use of different diagnostic criteria in different studies. However, differences among populations in sun exposure could also play a part.[25] Dysplastic nevi also appear to be more prevalent in younger populations (those less than 30 to 40 years of age) than in older groups.[5,8]

Clinically atypical nevi may evolve from normal-appearing nevi or may be dysplastic from their first appearance.[26] As dynamic lesions, dysplastic nevi can become progressively more or progressively less clinically atypical, but the majority either remain stable or regress over time.[5,27] New dysplastic nevi may develop after the age of 30 years.[5]

The predilection of atypical nevi for intermittently sun-exposed areas (especially the trunk), their positive association with a history of painful sunburn (in which the pain lasts more than two days) or blistering sunburn, and the finding that persons with clinically atypical nevi often have sun-sensitive skin types suggest that the development of dysplastic nevi could relate to acute, intense sun exposure.[3,18] Genetic factors also appear to be important; an autosomal dominant mode of inheritance has been reported in families with the dysplastic nevus–melanoma syndrome.[8]

Clinical Significance of Dysplastic Nevi

The clinical importance of dysplastic nevi lies in their association with the risk of melanoma. This has been demonstrated in several cohort and case–control studies.[17-24,27-35] In most of these studies, dysplastic nevi were defined according to clinical criteria, without histologic confirmation.[21-24,27,28,30-34] In some studies, the presence of large nevi without other atypical features was also found to be associated with an increased risk of melanoma.[22,24,35] The age-adjusted incidence of melanoma is approximately 15 times as high among patients with dysplastic nevi as among members of the general population (154 vs. 10 per 100,000 person-years, standardized to the population of Pennsylvania in 1985).[31]

The risk of melanoma in persons with dysplastic nevi increases with an increasing number of nevi and in the presence of a personal or family history of melanoma.[29-32,34] There is a 100-fold increase in the incidence of melanoma in patients who have previously had melanoma, a 200-fold increase in those with at least two family members with melanoma, and a more than 1200-fold increase in those with both a personal and family history of melanoma.[31] In persons with a family history of melanoma, the incidence of melanoma is highly concentrated in family members with dysplastic nevi, although melanoma may occur in those without this phenotype.[28] The presence of dysplastic nevi is an independent risk factor for the development of multiple primary melanomas.[28,36]

Melanoma has been shown to occur both in and separate from preexisting nevi (common or dysplastic). In cohort studies of persons with dysplastic nevi, melanoma appears to arise in contiguity with dysplastic nevi in 44 to 80 percent of subjects,[27,29,31,37] a rate much higher than that for melanoma in the general population.[38,39] Currently, there are no published data on the extent to which the presence of histologic melanocytic dysplasia predicts melanoma independently of other risk factors for melanoma, such as clinically atypical nevi and the total number of nevi.

Dysplastic nevi may be confused with melanoma, both clinically and histologically. In one study, lesions histologically diagnosed as dysplastic nevi by an expert panel were diagnosed by other pathologists as melanoma in 21 percent of the readings (in situ in 86 percent of the cases), and thin or in situ melanomas were misdiagnosed as dysplastic nevi in 12 percent of the readings.[40]

STRATEGIES AND EVIDENCE

Prophylactic Excision

According to the available evidence, the clinical diagnosis of dysplastic nevi (or dysplastic nevus syndrome) does not need to be confirmed histologically.[21-24,27,28,30-34] Despite the recognized association between dysplastic nevi and the risk of melanoma, the majority of dysplastic nevi will never progress to melanoma.[26] The relatively low absolute risk that a single dysplastic nevus will develop into melanoma is indicated by the following calculations: in a population of 10 million inhabitants in which the incidence of melanoma is 10 per 100,000 inhabitants per year, about 1 million people (10 percent of the population) will have one or more dysplastic nevi (with a mean of two such nevi). On the assumption that 20 percent of melanomas develop in contiguity with a dysplastic nevus, this calculation implies that only 1 in 10,000 dysplastic nevi per year will progress to melanoma. These estimates underscore the argument that prophylactic excision of dysplastic nevi is unlikely to be cost effective and might, in addition, give patients a false sense of security, since an increased risk of melanoma may remain after these nevi have been removed. Some have advocated the excision of dysplastic nevi that are difficult to follow because of their location; however, data are lacking to support this approach.[2]

Follow-up of Patients with Dysplastic Nevi

Melanoma of the skin offers the theoretical advantage of early detection by simple, noninvasive investigation (examination of the skin), and therefore regular dermatologic examinations are commonly recommended for persons with dysplastic nevi. In several studies, monitoring by trained dermatologists, with follow-up schedules ranging from once every three months to once a year, has been associated with high proportions of thin melanomas with a good prognosis,[27,29,31,32,37] although those studies did not include contemporaneous control groups. Serial photographs have also been proposed as a method of documenting changes in existing lesions or the development of new lesions.[29,31,32,41] In a historical, uncontrolled cohort study of patients with dysplastic nevi, 6 of 11 melanomas were excised because of change, relative to base line, in a preexisting nevus (in 5 cases) or development of a new lesion (in 1 case) on serial photographs; only 2 of the 11 lesions were diagnosed clinically as melanoma at the time of excision.[31]

Although close follow-up seems reasonable, it remains possible that close surveillance may preferentially detect slow-growing tumors with a good prognosis. In addition, it is uncertain whether the in situ melanomas (Clark level I) detected by such surveillance would have progressed to invasive melanoma if left in place. There are no prospective cohort studies comparing the survival of patients who are being closely monitored with those who are not. Proposed benefits of close surveillance include the opportunity to teach patients to identify suspicious lesions and possible improvements in the quality of life resulting from the reassurance of regular expert skin examinations; however, there are currently no data to support these possibilities.

Prospective studies have demonstrated that the risk of melanoma in members of families affected by the dysplastic nevus–melanoma syndrome is considerable, with an estimated cumulative risk of 49 percent for persons 10 to 50 years of age and 82 percent by the age of 72 years[27]; the benefit of close surveillance is likely to be higher among such persons than among those with one or more dysplastic nevi but no family history of melanoma (which is the more frequent scenario). No studies have assessed the cost effectiveness of surveillance programs for dysplastic nevi.

Self-Examination   No randomized, controlled trials have assessed the value of self-examination of the skin. One study, which included 650 patients with melanoma, suggested a survival benefit in patients who had performed self-examination of the skin, as compared with those who had not, although the investigators emphasized that longer follow-up was needed to confirm a beneficial effect of self-examinations.[42] In a survey of 816 patients with melanoma, the habit of skin self-examination was associated with thinner melanomas.[43] Since self-examination is relatively simple and inexpensive, it is routinely recommended, despite the limited supporting data.

Ocular Examination   Patients with dysplastic nevi may have an increased risk of ocular melanoma.[44] In a case–control study involving 211 patients with ocular melanoma, 16 percent had one or more dysplastic nevi, as compared with 7 percent of the controls (odds ratio, 24.1 [95 percent confidence interval, 4.8 to 119.8] among patients with four or more atypical nevi).[44] The estimated cumulative lifetime risk of eye melanoma in patients with the dysplastic nevus phenotype is 1 in 200.[44] A yearly ocular examination of patients with the dysplastic nevus syndrome has been recommended by some experts[45] but not by others.[46]

Genetic Screening

Germ-line *CDKN2A* mutations (on chromosome 9p21) have been found in 20 to 40 percent of families in which at least three first-degree relatives are affected by melanoma.[47] These germ-line mutations were three times as likely to be found in family members affected by the dysplastic nevus syndrome as in relatives who were unaffected; however, the presence or absence of the syndrome was not perfectly correlated with gene-carrier status.[48] Thus, a consortium recommended in a consensus statement that DNA testing not be performed in persons with the dysplastic nevus syndrome (familial or not) unless it is in the context of a defined research program, since the implications for management are currently unclear.[47]

AREAS OF UNCERTAINTY

Use of Sunscreens

Total nevus counts have been found to be higher in children protected by sunscreens than in those protected by clothing,[49] and a recent study[50] indicated that the use of broad-spectrum sunscreens was effective in reducing the development of nevi in white children with freckles. However, data are lacking on the relation between the use of sunscreens and dysplastic nevi, and it is not known whether the use of sunscreens reduces the risk of mela-

Table 1. Published Guidelines for the Management of Dysplastic Nevi.

Organization	Patient Characteristics	Surveillance	Self-Examination	Other Advice	Source
Melanoma Working Group, the Netherlands	History of melanoma in at least two of the following and a history of dysplastic nevus in at least one of the following: patient, children, parents, brothers, sisters, uncles, or aunts	At least once a year, starting at age 10 yr (absolute indication)	No recommendations	Oral and written information about alarming signs and sun protection should be offered	Bergman et al.[57]
	At least three dysplastic nevi and a family history of melanoma	Once a year (relative indication)	No recommendations	Oral and written information about alarming signs and sun protection should be offered	
	At least three dysplastic nevi and no family history of melanoma	Not recommended	No recommendations	Oral and written information about alarming signs and sun protection should be offered	
National Institutes of Health	Large numbers of moles (often more than 50), some of which are atypical and have certain distinct histologic features; family history of melanoma (in a first- or second-degree relative)	Intensive surveillance, initially at intervals of 4 to 6 mo; total-body photographs and dermoscopy in some cases	Once a month	Sun protection	NIH Consensus Conference[58]

noma.[50,51] A real concern is that sunscreen use may lead to increased sun exposure, which could increase the risk of melanoma. Patients should thus be advised to avoid sun exposure during the hours of peak intensity of ultraviolet (UV) B radiation (noon to 4 p.m.) and to use physical protection, such as clothing, in addition to a broad-spectrum sunscreen (sun protection factor [SPF] 15 or higher) on uncovered areas.

Dermoscopy

Dermoscopy, or dermatoscopy (epiluminescence or incident-light microscopy), is a non-invasive technique in which oil immersion and optical magnification are used to make the epidermis translucent and to allow the visualization of structures not visible to the naked eye. The use of this technique has been proposed as a means of distinguishing melanocytic from nonmelanocytic pigmented lesions and of differentiating benign, suspicious, and malignant melanocytic lesions.[52-56] Studies of images of skin lesions (including dysplastic nevi and early melanomas) extracted from image data bases have suggested that this technique improves the number of correct diagnoses over that achieved by clinical examination,[53] but its influence on the rate of excision of benign lesions or other clinical outcomes has not been studied.

GUIDELINES

Table 1 summarizes recommendations for the management of dysplastic nevi according to two published sets of guidelines.[57,58]

CONCLUSIONS AND RECOMMENDATIONS

When encountering a patient with clinically dysplastic nevi, as in the case described in the vignette, the physician should take a detailed personal history, including information on any history of skin or other cancer, prior excisions of nevi, episodes of sunburn, and UV-radiation exposure (e.g., during childhood while residing in a sunny region) and should ask whether any family members have or have had melanoma or dysplastic nevi. All first-degree relatives should be encouraged to undergo a skin examination. During the complete examination of the skin at base line (which should include examination of the doubly protected areas and the scalp), the total number of nevi should be evaluated and the presence or absence of atypical nevi assessed.

Although the role of dermoscopy remains controversial, we use this technique to evaluate lesions that look suspicious clinically, in particular to rule out the presence of non-melanocytic pigmented lesions. A lesion should be excised if, after careful examination, the dermatologist believes that melanoma cannot be ruled out; in such cases, we excise the lesion with a 2-mm margin. Prophylactic excision is not warranted for lesions diagnosed clinically as dysplastic nevi, since the probability that a single lesion will develop into melanoma is very low and since excision does not clearly reduce the overall risk of melanoma.

Patients should be educated about the risk of melanoma and should be advised to watch for alarming signs (changes in a mole or findings according to the "ABCD" rule for melanoma detection [asymmetry, border irregularity, color variation, or a diameter greater than 6 mm]). Avoidance of sun exposure during the hours of peak UV intensity (noon to 4 p.m.) and routine use of sun-protective clothing, sunglasses, and broad-spectrum sunscreens (SPF 15 or higher) should be routinely advised.

Although data to guide follow-up are lacking, we follow patients with the use of serial, standardized (digital), total-body photographs and close-up photographs of prominent atypical nevi (with a ruler placed next to the nevus). We recommend reevaluation six months after the base-line examination and then once a year, or more frequent follow-up if there is a personal history of melanoma. Patients should be advised to request an earlier visit if they judge a newly appearing lesion to be suspicious or a change in an existing lesion to be suspicious, according to the information they have received.

This article first appeared in the December 4, 2003, issue of the New England Journal of Medicine.

REFERENCES

1. Clark WH, Reimer RR, Greene MH, Ainsworth AM, Mastrangelo MJ. Origin of familial malignant melanomas from heritable melanocytic lesions: 'the B-K mole syndrome.' Arch Dermatol 1978;114:732-8.

2. Tsao H, Sober AJ. Atypical melanocytic nevi. In: Freedberg IM, Eisen AZ, Wolff K, Austen KF, Goldsmith LA, Katz SI, eds. Fitzpatrick's dermatology in general medicine. 6th ed. New York: McGraw-Hill, 2003:906-16.

3. Richard MA, Grob JJ, Gouvernet J, et al. Role of sun exposure on nevus: first study in age-sex phenotype-controlled populations. Arch Dermatol 1993;129:1280-5.

4. Tucker MA, Greene MH, Clark WH Jr, Kraemer KH, Fraser MC, Elder DE. Dysplastic nevi on the scalp of prepubertal children from melanoma-prone families. J Pediatr 1983;103:65-9.

5. Halpern AC, Guerry D IV, Elder DE, Trock B, Synnestvedt M, Humphreys T. Natural history of dysplastic nevi. J Am Acad Dermatol 1993;29:51-7.

6. Elder DE, Goldman LI, Goldman SC, Greene MH, Clark WH Jr. Dysplastic nevus syndrome: a phenotypic association of sporadic cutaneous melanoma. Cancer 1980;46:1787-94.

7. Kopf AW, Friedman RJ, Rigel DS. Atypical mole syndrome. J Am Acad Dermatol 1990;22:117-8.

8. Crijns MB, Vink J, Van Hees CLM, Bergman W, Vermeer BJ. Dysplastic nevi: occurrence in first- and second-degree relatives of patients with 'sporadic' dysplastic nevus syndrome. Arch Dermatol 1991;127:1346-51. [Erratum, Arch Dermatol 1992;128:513.]

9. Bishop JA, Bradburn M, Bergman W, et al. Teaching non-specialist health care professionals how to identify the atypical mole syndrome phenotype: a multinational study. Br J Dermatol 2000;142:331-7.

10. Clemente C, Cochran AJ, Elder DE, et al. Histopathologic diagnosis of dysplastic nevi: concordance among pathologists convened by the World Health Organisation Melanoma Programme. Hum Pathol 1991;22:313-9.

11. de Wit PEJ, van't Hof-Grootenboer B, Ruiter DJ, et al. Validity of the histopathological criteria used for diagnosing dysplastic naevi: an interobserver study by the pathology subgroup of the EORTC Malignant Melanoma Cooperative Group. Eur J Cancer 1993;29A:831-9.

12. Duncan LM, Berwick M, Bruijn JA, Byers HR, Mihm MC, Barnhill RL. Histopathologic recognition and grading of dysplastic melanocytic nevi: an interobserver agreement study. J Invest Dermatol 1993;100:318S-321S.

13. Duray PH, DerSimonian R, Barnhill R, et al. An analysis of interobserver recognition of the histopathologic features of dysplastic nevi from a mixed group of nevomelanocytic lesions. J Am Acad Dermatol 1992;27:741-9.

14. Grob JJ, Andrac L, Romano MH, et al. Dysplastic naevus in non-familial melanoma: a clinicopathological study of 101 cases. Br J Dermatol 1988;118:745-52.

15. Klein LJ, Barr RJ. Histologic atypia in clinically benign nevi: a prospective study. J Am Acad Dermatol 1990;22:275-82.

16. Piepkorn M, Meyer LJ, Goldgar D, et al. The dysplastic melanocytic nevus: a prevalent lesion that correlates poorly with clinical phenotype. J Am Acad Dermatol 1989;20:407-15.

17. Halpern AC, Guerry D IV, Elder DE, et al. Dysplastic nevi as risk markers of sporadic (nonfamilial) melanoma: a case-control study. Arch Dermatol 1991;127:995-9.

18. Augustsson A, Stierner U, Rosdahl I, Suurküla M. Common and dysplastic naevi as risk factors for cutaneous malignant melanoma in a Swedish population. Acta Derm Venereol 1991;71:518-24.

19. Piepkorn MW, Barnhill RL, Cannon-Albright LA, et al. A multiobserver, population-based analysis of histologic dysplasia in melanocytic nevi. J Am Acad Dermatol 1994;30:707-14.

20. Steijlen PM, Bergman W, Hermans J, Scheffer E, Van Vloten WA, Ruiter DJ. The efficacy of histopathological criteria required for diagnosing dysplastic naevi. Histopathology 1988;12:289-300.

21. Holly EA, Kelly JW, Shpall SN, Chiu SH. Number of melanocytic nevi as a major risk factor for malignant melanoma. J Am Acad Dermatol 1987;17:459-68.

22. Grob JJ, Gouvernet J, Aymar D, et al. Count of benign melanocytic nevi as a major indicator of risk for nonfamilial nodular and superficial spreading melanoma. Cancer 1990;66:387-95.

23. Garbe C, Büttner P, Weiss J, et al. Risk factors for developing cutaneous melanoma and criteria for identifying persons at risk: multicenter case-control study of the Central Malignant Melanoma Registry of the German Dermatological Society. J Invest Dermatol 1994;102:695-9.

24. Tucker MA, Halpern A, Holly EA, et al. Clinically recognized dysplastic nevi: a central risk factor for cutaneous melanoma. JAMA 1997;277:1439-44.

25.
Bataille V, Grulich A, Sasieni P, et al. The association between naevi and melanoma in populations with different levels of sun exposure: a joint case-control study of melanoma in the UK and Australia. Br J Cancer 1998;77:505-10.

26.
Clark WH Jr, Elder DE, Guerry D IV, Epstein MN, Greene MH, Van Horn M. A study of tumor progression: the precursor lesions of superficial spreading and nodular melanoma. Hum Pathol 1984;15:1147-65.

27.
Tucker MA, Fraser MC, Goldstein AM, Elder DE, Guerry D IV, Organic SM. The risk of melanoma and other cancers in melanoma-prone families. J Invest Dermatol 1993;100:350S-355S.

28.
Carey WP Jr, Thompson CJ, Synnestvedt M, et al. Dysplastic nevi as a melanoma risk factor in patients with familial melanoma. Cancer 1994;74:3118-25.

29.
Rigel DS, Rivers JK, Kopf AW, et al. Dysplastic nevi: markers of increased risk for melanoma. Cancer 1989;63:386-9.

30.
Tiersten AD, Grin CM, Kopf AW, et al. Prospective follow-up for malignant melanoma in patients with atypical-mole (dysplastic-nevus) syndrome. J Dermatol Surg Oncol 1991;17:44-8.

31.
Halpern AC, Guerry D IV, Elder DE, Trock B, Synnestvedt M. A cohort study of melanoma in patients with dysplastic nevi. J Invest Dermatol 1993;100:346S-349S.

32.
MacKie RM, McHenry P, Hole D. Accelerated detection with prospective surveillance for cutaneous malignant melanoma in high-risk groups. Lancet 1993;341:1618-20.

33.
Kang S, Barnhill RL, Mihm MC Jr, Fitzpatrick TB, Sober AJ. Melanoma risk in individuals with clinically atypical nevi. Arch Dermatol 1994;130:999-1001.

34.
Marghoob AA, Kopf AW, Rigel DS, et al. Risk of cutaneous malignant melanoma in patients with 'classic' atypical-mole syndrome: a case-control study. Arch Dermatol 1994;130:993-8.

35.
Swerdlow AJ, English J, MacKie RM, et al. Benign melanocytic naevi as a risk factor for malignant melanoma. Br Med J (Clin Res Ed) 1986;292:1555-9.

36.
Burden AD, Newell J, Andrew N, Kavanagh G, Connor JM, MacKie RM. Genetic and environmental influences in the development of multiple primary melanoma. Arch Dermatol 1999;135:261-5.

37.
Masri GD, Clark WH Jr, Guerry D IV, Halpern A, Thompson CJ, Elder DE. Screening and surveillance of patients at high risk for malignant melanoma result in detection of earlier disease. J Am Acad Dermatol 1990;22:1042-8.

38.
Sagebiel RW. Melanocytic nevi in histological association with primary cutaneous melanoma of superficial spreading and nodular types: effect of tumour thickness. J Invest Dermatol 1993;100:322S-325S.

39.
Rhodes AR, Harrist TJ, Day CL, Mihm MC Jr, Fitzpatrick TB, Sober AJ. Dysplastic melanocytic nevi in histologic association with 234 primary cutaneous melanomas. J Am Acad Dermatol 1983;9:563-74.

40.
Brochez J, Verhaeghe E, Grosshans E, et al. Interobserver variation in the histopathological diagnosis of clinically suspicious pigmented skin lesions. J Pathol 2002;196:459-66.

41.
Rhodes AR. Intervention strategy to prevent lethal cutaneous melanoma: use of dermatologic photography to aid surveillance of high-risk persons. J Am Acad Dermatol 1998;39:262-7.

42.
Berwick M, Begg CB, Fine JA, Roush GC, Barnhill RL. Screening for cutaneous melanoma by skin self-examination. J Natl Cancer Inst 1996;88:17-23.

43.
Carli P, De Giorgi V, Palli D, et al. Dermatologist detection and skin self-examination are associated with thinner melanomas: results from a survey of the Italian Multidisciplinary Group on Melanoma. Arch Dermatol 2003;139:607-12.

44.
Bataille V, Sasieni P, Cuzick J, Hungerford JL, Swerdlow A, Bishop JA. Risk of ocular melanoma in relation to cutaneous and iris naevi. Int J Cancer 1995;60:622-6.

45.
Vink J, Crijns MB, Mooy CM, Bergman W, Oosterhuis JA, Went LN. Ocular melanoma in families with dysplastic nevus syndrome. J Am Acad Dermatol 1990;23:858-62.

46.
Taylor MR, Guerry D IV, Bondi EE, et al. Lack of association between intraocular melanoma and cutaneous dysplastic nevi. Am J Ophthalmol 1984;98:478-82.

47.
Kefford RF, Newton Bishop JA, Bergman W, Tucker MA. Counseling and DNA testing for individuals perceived to be genetically predisposed to melanoma: a consensus statement of the Melanoma Genetics Consortium. J Clin Oncol 1999;17:3245-51.

48.
Bishop JA, Wachsmuth RC, Harland M, et al. Genotype/phenotype and penetrance studies in melanoma families with germline CDKN2A mutations. J Invest Dermatol 2000;114:28-33.

49.
Autier P, Doré JF, Cattaruzza MS, et al. Sunscreen use, wearing clothes, and number of nevi in 6- to 7-year-old European children. J Natl Cancer Inst 1998;90:1873-80.

50.
Gallagher RP, Rivers JK, Lee TK, Bajdik CD, McLean DI, Coldman AJ. Broad-spectrum sunscreen use and the development of new nevi in white children: a randomized controlled trial. JAMA 2000;283:2955-60.

51.
Autier P. Sunscreen and melanoma revisited. Arch Dermatol 2000;136:423.

52.
Stolz W, Semmelmayer U, Johow K, Burgdorf WH. Principles of dermatoscopy of pigmented skin lesions. Semin Cutan Med Surg 2003;22:9-20.

53.
Pehamberger H, Binder M, Steiner A, Wolff K. In vivo epiluminescence microscopy: improvement of early diagnosis of melanoma. J Invest Dermatol 1993;100:356S-362S.

54.
Menzies SW, Ingvar C, Crotty KA, McCarthy WH. Frequency and morphologic characteristics of invasive melanomas lacking specific surface microscopic features. Arch Dermatol 1996;132:1178-82.

55.
Argenziano G, Fabbrocini G, Carli P, De Giorgi V, Sammarco E, Delfino M. Epiluminescence microscopy for the diagnosis of doubtful melanocytic skin lesions: comparison of the ABCD rule of dermatoscopy and a new 7-point checklist based on pattern analysis. Arch Dermatol 1998;134:1563-70.

56.
Dal Pozzo V, Benelli C, Roscetti E. The seven features for melanoma: a new dermoscopic algorithm for the diagnosis of malignant melanoma. Eur J Dermatol 1999;9:303-8.

57.
Bergman W, Van Voorst Vader PC, Ruiter DJ. Dysplastic naevi and the risk of melanoma: a guideline for patient care. Ned Tijdschr Geneeskd 1997;141:2010-4.

58.
NIH Consensus Conference: diagnosis and treatment of early melanoma. JAMA 1992;268:1314-9.

Genital Chlamydial Infections

JEFFREY F. PEIPERT, M.D., M.P.H.

A 19-year-old woman visits her primary care provider for counseling about contraception. She became sexually active one year previously and has had a new sexual partner for the past three months. Her partner currently uses a condom intermittently for contraception, and she inquires about oral contraceptives. She reports no medical problems and is in good health. Her physical examination is unremarkable. Is testing for *Chlamydia trachomatis* indicated?

THE CLINICAL PROBLEM

*C*hlamydia trachomatis is the most common bacterial cause of sexually transmitted infections in the United States, responsible for an estimated 3 million new infections each year.[1,2] The cost of care for untreated chlamydial infections and their complications is estimated to exceed $2 billion annually.[3]

Clinical Presentation

As many as 85 to 90 percent of *C. trachomatis* infections in men and women are asymptomatic.[4,5] Asymptomatic infections can persist for several months.[5] Despite the frequent absence of symptoms, at least one third of women have local signs of infection on examination.[5] The two most commonly reported signs are mucopurulent discharge from the cervix and hypertrophic cervical ectopy (Figure 1). Signs and symptoms in men include urethral discharge of mucopurulent or purulent material, dysuria, or urethral pruritus.

Clinical manifestations of *C. trachomatis* infections in women include acute urethral syndrome, urethritis, bartholinitis, cervicitis, upper genital tract infection (endometritis, salpingo-oophoritis, or pelvic inflammatory disease), perihepatitis (Fitz-Hugh–Curtis syndrome), and reactive arthritis.[5] Symptoms depend on the site of infection. Infection of the urethra and lower genital tract may cause dysuria, abnormal vaginal discharge, or postcoital bleeding, whereas infection of the upper genital tract (e.g., endometritis or salpingitis) may be manifested as irregular uterine bleeding and abdominal or pelvic discomfort.

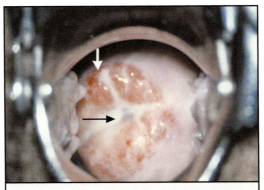

Figure 1. Cervical Ectropion (White Arrow) with Muco-purulent Cervicitis (Black Arrow).

Photograph courtesy of Dr. Marc Steben.

In women, untreated chlamydial infection can lead to severe reproductive complications. *C. trachomatis* is an important causal agent in pelvic inflammatory disease, with sequelae including infertility, ectopic pregnancy, and chronic pelvic pain.[6] Up to two thirds of cases of tubal-factor infertility and one third of cases of ectopic pregnancy may be attributable to *C. trachomatis* infection.[7] Chlamydial infection during pregnancy is associated with a number of adverse outcomes of pregnancy including preterm labor, premature rupture of the membranes, low birth weight, neonatal death, and postpartum endometritis.[8,9]

Chlamydial infection during pregnancy may be transmitted to the infant during delivery.[10] An infant born to a mother with active infection has a risk of acquiring infection at any anatomical site of 50 to 75 percent. Approximately 30 to 50 percent of infants born to chlamydia-positive mothers will have conjunctivitis, and at least 50 percent of infants with chlamydial conjunctivitis will also have nasopharyngeal infection. Chlamydial pneumonia develops in about 30 percent of infants with nasopharyngeal infection.[5]

In men, the most common clinical manifestation of *C. trachomatis* infection is nongonococcal urethritis. In fact, *C. trachomatis* causes approximately 35 to 50 percent of all cases of nongonococcal urethritis in heterosexual men. Symptoms of nongonococcal urethritis may develop after an incubation period of 7 to 21 days and include dysuria and mild-to-moderate whitish or clear urethral discharge. In most cases, physical examination reveals no abnormalities other than the discharge. Other clinical syndromes in men include acute epididymitis, acute proctitis, acute proctocolitis, conjunctivitis, and Reiter's syndrome.[5] Male infertility, chronic prostatitis, and urethral strictures are possible results of infection.

Both Reiter's syndrome (urethritis, conjunctivitis, arthritis, and mucocutaneous lesions) and reactive tenosynovitis or arthritis (without the other components of Reiter's syndrome) have been associated with genital *C. trachomatis* infection.[5] Infection with *C. trachomatis* is also believed to be a cofactor for the transmission of human immunodeficiency virus in both men and women.[11]

Epidemiology of Chlamydial Infections

The prevalence of chlamydia depends on the characteristics of the population studied. Reported prevalence rates in the United States have ranged from 2 to 7 percent among female college students and 4 to 12 percent among women attending a family planning clinic to 6 to 20 percent among men and women attending a clinic for sexually transmitted diseases or persons entering correctional facilities.[5,12] In the United Kingdom, recent data suggest that the rate of infection among young women exceeds 10 percent.[13] The prevalence of *C. trachomatis* infection is highest in groups of persons who are the least likely to see a clinician. Prevalence rates have declined in geographic areas where screening programs have been implemented.[14]

Risk factors for chlamydial infection in sexually active women include a young age (less than 25 years and, in particular, less than 20 years), intercourse at an early age, having more than one sexual partner, involvement with a new sexual partner, being unmarried, black race, a history of or coexistent sexually transmitted infection, cervical ectopy, and inconsistent use of barrier contraceptive methods.[15,16] Young age is the factor that is most strongly associated with infection (relative risk among women younger than 25 years as compared with older women, 2.0 to 3.5).[17] This association is largely attributable to the higher level of sexual activity among younger women. Also, in younger women, the squamocolumnar junction of the cervix often lies well out on the ectocervix, forming a bright red central zone of ectopic columnar epithelium called an ectropion (Figure 1); this ectopy provides a larger target area for chlamydial infection than is present in older women.[18]

STRATEGIES AND EVIDENCE

Screening

Screening in Women   There is good evidence that screening women who are at risk for *C. trachomatis* infection can prevent reproductive sequelae by reducing the rate of pelvic inflammatory disease.[15] The strongest evidence supporting screening in women comes from a large randomized trial of screening and treatment at a health maintenance organization in Seattle.[19] Participants were unmarried, asymptomatic women (18 to 34 years of age) who were considered to have a high risk of *C. trachomatis* infection on the basis of a scoring system that included as risk factors a young age (less than 25 years), black race, nulligravidity, douching, and two or more sexual partners during the previous 12 months. By the end of the follow-up period, there were 9 verified cases of pelvic inflammatory disease in the screened group (8 per 10,000 woman-months of follow-up) and 33 cases in the usual-care group (18 per 10,000 woman-months; relative risk in the screened group, 0.44; 95 percent confidence interval, 0.20 to 0.90). Long-term adverse outcomes of chlamydial infection were not addressed in this study.

In addition, two ecologic studies (studies evaluating associations between types of exposure and outcomes in populations rather than individual persons), conducted in Sweden, showed that the rates of both ectopic pregnancies and pelvic inflammatory disease were reduced in communities after screening for chlamydial infection was adopted.[20,21] However, it is possible that the lower prevalence of adverse outcomes in these studies was due to factors other than screening, such as increased use of barrier contraceptives and reductions in risk-taking behavior.

Although data from randomized trials of screening for chlamydial infection during pregnancy are lacking, there is some evidence that screening high-risk women for *C. trachomatis* during pregnancy can reduce the rate of adverse outcomes of pregnancy. Two observational studies showed associations between the treatment of chlamydial infections during pregnancy and improved outcomes of pregnancy, including lower rates of premature rupture of the membranes, low birth weight, births of infants who were small for their gestational age, and neonatal death.[22,23]

Screening in Men   The U.S. Preventive Services Task Force found no direct evidence to determine whether screening asymptomatic men is effective for reducing the incidence of new infections in women, and it could not determine the balance of the harms and benefits of screening men.[15]

Testing Methods   The gold standard for the diagnosis of *C. trachomatis* infection was traditionally a culture of a swab from the endocervix in women or the urethra in men. However, the methodologic challenges of culturing this organism led to the development of non–culture-based tests. Whereas early non–culture-based tests, including antigen-detection tests and nonamplified nucleic acid hybridization, were limited by their failure to detect a substantial proportion of infections,[24] newer tests that amplify and detect *C. trachomatis*–specific DNA or RNA sequences[25] (including polymerase chain reaction, ligase chain reaction, and transcription-mediated amplification of RNA) are substantially more sensitive than the first-generation non–culture-based tests (80 to 91 percent, depending

Table 1. Common Clinical Syndromes and Their Treatment.

Syndrome	Recommended Regimens
Men	
Nongonococcal urethritis	Azithromycin, 1 g orally (single dose), or doxycycline, 100 mg orally 2 times a day for 7 days
Recurrent or persistent urethritis	Metronidazole, 2 g orally (single dose), plus erythromycin base, 500 mg orally 4 times a day for 7 days, or erythromycin ethylsuccinate, 800 mg orally 4 times a day for 7 days
Epididymitis	Ceftriaxone, 250 mg intramuscularly (single dose), plus doxycycline, 100 mg orally 2 times a day for 10 days
Women	
Mucopurulent cervicitis	Azithromycin, 1 g orally (single dose), or doxycycline, 100 mg orally 2 times a day for 7 days
Chlamydia during pregnancy	Erythromycin base, 500 mg orally 4 times a day for 7 days, or amoxicillin, 500 mg orally 3 times a day for 7 days, or azithromycin, 1 g orally (single dose)
Pelvic inflammatory disease*	
Outpatient	Ofloxacin, 400 mg orally 2 times a day for 14 days, or levofloxacin, 500 mg orally once a day for 14 days, with or without metronidazole, 500 mg orally 2 times a day for 14 days; otherwise, ceftriaxone, 250 mg intramuscularly (single dose), or cefoxitin, 2 g intramuscularly (single dose), plus probenecid, 1 g orally, plus doxycycline, 100 mg orally 2 times a day for 14 days, with or without metronidazole, 500 mg orally 2 times a day for 14 days
Inpatient	Cefotetan, 2 g intravenously every 12 hours, or cefoxitin, 2 g intravenously every 6 hours, plus doxycycline, 100 mg orally or intravenously every 12 hours; otherwise, clindamycin, 900 mg intravenously every 8 hours, plus gentamicin, 2 mg per kg of body weight loading dose intravenously, then 1.5 mg per kg every 8 hours; daily administration of a single dose may be substituted

* Therapy for pelvic inflammatory disease should be continued for 24 to 48 hours after clinical improvement occurs and should consist of continuous oral therapy with doxycycline, 100 mg orally twice a day, or clindamycin, 450 mg orally 4 times a day, for a total of 14 days.

on the site from which the specimen is obtained, vs. 62 to 75 percent), when culture is used as the gold standard.[25] The sensitivity is slightly lower when these newer tests are performed on urine specimens rather than endocervical specimens, but the specificity is high for all types of specimens (range, 94 to nearly 100 percent).[25] The majority of nucleic acid–amplification tests have been approved by the Food and Drug Administration for the detection of *C. trachomatis* (and *Neisseria gonorrhoeae*) in urine from both men and women, providing a noninvasive testing method.[25] Limitations of nucleic acid–amplification tests include their relatively high cost and the requirement for a suitable laboratory.[25]

The most recent addition to the testing armamentarium is the use of specimens collected by patients.[26,27] Amplification testing of vaginal or urethral swab specimens collected by patients has a sensitivity and specificity similar to those of amplification testing of specimens collected by clinicians, and studies indicate that patients prefer this method to the standard collection methods.[28,29]

Treatment

The treatment of chlamydial infection depends on the clinical syndrome (Table 1).[2] Effective and low-cost treatments for genital chlamydial infection are available for the most common clinical syndromes (nongonococcal urethritis in men and mucopurulent cervicitis in women). In a randomized trial, the efficacy of a seven-day course of doxycycline was equivalent to that of a single dose of azithromycin; both resulted in cure rates of more than 95 percent among men and nonpregnant women.[30] Sexual partners should be notified, examined, and treated for chlamydia and any other identified or suspected sexually transmitted disease. Patients and their partners should be instructed to refrain from sexual intercourse until therapy is completed (specifically, until seven days after a single-dose regimen or until the completion of a seven-day regimen).[2]

Infection during Pregnancy   A Cochrane review of 11 randomized trials for the treatment of chlamydia during pregnancy concluded that amoxicillin was as effective as oral erythromycin.[31] Several small trials comparing oral azithromycin with these therapies have shown similar cure rates and acceptability for azithromycin.[32,33]

Pelvic Inflammatory Disease   Although pelvic inflammatory disease is thought to be a polymicrobial infection, *C. trachomatis* is one of the more common pathogens involved. The minimal criteria for a diagnosis of pelvic inflammatory disease include uterine–adnexal tenderness or cervical-motion tenderness.[2] Some studies suggest that atypical presentations of pelvic inflammatory disease, including discomfort without appreciable tenderness, abnormal uterine bleeding, and abnormal vaginal discharge, are often associated with infection and inflammation in the upper genital tract (i.e., endometritis and salpingitis).[34,35] Chlamydial pelvic inflammatory disease tends to have a more insidious onset than pelvic inflammatory disease caused by *N. gonorrhoeae* or other more virulent organisms. However, the damage to the fallopian tube can be as great or greater with chlamydia, especially with repeated infections.[36]

Because of the risks of infertility and other sequelae of pelvic inflammatory disease, clinicians should have a low threshold for the prompt institution of treatment in women who are at risk for chlamydial infection. The delay of antibiotic therapy is associated with an increased risk of adverse outcomes.[37] The PID [Pelvic Inflammatory Disease] Evaluation and Clinical Health (PEACH) study, a randomized trial comparing inpatient therapy consisting of cefoxitin and doxycycline with similar outpatient therapy, demonstrated that outpatient therapy for uncomplicated pelvic inflammatory disease (without tubo-ovarian abscess or severe illness) was as effective as intravenous inpatient therapy in terms of fertility and other long-term health outcomes, including the prevention of ectopic pregnancy and chronic pelvic pain.[38]

AREAS OF UNCERTAINTY

There continues to be uncertainty regarding whom to screen and how frequently to do so. There is little evidence of the effectiveness of screening in asymptomatic women who are not in high-risk groups.[15] Screening on the basis of age (less than 25 years) appears to be effective even in areas where the prevalence of chlamydial infection is low to moderate (3 to 6 percent). In a longitudinal cohort study of screening in 3202 high-risk, inner-city young women, chlamydial infection was detected in 24.1 percent; the median time to new infection was slightly more than 7 months, and the median time to a repeated positive test was 6.3 months. On the basis of these results, it was recommended that all young, sexually active women be screened every six months.[39] It is unclear, however, whether these findings can be generalized to populations with a lower prevalence of infection.

Level I evidence (from randomized trials) is also lacking regarding the effectiveness of the screening and treatment of pregnant women in populations with a low prevalence of chlamydial infection. In addition, the balance of benefits and harms (including false-positive test results and the inappropriate use of antibiotics) has not been assessed.[15]

Given the high prevalence of asymptomatic infections in the population, some experts advocate for the routine screening of young men as the next important step toward reduced rates of infections and complications.[40,41] Although there is strong evidence that treatment can eradicate *C. trachomatis* infection in men, there are no studies demonstrating that the screening of asymptomatic men can reduce the rates of acute infection and adverse outcomes in men or in women. Cost-effectiveness analyses have suggested that there is an economic benefit to society of screening for *C. trachomatis*, as compared with not screening, in high-risk women.[42,43] However, the cost effectiveness of the screening of men and low-risk women is debatable and will depend on the prevalence of infections, the ease and cost of specimen collection, the cost of testing, the characteristics of the diagnostic tests (e.g., their sensitivity and specificity), and the short- and long-term adverse outcomes that are prevented. Additional research is needed to determine the optimal interval between screenings and to compare the universal screening of all sexually active women younger than 25 years of age with screening based on the presence of additional risk factors in populations with a range of prevalence rates.

It remains uncertain whether the routine use of urine specimens or specimens collected by patients would improve compliance with testing and treatment. Also, it is unclear whether the empirical treatment of the sexual partners of patients with chlamydial infections is preferable to the screening of these partners. Some experts suggest that providing patients with prescriptions for empirical treatment to deliver to their sexual partners will reduce the rate of reinfection,[44] but this hypothesis remains unproven. In a recent trial in which patients were randomly assigned to either patient-delivered treatment for partners (patients were asked to deliver a dose of azithromycin to each of their sexual partners) or self-referral (patients were asked to refer their sexual partners for treatment), the risk of reinfection was nonsignificantly lower in the group assigned to patient-delivered treatment (odds ratio for reinfection, 0.8; 95 percent confidence interval, 0.6 to 1.1).[45]

GUIDELINES

Guidelines from several professional societies, the Centers for Disease Control and Prevention, and the U.S. Preventive Services Task Force are summarized in Table 2.[46-50]

Table 2. Guidelines from Professional Societies and Federal Agencies.		
Organization	Who Should Be Screened	Timing or Frequency of Screening
American Academy of Pediatrics[46]	All young, sexually active women	Perform annually
American College of Obstetricians and Gynecologists[47]	All young sexually active women and other women at high risk for infection	Perform routinely (interval not specified)
American College of Preventive Medicine[48]	All sexually active women with risk factors (age ≤25 yr, new male sexual partner or two or more sexual partners in previous year, inconsistent use of barrier contraceptives, history of sexually transmitted disease, black race, cervical ectopy)	Perform annually
	Pregnant women	Perform during first trimester in all women, third trimester if risk factors present
American Medical Association[49]	All young, sexually active women	Perform annually
Canadian Task Force on Preventive Health Care[50]	Persons in high-risk groups (sexually active women <25 yr of age, men and women with a new sexual partner or more than one partner in the previous year, women who use nonbarrier contraceptive methods)	Not specified
	Pregnant women	Perform during first trimester in all women
Centers for Disease Control and Prevention[2]*	All sexually active women <20 yr of age; women 20–24 yr of age if one of the following risk factors is present: inconsistent use of barrier contraceptives or a new sexual partner or multiple sexual partners during the previous 3 mo; women >24 yr of age if both risk factors are present	Perform annually
	Pregnant women	Perform during first prenatal visit in all women, third trimester if high risk (<25 yr of age or other risk factors)
U.S. Preventive Services Task Force[15]†	All sexually active women ≤25 yr of age and other asymptomatic women at increased risk for infection	Perform routinely, optimal interval uncertain
	All asymptomatic pregnant women ≤25 yr of age and others at increased risk for infection	Perform routinely, optimal interval uncertain

* The guidelines of the Centers for Disease Control and Prevention are available at http://www.cdc.gov/std/treatment/rr5106.pdf.
† The guidelines of the U.S. Preventive Services Task Force are available at http://www.ahrq.gov/clinic/uspstf/uspschlm.htm. The task force recommends routine screening in the groups listed and notes that there is insufficient evidence to make a recommendation for or against screening in asymptomatic men.

All groups suggest that clinicians screen routinely for *C. trachomatis* in all sexually active women less than 25 years of age and in other asymptomatic women who are at increased risk for infection.

CONCLUSIONS AND RECOMMENDATIONS

Screening for *C. trachomatis* infection is indicated in sexually active women with risk factors for this infection, including an age of less than 25 years, inconsistent use of barrier contraceptives, a new sexual partner, more than one sexual partner, cervical ectopy, and a history of or coexisting sexually transmitted disease. The patient described in the vignette has some of these risk factors. Electing not to screen her would place her at risk for adverse outcomes, including ascending infection (pelvic inflammatory disease) and infertility, chronic pelvic pain, and ectopic pregnancy. Annual screening is reasonable, although more frequent testing may be indicated in areas of high prevalence or in women with several risk factors. Information on prevalence (the rates of positive tests) can often be obtained from microbiology laboratories. The use of barrier contraception (e.g., condoms) as a method of prevention should be discussed with all patients. If a screening test is positive for *C. trachomatis*, I would treat the patient with doxycycline or azithromycin. Retesting (a "test of cure") after treatment with recommended regimens is not indicated unless compliance is in question, symptoms are present, or reinfection is suspected.[2] Rescreening for chlamydia is recommended when patients present for care within 12 months after a positive test.[2]

The timely treatment of the patient's sexual partners is also essential in order to reduce the risk of reinfection. The sexual partners should be evaluated, tested, and treated if they have had sexual contact with the patient during the 60 days preceding the diagnosis. Treatment for sexual partners that is delivered by the patient for the prevention of repeated infection has efficacy similar to that of self-referral and is a reasonable approach.

Supported in part by a Midcareer Investigator Award in Women's Health Research from the National Institute of Child Health and Human Development (K24 HD01298-03).

This article first appeared in the December 18, 2003, issue of the New England Journal of Medicine.

REFERENCES

1.
Sexually transmitted disease surveillance, 2001. Atlanta: Centers for Disease Control and Prevention, September 2002.

2.
Sexually transmitted diseases treatment guidelines 2002. MMWR Recomm Rep 2002;51(RR-6):30-6.

3.
Eng Tr, Butler WT, eds. The hidden epidemic: confronting sexually transmitted diseases. Washington, D.C.: National Academy Press, 1997.

4.
Cecil JA, Howell MR, Tawes JJ, et al. Features of Chlamydia trachomatis and Neisseria gonorrhoeae infection in male army recruits. J Infect Dis 2001;184:1216-9.

5.
Stamm WE. Chlamydia trachomatis infections of the adult. In: Holmes KK, Mårdh P-A, Sparling PF, et al., eds. Sexually transmitted diseases. 3rd ed. New York: Mc-Graw-Hill, 1999:407-22.

6.
Westrom L, Joesoef R, Reynolds G, Hagdu A, Thompson SE. Pelvic inflammatory disease and fertility: a cohort study of 1,844 women with laparoscopically verified disease and 657 control women with normal laparoscopic results. Sex Transm Dis 1992;19:185-92.

7.
Paavonen J, Eggert-Kruse W. Chlamydia trachomatis: impact on human reproduction. Hum Reprod Update 1999;5:433-47.

8.
Mardh PA. Influence of infection with Chlamydia trachomatis on pregnancy outcome, infant health and life-long sequelae in infected offspring. Best Pract Res Clin Obstet Gynaecol 2002;16:847-64.

9.
Andrews WW, Goldenberg RL, Mercer B, et al. The Preterm Prediction Study: association of second-trimester genitourinary chlamydia infection with subsequent spontaneous preterm birth. Am J Obstet Gynecol 2000;183:662-8.

10.
Jain S. Perinatally acquired Chlamydia trachomatis associated morbidity in young infants. J Matern Fetal Med 1999;8:130-3.

11.
Fleming DT, Wasserheit JN. From epidemiological synergy to public health policy and practice: the contribution of other sexually transmitted diseases to sexual transmission of HIV infection. Sex Transm Infect 1999;75:3-17.

12.
Hardick J, Hsieh Y, Tulloch S, Kus J, Tawes J, Gaydos CA. Surveillance of Chlamydia trachomatis and Neisseria gonorrhoeae infections in women in detention in Baltimore, Maryland. Sex Transm Dis 2003;30:64-70.

13.
Tobin JM. Chlamydia screening in primary care: is it useful, affordable and universal? Curr Opin Infect Dis 2002;15:31-6.

14.
Herrmann B, Egger M. Genital Chlamydia trachomatis infections in Uppsala County, Sweden, 1985-1993: declining rates for how much longer? Sex Transm Dis 1995;22:253-60.

15.
U.S. Preventive Services Task Force. Screening for chlamydial infection: recommendations and rationale. Am J Prev Med 2001;20: Suppl:90-4.

16.
Gaydos CA, Howell R, Pare B, et al. Chlamydia trachomatis infections in female military recruits. N Engl J Med 1998;339:739-44.

17.
Gaydos CA, Howell MR, Quinn TC, McKee KT Jr, Gaydos JC. Sustained high prevalence of Chlamydia trachomatis infections in female Army recruits. Sex Transm Dis 2003;30:539-44.

18.
Faro S, Soper DE, eds. Infectious diseases in women. Philadelphia: W.B. Saunders, 2001:261-2.

19.
Scholes D, Stergachis A, Heidrich FE, Andrilla H, Holmes KK, Stamm WE. Prevention of pelvic inflammatory disease by screening for cervical chlamydial infection. N Engl J Med 1996;334:1362-6.

20.
Kamwendo F, Forslin L, Bodin L, Danielsson D. Decreasing incidences of gonorrhea- and chlamydia-associated acute pelvic inflammatory disease: a 25-year study from an urban area of central Sweden. Sex Transm Dis 1996;23:384-91.

21.
Egger M, Low N, Smith GD, Lindblom B, Herrmann B. Screening for chlamydial infections and the risk of ectopic pregnancy in a county in Sweden: ecological analysis. BMJ 1998;316:1776-80.

22.
Ryan GM Jr, Abdella TN, McNeeley SG, Baselski VS, Drummond DE. Chlamydia trachomatis infection in pregnancy and effect of treatment on outcome. Am J Obstet Gynecol 1990;162:34-9.

23.
Cohen I, Veille J-C, Calkins BM. Improved pregnancy outcomes following successful treatment of chlamydial infection. JAMA 1990;263:3160-3.

24.
Guaschino S, De Seta F. Update on Chlamydia trachomatis. Ann N Y Acad Sci 2000;900:293-300.

25.
Johnson RE, Newhall WJ, Papp JR, et al. Screening tests to detect Chlamydia trachomatis and Neisseria gonorrhoeae infections — 2002. MMWR Recomm Rep 2002;51(RR-15): 1-38.

26.
Wiesenfeld HC, Lowry DL, Heine RP, et al. Self-collection of vaginal swabs for the detection of Chlamydia, gonorrhea, and trichomoniasis: opportunity to encourage sexually transmitted disease testing among adolescents. Sex Transm Dis 2001;28:321-5.

27.
Gaydos CA, Rompalo AM. The use of urine and self-obtained vaginal swabs for the diagnosis of sexually transmitted diseases. Curr Infect Dis Rep 2002;4:148-57.

28.
Verhoeven V, Avonts D, Van Royen P, Denekens J. Self-collection of vaginal swab specimens: the patient's perception. Sex Transm Dis 2002;29:426.

29.
Newman SM, Nelson MB, Gaydos CA, Friedman HB. Female prisoners' preferences of collection methods for testing for Chlamydia trachomatis and Neisseria gonorrhoeae infection. Sex Transm Dis 2003;30:306-9.

30.
Martin DH, Mroczkowski TF, Dalu ZA, et al. A controlled trial of a single dose of azithromycin for the treatment of chlamydial urethritis and cervicitis. N Engl J Med 1992; 327:921-5.

31.
Brocklehurst P, Rooney G. Interventions for treating genital chlamydia trachomatis infection in pregnancy. Cochrane Database Syst Rev 2000;2:CD000054.

32.
Jacobson GF, Autry AM, Kirby RS, Liverman EM, Motley RU. A randomized controlled trial comparing amoxicillin and azithromycin for the treatment of Chlamydia trachomatis in pregnancy. Am J Obstet Gynecol 2001;184:1352-4.

33.
Kacmar J, Cheh E, Montagno A, Peipert JF. A randomized trial of azithromycin versus amoxicillin for the treatment of Chlamydia trachomatis in pregnancy. Infect Dis Obstet Gynecol 2001;9:197-202.

34.
Wiesenfeld HC, Hillier SL, Krohn MA, et al. Lower genital tract infection and endometritis: insight into subclinical pelvic inflammatory disease. Obstet Gynecol 2002;100:456-63.

35.
Korn AP, Bolan G, Padian N, Ohn-Smith M, Schachter J, Landers DV. Plasma cell endometritis in women with symptomatic bacterial vaginosis. Obstet Gynecol 1995;85:387-90.

36.
Hillis SD, Owens LM, Marchbanks PA, Amsterdam LF, Mac Kenzie WR. Recurrent chlamydial infections increase the risks of hospitalization for ectopic pregnancy and pelvic inflammatory disease. Am J Obstet Gynecol 1997;176:103-7.

37.
Hillis SD, Joesoef R, Marchbanks PA, Wasserheit JN, Cates W Jr, Westrom L. Delayed care of pelvic inflammatory disease as a risk factor for impaired fertility. Am J Obstet Gynecol 1993;168:1503-9.

38.
Ness RB, Soper DE, Holley RL, et al. Effectiveness of inpatient and outpatient treatment strategies for women with pelvic inflammatory disease: results from the Pelvic Inflammatory Disease Evaluation and Clinical Health (PEACH) Randomized Trial. Am J Obstet Gynecol 2002;186:929-37.

39.
Burstein GR, Gaydos CA, Diener-West M, Howell MR, Zenilman JM, Quinn TC. Incident Chlamydia trachomatis infections among inner-city adolescent females. JAMA 1998;280:521-6.

40.
LaMontagne DS, Fine DN, Marrazzo JM. Chlamydia trachomatis infection in asymptomatic men. Am J Prev Med 2003;24:36-42.

41.
Turner CF, Rogers SM, Miller HG, et al. Untreated gonococcal and chlamydial infection in a probability sample of adults. JAMA 2002;287:726-33.

42.
Howell MR, Gaydos JC, McKee KT Jr, Quinn TC, Gaydos CA. Control of Chlamydia trachomatis infection in female Army recruits: cost-effective screening and treatment in training cohorts to prevent pelvic inflammatory disease. Sex Transm Dis 1999;26:519-26.

43.
Paavonen J, Puolakkainen M, Paukku M, Sintonen H. Cost-benefit analysis of first-void urine Chlamydia trachomatis screening program. Obstet Gynecol 1998;92:292-8.

44.
Klausner JD, Chaw JK. Patient-delivered therapy for chlamydia: putting research into practice. Sex Transm Dis 2003;30:509-11.

45.
Schillinger JA, Kissinger P, Calvet H, et al. Patient-delivered partner treatment with azithromycin to prevent repeated Chlamydia trachomatis infection among women: a randomized, controlled trial. Sex Transm Dis 2003;30:49-56.

46.
Committee on Practice and Ambulatory Medicine. Recommendations for preventive pediatric health care. Pediatrics 2000;105:645-6.

47.
Screening for chlamydia and gonorrhea in adolescents. In: Health care for adolescents. Washington, D.C.: American College of Obstetricians and Gynecologists, 2003.

48.
Hollblad-Fadiman K, Goldman SM. American College of Preventive Medicine practice policy statement: screening for Chlamydia trachomatis. Am J Prev Med 2003;24:287-92.

49.
Guidelines for adolescent preventive services. Chicago: American Medical Association, 1997. (Accessed August 29, 2005, at http://www.ama-assn.org/ama/upload/mm/39/gapsmono.pdf.)

50.
Davies HD, Wang EE. Periodic health examination, 1996 update. 2. Screening for chlamydial infections. CMAJ 1996;154:1631-44.

Prevention of Hepatitis A with the Hepatitis A Vaccine

ALLEN S. CRAIG, M.D., AND WILLIAM SCHAFFNER, M.D.

A 34-year-old man presented to the emergency department two weeks after returning from a trip to India, reporting a six-day history of anorexia, vomiting, malaise, fatigue, and dark urine. His alanine aminotransferase level was 7330 U per liter, the bilirubin level was 8 mg per deciliter (137 μmol per liter), and a test of the serum for hepatitis A IgM antibodies was positive. He was admitted for observation and hydration. Should he have been vaccinated against hepatitis A before his departure, and should his household contacts receive vaccine?

THE CLINICAL AND PUBLIC HEALTH PROBLEMS

The hepatitis A virus occurs throughout the world, and humans are thought to be its principal host.[1] The virus replicates in the liver and is transported through the bile to the stool, where it is shed beginning one to three weeks before the onset of illness and continuing for a week or more after the onset of jaundice. The virus is transmitted from person to person through the fecal–oral route and through the ingestion of contaminated food or drink. Although more than 75 percent of adults with hepatitis A infection have symptoms,[2] 70 percent of infections in children younger than six years of age are asymptomatic. These biologic characteristics contribute to the stealthy and efficient spread of the virus. The virus is spread easily from asymptomatic young children to other young children and to adult contacts. Young children are thus considered to be a principal reservoir and the dominant source of transmission in the community. The virus may also be transmitted by adults before symptoms occur, given that the virus appears in the stool substantially before the onset of illness. Thus, the source of a patient's infection often remains unknown.

After an average incubation period of 28 days (range, 15 to 50), an illness characterized by nausea, abdominal pain, fever, fatigue, dark urine, and jaundice occurs. Although

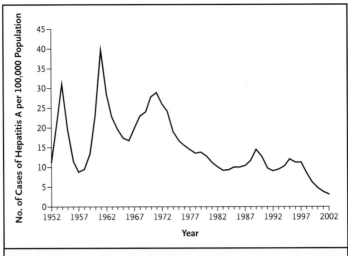

Figure 1. Rates of Reported Cases of Hepatitis A per 100,000 Population in the United States, 1952 through 2002.

Data are from the National Notifiable Disease Surveillance Systems, Centers for Disease Control and Prevention.

most patients recover completely and uneventfully, the potential seriousness of hepatitis A in adults is generally underappreciated.[3] Coagulopathy, encephalopathy, renal failure, a prolonged duration of disease, and occasional relapses are among its complications. Overall, 13 percent of patients require hospitalization, with a range from 7 percent of children younger than 15 years of age to 27 percent of adults 45 years of age or older.[4] Each year, approximately 100 deaths in the United States are attributed to fulminant hepatitis A infection.

Enhanced surveillance for hepatitis, conducted since 1981 by the Centers for Disease Control and Prevention (CDC) in four sentinel counties, has demonstrated that the epidemiology of hepatitis A in the United States is heterogeneous.[4] The CDC surveillance program showed that 52 percent of patients could not identify the source of their infection. Household or sexual contact with a person with hepatitis A (in 12 percent of patients) and a history of injection-drug use within the six months before the onset of illness (in 14 percent of patients) were the two most commonly recognized risk factors. Whether the latter risk factor reflected actual transmission through the sharing of blood-contaminated needles[5] or simply close contact could not be ascertained. Other reported risk factors included attendance or employment at a day-care center (in 11 percent of patients), a history of male homosexual activity within the previous six months (in 7 percent), and recent international travel to countries where hepatitis A is endemic (in 4 percent). Contrary to common belief, outbreaks of hepatitis A associated with restaurants are infrequent[6]; their notoriety probably stems from the extensive publicity surrounding these events.

There have been cyclic communitywide outbreaks of hepatitis A every 5 to 10 years in the United States for decades. More than 10,000 cases were reported in this country in 2001.[7] The actual number of cases of hepatitis A was probably 5 times that reported, and the number of new asymptomatic infections was probably 10 times the number of reported symptomatic cases. The incidence is highest in the western states and among persons 5 to 39 years of age.[8] One third of the U.S. population has serologic evidence of previous hepatitis A infection, with a prevalence ranging from 9 percent among children 6 to 11 years of age to 75 percent among persons 70 years of age or older.[6]

Periodic community epidemics notwithstanding, the rates of hepatitis A infection in the United States have been decreasing gradually during the past several decades (Figure 1). This decrease probably reflects advances in hygiene, including improved water supplies, enhanced sewage disposal, reduced crowding, augmented food safety, and other factors. The use of hepatitis A vaccine since 1995 in many communities where the rate of infection had been high has most likely accelerated this downward trend. Rates of hepatitis A infection are similar in Europe and in most developed countries. In developing countries, nearly all people have had hepatitis A infection by early adulthood.[9]

STRATEGIES AND EVIDENCE

Two biologic products, hepatitis A vaccine and immune globulin, have been used successfully to prevent hepatitis A infection.

Hepatitis A Vaccine

In the mid-1990s two formalin-inactivated hepatitis A virus vaccines were licensed by the Food and Drug Administration (FDA) for use in preventing disease in persons two years of age or older. Both vaccines are highly immunogenic; neutralizing antibodies are present in more than 94 percent of vaccinees one month after the first dose has been given, and essentially all recipients have a response after the second dose.[10-12] Two large efficacy trials were conducted, one in Thai villages and the other in a religious community in New York, all of which had sustained high rates of transmission of hepatitis A. Vaccination efficacy rates of 94 to 100 percent were recorded in these challenging circumstances.[13,14] The available data suggest that the vaccine is less immunogenic in patients with chronic liver disease (seroconversion rate, 93 percent),[15,16] immunocompromised persons (88 percent),[17] and transplant recipients (26 percent).[18] The immunogenicity also appears to be lower in the elderly (65 percent).[19]

Table 1. Recommended Doses of Hepatitis A Vaccine and Immune Globulin.*			
Agent and Age Group	**Dose**	**Volume**	**Dose Schedule**
		ml	
Havrix			
2–18 Yr	720 ELISA units	0.5	2 doses, 6–12 mo apart
>18 Yr	1440 ELISA units	1.0	2 doses, 6–12 mo apart
Vaqta			
2–18 Yr	25 U	0.5	2 doses, 6–18 mo apart
>18 Yr	50 U	1.0	2 doses, 6–12 mo apart
Twinrix (>17 yr)†	720 ELISA units	1.0	3 doses, at 0, 1, and 6 mo
Immune globulin (any age)	—	0.02 per kg of body weight	1 dose

* ELISA denotes enzyme-linked immunosorbent assay.
† Twinrix is a combination hepatitis A–hepatitis B vaccine.

Hepatitis A vaccine is not approved for use in children younger than two years of age because of concern that children who have passively acquired maternal antibody will have a diminished response to the vaccine.[20,21] In spite of a lower antibody response, an anamnestic response occurred in children who were vaccinated at two, four, and six months of age and then revaccinated several years later.[20]

The vaccine is considered to be very safe. Reported adverse events have included soreness at the injection site in 18 to 39 percent of persons, headache (in 15 percent), and fever (in less than 10 percent).[10-14,22] By 1999, more than 65 million doses of hepatitis A vaccine had been administered worldwide; investigators who reviewed data from multiple sources could not identify any serious adverse events that could be attributed to the vaccines with certainty.[6,23] The only contraindication to vaccination is a previous allergic reaction to either of the vaccines or sensitivity to any vaccine component. Although the vaccines have not been studied in pregnant women, it is likely that they would be safe during pregnancy, given their inactivated formulation. Both vaccines are classified in pregnancy category C (studies in animals and humans have not been conducted). Pregnant women who are at risk for hepatitis A, such as those traveling to developing countries, should be vaccinated only if there is a clear indication; immune globulin (discussed below) is a reasonable alternative for such women.

A two-dose schedule is recommended for both vaccines, with the second dose given 6 to 18 months after the first (Table 1). If the second dose is delayed, it can still be given without the need to repeat the primary dose.[24] Because of the high rate of seroconversion,

Table 2. Persons Currently Considered to Have an Indication for Hepatitis A Vaccine or Immune Globulin.

Hepatitis A vaccine

Children at least 2 years of age living in a state (Alaska, Arizona, California, Idaho, Nevada, New Mexico, Oklahoma, Oregon, South Dakota, Utah, or Washington) or a county with a high rate of infection (≥20 cases per 100,000 population from 1987 through 1997)*

Travelers at least 2 years of age to countries with high or intermediate rates of disease†

Men who have sex with men

Users of illicit drugs

Persons who have chronic liver disease or who have received or will receive a liver transplant

Persons who use clotting-factor concentrates

Laboratory personnel who work with the hepatitis A virus or with nonhuman primates that are infected with hepatitis A

Immune globulin

Persons who will be traveling to countries with high or intermediate rates of disease within the next 2 weeks

Children younger than 2 years of age who will be traveling to countries with high rates of disease

For postexposure prophylaxis, within 14 days after exposure: persons who have been exposed to food that was handled by someone with acute hepatitis A who had either poor hygiene or diarrhea or persons exposed to a family member with acute hepatitis A

* Further information is available at http://www.cdc.gov/ncidod/diseases/hepatitis/a/vax/index.htm.
† Further information is available at http://www.cdc.gov/ncidod/diseases/hepatitis/a/prevalence.htm.

testing for antibodies after vaccination is not required. Pediatric and adult formulations are available for both vaccines. The vaccines are given in the deltoid muscle and can be administered concurrently with other vaccines. They can also be given with immune globulin, at different anatomical sites, if immediate protection is required. The two brands of vaccine are considered to be interchangeable; if necessary, the two doses of vaccine can be of two different brands.[6] Serologic testing for hepatitis A before vaccination is likely to be cost effective only among persons who have a high likelihood of previous infection. Three additional hepatitis A vaccines have been licensed for use in Europe, Latin America, and other parts of the world. Routine vaccination programs are in place in Israel[25] and in regions of Italy and Spain.

Recently, a combination hepatitis A–hepatitis B vaccine was licensed in the United States for use in persons older than 17 years of age. This vaccine appears to be both as safe and as effective as individual vaccines for the two viruses given separately.[26] The 1-ml dose is given in a three-dose schedule at 0, 1, and 6 months (Table 1). Studies suggest that the combination vaccine is highly immunogenic in children 1 to 15 years of age.[27]

Strategies for the Use of Hepatitis A Vaccine

One strategy is to immunize people who are recognized to be at high risk for hepatitis A, in order to protect them. Vaccination should be offered to all high-risk persons two years of age or older (Table 2).[6] Such an approach, however, would be expected to have only a marginal effect on the occurrence of disease nationwide, because most persons who become infected with hepatitis A do not have identifiable risk factors.[4]

In addition to protecting the individual vaccinee, immunization has the public health goal of protecting the entire community. The achievement of this goal requires interruption of the transmission of the hepatitis A virus, which extends protection to immunocompromised persons (who have an insufficient response to the vaccine and who may be at particular risk for severe disease) and to persons who, for whatever reason, have not been immunized. The effectiveness of immunization strategies is also influenced by practical realities, such as the acceptance of the vaccine by the public and providers, competing priorities, and costs.

An initial approach to protecting the community involved the use of hepatitis A vaccine during large community outbreaks. Although small outbreaks in rural communities could be aborted by use of hepatitis A vaccine,[28] the strategy was less successful for epidemics occurring in larger urban centers,[29-31] reflecting the difficulty of attaining high rates of vaccine coverage in the target population. Moreover, by the time mass vaccination campaigns were initiated in urban centers, the outbreaks had begun to wane.

These experiences led to a shift in strategy to classic preexposure prevention: the areas of the country with the highest rates of cases were identified, and routine childhood immunization against hepatitis A was recommended in the identified communities. The intent was to reduce the rates of hepatitis A infection and disease among immunized children and — because children had been the primary sources of the spread of hepatitis A virus in these settings — to curtail the transmission of the virus and the incidence of disease among older children and adults through a herd-immunity effect. The introduction of routine immunization of young children in selected areas with high rates of infection, including a California county,[32] a community in New York,[33] and Indian reservations,[34] has demonstrated that universal childhood immunization against hepatitis A is feasible and that it can be sustained. Furthermore, after the introduction of hepatitis A vaccine in these communities, the incidence of disease rapidly decreased to rates that were similar to the national average or even lower. As anticipated, the rates of disease were also reduced among older persons who were not targeted for immunization.[35] It is likely that a sustained reduction in the national incidence of hepatitis A will require universal routine immunization, just as the elimination of measles and other diseases has been achieved by means of childhood vaccination.

Immune Globulin for Passive Immunoprophylaxis

Immune globulin is a preparation of concentrated antibodies derived from pooled human plasma. In 1945, Stokes and Neefe demonstrated that immune globulin provided protection against illness among children at a summer camp who had been exposed to hepatitis A.[36] Since then, immune globulin has been used widely for postexposure prophylaxis. The administration of a dose of 0.02 ml per kilogram of body weight intramuscularly in the gluteus within the first two weeks after exposure prevents disease in more than 85 percent of persons.[37] Prophylaxis given later during the incubation period may not prevent disease entirely but does result in reductions in the severity of symptoms and the duration of illness.[36] There is no need to perform serologic testing for antibody against hepatitis A before administering immune globulin.

Immune globulin remains an effective intervention for preventing the transmission of hepatitis A to family members and other close contacts of patients who have recently become ill. Immune globulin has also been used widely for preexposure prophylaxis in persons planning short-term or long-term travel to developing countries, as well as in persons exposed to food prepared by someone who was infected with hepatitis A. The use of immune globulin in travelers has been largely superceded by the use of hepatitis A vaccine, except when the traveler's departure is imminent and immediate protection must be provided or the traveler is younger than two years of age (Table 2), or possibly when the traveler is pregnant. The most common adverse event is pain at the injection site.

AREAS OF UNCERTAINTY

Although experience has been limited, hepatitis A vaccination appears likely to provide long-term protection. Follow-up five to six years after vaccination has demonstrated protective levels of antibody,[33] and clinical efficacy has been maintained for seven to nine years.[38,39] Models based on the kinetics of antibody against hepatitis A virus suggest that immunity will persist for at least 20 years, without the need for periodic boosters.[38-42]

The question of whether hepatitis A vaccine can be used for postexposure prophylaxis is unresolved. One study suggests that it may be effective when given after exposure,[43] but this study was small and did not involve a comparison with immune globulin, and its observations remain unconfirmed.

Fulminant infection may develop in patients with chronic liver disease if they are exposed to hepatitis A virus. There has been some debate about the cost effectiveness of hepatitis A vaccination in this population.[44-47] We believe that hepatitis A vaccine should be given to persons who have evidence of chronic liver disease and those who are awaiting or have received a liver transplant; these groups are at high risk for complications from a superimposed insult to the liver.

Although the FDA has approved these vaccines only for use one month or more before international travel, the vaccine is protective in most persons two weeks after the administration of the first dose, and many travel clinics administer it up to two weeks before departure.[48]

GUIDELINES

The Advisory Committee on Immunization Practices of the CDC[6] recommends the vaccination of high-risk persons two years of age or older, as outlined in Table 2. The advisory committee also recommends the routine immunization of all children in states or counties with high rates of infection, beginning at two years of age. The cases of hepatitis A reported in the 11 states that have high infection rates, most of which are in the West, accounted for half the total number of cases in the United States between 1987 and 1997, yet these states contained only 22 percent of the U.S. population (Table 2).[6]

CONCLUSIONS AND RECOMMENDATIONS

The patient described in the vignette clearly should have been vaccinated when he was planning his journey to a country that is known to have a high rate of hepatitis A. His family members should now receive immune globulin as postexposure prophylaxis against infection. The new combination hepatitis A–hepatitis B vaccine is an option for adults who are at risk for either infection and have not previously been vaccinated.

Routine vaccination is currently recommended for all young children in states with high rates of hepatitis A infection. Nevertheless, large community-wide outbreaks of hepatitis A continue to occur throughout the United States, with consequent disruption, hospitalizations, and deaths. Although it is not current policy, we propose that the universal vaccination of children for hepatitis A be extended to the entire United States, starting at two years of age, with catch-up immunization for all older children through adolescence.[49,50]

This article first appeared in the January 29, 2004, issue of the New England Journal of Medicine.

REFERENCES

1.
Cuthbert JA. Hepatitis A: old and new. Clin Microbiol Rev 2001;14:38-58. [Erratum, Clin Microbiol Rev 2001;14:642.]

2.
Lednar WM, Lemon SM, Kirkpatrick JW, Redfield RR, Fields ML, Kelley PW. Frequency of illness associated with epidemic hepatitis A virus infections in adults. Am J Epidemiol 1985;122:226-33.

3.
Willner IR, Uhl MD, Howard SC, Williams EQ, Riely CA, Waters B. Serious hepatitis A: an analysis of patients hospitalized during an urban epidemic in the United States. Ann Intern Med 1998;128:111-4.

4.
Bell BP, Shapiro CN, Alter MJ, et al. The diverse patterns of hepatitis A epidemiology in the United States — implications for vaccination strategies. J Infect Dis 1998;178:1579-84.

5.
Bower WA, Nainan OV, Han X, Margolis HS. Duration of viremia in hepatitis A virus infection. J Infect Dis 2000;182:12-7.

6.
Prevention of hepatitis A through active or passive immunization: recommendations of the Advisory Committee on Immunization Practices (ACIP). MMWR Recomm Rep 1999;48 (RR-12):1-37.

7.
Disease burden from viral hepatitis A, B, and C in the United States. Atlanta: Centers for Disease Control and Prevention, 2002. (Accessed August 29, 2004, at http://www.cdc.gov/ncidod/diseases/hepatitis/resource/dz_burden02.htm.)

8.
Hepatitis surveillance. Report no. 57. Atlanta: Centers for Disease Control and Prevention, September 2000.

9.
Bell BP, Feinstone SM. Hepatitis A vaccine. In: Plotkin SA, Orenstein WA, eds. Vaccines. 4th ed. Philadelphia: Saunders, 2004:269-97.

10.
Clemens R, Safary A, Hepburn A, Roche C, Stanbury WJ, Andre FE. Clinical experience with an inactivated hepatitis A vaccine. J Infect Dis 1995;171: Suppl 1:S44-S49.

11.
Ashur Y, Adler R, Rowe M, Shouval D. Comparison of immunogenicity of two hepatitis A vaccines — VAQTA and HAVRIX — in young adults. Vaccine 1999;17:2290-6.

12.
McMahon BJ, Williams J, Bulkow L, et al. Immunogenicity of an inactivated hepatitis A vaccine in Alaska Native children and Native and non-Native adults. J Infect Dis 1995;171:676-9.

13.
Innis BL, Snitbhan R, Kunasol P, et al. Protection against hepatitis A by an inactivated vaccine. JAMA 1994;271:1328-34.

14.
Werzberger A, Mensch B, Kuter B, et al. A controlled trial of a formalin-inactivated hepatitis A vaccine in healthy children. N Engl J Med 1992;327:453-7.

15.
Lee SD, Chan CY, Yu MI, et al. Safety and immunogenicity of inactivated hepatitis A vaccine in patients with chronic liver disease. J Med Virol 1997;52:215-8.

16.
Keeffe EB, Iwarson S, McMahon BJ, et al. Safety and immunogenicity of hepatitis A vaccine in patients with chronic liver disease. Hepatology 1998;27:881-6.

17.
Neilsen GA, Bodsworth NJ, Watts N. Response to hepatitis A vaccination in human immunodeficiency virus-infected and uninfected homosexual men. J Infect Dis 1997;176:1064-7.

18.
Arslan M, Wiesner RH, Poterucha JJ, Zein NN. Safety and efficacy of hepatitis A vaccination in liver transplantation recipients. Transplantation 2001;72:272-6.

19.
Wolters B, Junge U, Dziuba S, Roggendorf M. Immunogenicity of combined hepatitis A and B vaccine in elderly persons. Vaccine 2003;21:3623-8.

20.
Fiore AE, Shapiro CN, Sabin K, et al. Hepatitis A vaccination of infants: effect of maternal antibody status on antibody persistence and response to a booster dose. Pediatr Infect Dis J 2003;22:354-9.

21.
Piazza M, Safary A, Vegnente A, et al. Safety and immunogenicity of hepatitis A vaccine in infants: a candidate for inclusion in the childhood vaccination programme. Vaccine 1999;17:585-8.

22.
Hoke CH Jr, Binn LN, Egan JE, et al. Hepatitis A in the US Army: epidemiology and vaccine development. Vaccine 1992;10:Suppl 1: S75-S79.

23.
Niu MT, Salive M, Krueger C, Ellenberg SS. Two-year review of hepatitis A vaccine safety: data from the Vaccine Adverse Event Reporting System (VAERS). Clin Infect Dis 1998;26:1475-6.

24.
Landry P, Tremblay S, Darioli R, Genton B. Inactivated hepatitis A vaccine booster given >/=24 months after the primary dose. Vaccine 2000;19:399-402.

25.
Dagan R, Leventhal A, Anis E, Slater P, Shouval D. National Hepatitis A Virus (HAV) immunization program aimed exclusively at toddlers in an endemic country resulting in >90% reduction in morbidity rate in all ages. In: Abstracts of the 40th Annual Meeting of the Infectious Diseases Society of America, Chicago, October 24–27, 2002. Alexandria, Va.: Infectious Diseases Society of America, 2002:189. abstract. (Also available at http://www.journals.uchicago.edu/CID/2002Abstracts.html.)

26.
Tsai IJ, Chang MH, Chen HL, et al. Immunogenicity and reactogenicity of the combined hepatitis A and B vaccine in young adults. Vaccine 2000;19:437-41.

27.
Diaz-Mitoma F, Law B, Parsons J. A combined vaccine against hepatitis A and B in children and adolescents. Pediatr Infect Dis J 1999;18:109-14.
28.
McMahon BJ, Beller M, Williams J, Schloss M, Tanttila H, Bulkow L. A program to control an outbreak of hepatitis A in Alaska by using an inactivated hepatitis A vaccine. Arch Pediatr Adolesc Med 1996;150:733-9.
29.
Craig AS, Sockwell DC, Schaffner W, et al. Use of hepatitis A vaccine in a community-wide outbreak of hepatitis A. Clin Infect Dis 1998;27:531-5.
30.
Allard R, Beauchemin J, Bedard L, Dion R, Tremblay M, Carsley J. Hepatitis A vaccination during an outbreak among gay men in Montreal, Canada, 1995-1997. J Epidemiol Community Health 2001;55:251-6.
31.
Averhoff F, Shapiro C, Hyams I, et al. Use of inactivated hepatitis A vaccine to interrupt a communitywide hepatitis A outbreak. In: Program and abstracts of the 36th Interscience Conference on Antimicrobial Agents and Chemotherapy, New Orleans, September 15–18, 1996. Washington, D.C.: American Society for Microbiology, 1996:176. abstract.

32.
Averhoff F, Shapiro CN, Bell BP, et al. Control of hepatitis A through routine vaccination of children. JAMA 2001;286:2968-73.
33.
Werzberger A, Kuter B, Nalin D. Six years' follow-up after hepatitis A vaccination. N Engl J Med 1998;338:1160.
34.
Bialek SR, Thoroughman DA, Hu D, et al. Hepatitis A incidence and hepatitis A vaccination among American Indians and Alaska natives, 1990–2001. Am J Public Health 2004; 94:996-1001.
35.
Armstrong GL, Bell BP. Hepatitis A virus infections in the United States: model-based estimates and implications for childhood immunizations. Pediatrics 2002;109:839-45.
36.
Stokes J Jr, Neefe JR. The prevention and attenuation of infectious hepatitis by gamma globulin: preliminary note. JAMA 1945;127:144-5.
37.
Mosley JW, Reisler DM, Brachott D, Roth D, Weiser J. Comparison of two lots of immune serum globulin for prophylaxis of infectious hepatitis. Am J Epidemiol 1968;87:539-50.
38.
Wiedermann G, Kundi M, Ambrosch F. Estimated persistence of anti-HAV antibodies after single dose and booster hepatitis A vaccination (0-6 schedule). Acta Trop 1998;69:121-5.

39.
Werzberger A, Mensch B, Nalin DR, Kuter BJ. Effectiveness of hepatitis A vaccine in a former frequently affected community: 9 years' followup after the Monroe field trial of VAQTA. Vaccine 2002;20:1699-701.
40.
Van Damme P, Banatvala J, Fay O, et al. Hepatitis A booster vaccination: is there a need? Lancet 2003;362:1065-71.
41.
Van Herckk, Van Damme P. Inactivated hepatitis A vaccine-induced antibodies: follow-up and estimates of long-term persistence. J Med Virol 2001;63:1-7.
42.
Van Damme P, Thoelen S, Cramm M, De Groote K, Safary A, Meheus A. Inactivated hepatitis A vaccine: reactogenicity, immunogenicity, and long-term antibody persistence. J Med Virol 1994;44:446-51.
43.
Sagliocca L, Amoroso P, Stroffolini T, et al. Efficacy of hepatitis A vaccine in prevention of secondary hepatitis A infection: a randomised trial. Lancet 1999;353:1136-9. [Erratum, Lancet 1999;353:2078.]
44.
Vento S. Fulminant hepatitis associated with hepatitis A virus superinfection in patients with chronic hepatitis C. J Viral Hepat 2000;7:Suppl 1:7-8.

45.
Battegay M, Naef M, Bucher HC. Hepatitis associated with hepatitis A superinfection in patients with chronic hepatitis C. N Engl J Med 1998;338:1771-2.
46.
Jacobs RJ, Koff RS, Meyerhoff AS. The cost-effectiveness of vaccinating chronic hepatitis C patients against hepatitis A. Am J Gastroenterol 2002;97:427-34.
47.
Arguedas MR, Heudebert GR, Fallon MB, Stinnett AA. The cost-effectiveness of hepatitis A vaccination in patients with chronic hepatitis C viral infection in the United States. Am J Gastroenterol 2002;97:721-8.
48.
Connor BA, Van Herck K, Van Damme P. Rapid protection and vaccination against hepatitis A for travellers. Biodrugs 2003;17:Suppl 1:19-21.
49.
Koff RS. The case for routine childhood vaccination against hepatitis A. N Engl J Med 1999;340:644-5.
50.
Jacobs RJ, Greenberg DP, Koff RS, Saab S, Meyerhoff AS. Regional variation in the cost effectiveness of childhood hepatitis A immunization. Pediatr Infect Dis J 2003;22:904-14.

Cellulitis

MORTON N. SWARTZ, M.D.

An otherwise healthy 40-year-old man felt feverish and noted pain and redness over the dorsum of his foot. Tender edema and erythema extended up the pretibial area. Fissures were present between the toes. What diagnostic procedures and treatment are indicated?

THE CLINICAL PROBLEM

Cellulitis is an acute, spreading pyogenic inflammation of the dermis and subcutaneous tissue, usually complicating a wound, ulcer, or dermatosis. The area, usually on the leg, is tender, warm, erythematous, and swollen. It lacks sharp demarcation from uninvolved skin. Erysipelas is a superficial cellulitis with prominent lymphatic involvement, presenting with an indurated, "peau d'orange" appearance with a raised border that is demarcated from normal skin. The distinctive features, including the anatomical location of cellulitis and the patient's medical and exposure history, should guide appropriate antibiotic therapy (Table 1).

Anatomical Features

Periorbital cellulitis involves the eyelid and periocular tissues anterior to the orbital septum. Periorbital cellulitis should be distinguished from orbital cellulitis because of the potential complications of the latter: decreased ocular motility, decreased visual acuity, and cavernous-sinus thrombosis.

Before young children began to be immunized with conjugated *Haemophilus influenzae* type b vaccine, buccal cellulitis due to *H. influenzae* type b was responsible for up to 25 percent of cases of facial cellulitis in children 3 to 24 months of age; now such cellulitis is rare. Infection originates in the upper respiratory tract.

Perianal cellulitis occurs mainly in young children and is generally caused by group A streptococci.[1] Manifestations include perianal pruritus and erythema, anal fissures, purulent secretions, and rectal bleeding.

Types of Exposure That Predispose Patients to Cellulitis

Severe bacterial cellulitis has been known to occur as a complication of liposuction. The subcutaneous injection of illicit drugs ("skin popping") can result in cellulitis due to unusual bacterial species.[2,3]

A distinctive form of cellulitis, sometimes recurrent, may occur weeks to months after breast surgery for cancer. Cellulitis in the ipsilateral arm has been well described after radical mastectomy,[4] where it occurs because of associated lymphedema; cellulitis in the ipsilateral breast is more common now, occurring after breast-conservation therapy.[5,6] Local lymphedema from the combination of partial mastectomy, axillary lymph-node dissection, and breast irradiation is a predisposing factor.

Cellulitis also occurs in the legs of patients whose saphenous veins have been harvested for coronary-artery bypass.[7] Lymphatic disruption and edema occur on the removal of the vein.

Unusual Manifestations of Cellulitis

Crepitant cellulitis is produced by either clostridia or non–spore-forming anaerobes (bacteroides species, peptostreptococci, and peptococci) — either alone or mixed with facultative bacteria, particularly *Escherichia coli*, klebsiella, and aeromonas.

Table 1. Specific Anatomical Variants of Cellulitis and Causes of Predisposition to the Condition.

Anatomical Variant or Cause of Predisposition	Location	Likely Bacterial Cause
Periorbital cellulitis	Periorbital	*Staphylococcus aureus*, pneumococcus, group A streptococcus
Buccal cellulitis	Cheek	*Haemophilus influenzae*
Cellulitis complicating body piercing	Ear, nose, umbilicus	*S. aureus*, group A streptococcus
Mastectomy (with axillary-node dissection) for breast cancer	Ipsilateral arm	Non–group A hemolytic streptococcus
Lumpectomy (with limited axillary-node dissection, breast radiotherapy)	Ipsilateral breast	Non–group A hemolytic streptococcus
Harvest of saphenous vein for coronary-artery bypass	Ipsilateral leg	Group A or non–group A hemolytic streptococcus
Liposuction	Thigh, abdominal wall	Group A streptococcus, peptostreptococcus
Postoperative (very early) wound infection	Abdomen, chest, hip	Group A streptococcus
Injection-drug use ("skin popping")	Extremities, neck	*S. aureus*; streptococci (groups A, C, F, G)*
Perianal cellulitis	Perineum	Group A streptococcus
Crepitant cellulitis	Trunk, extremities	See text
Gangrenous cellulitis	Trunk, extremities	See text
Erythema migrans (bright red, circular lesion at initial sites; secondary annular lesions may develop elsewhere several days later because of hematogenous spread)	Extremities, trunk	*Borrelia burgdorferi* (agent of Lyme disease)

* Other bacteria to consider on the basis of isolation from skin or abscesses in this setting include *Enterococcus faecalis*, viridans-group streptococci, coagulase-negative staphylococci, anaerobes (including bacteroides and clostridium species), and Enterobacteriaceae.

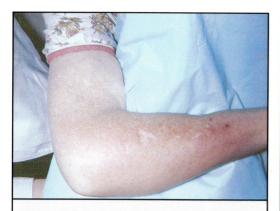

Figure 1. Cellulitis Due to *Pasteurella multocida* after a Cat Bite.

Bite marks are evident, as are adjacent swelling and edema.

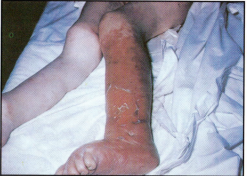

Figure 2. Cellulitis Due to Group A Beta-Hemolytic Streptococci in Leg (Previously Mildly Edematous) of a Patient with Paraplegia.

Some of the superficial skin is eroded. The initiating event was an abrasion on the lower leg.

Gangrenous cellulitis produces necrosis of the subcutaneous tissues and overlying skin. Skin necrosis may complicate conventional cellulitis or may occur with distinctive clinical features (including necrotizing cutaneous mucormycosis in immunocompromised patients).

Initiating Sources of Infection

Identifying the source of cellulitis — whether it is cutaneous, subjacent, or bacteremic — can provide clues as to the causative microorganism and the identity of a process that requires additional intervention. Most commonly, the source is skin trauma or an underlying lesion (an ulcer or fissured toe webs, for example). Animal or human bites can cause cellulitis due to the skin flora of the recipient of the bite or the oral flora of the biter (Figure 1). Specific pathogens are suggested when infection follows exposure to seawater (*Vibrio vulnificus*), fresh water (*Aeromonas hydrophila*), or aquacultured fish (*Streptococcus iniae*).

Edema predisposes patients to cellulitis (Figure 2). Some lymphedema persists after recovery from cellulitis or erysipelas and predisposes patients to recurrences,[8] which may be of longer duration than the initial inflammation.[9]

Occasionally, cellulitis may be caused by the spread of subjacent osteomyelitis. Rarely, infection may emerge as apparent cellulitis, sometimes distant from the initial site. Crepitant cellulitis on the left thigh, for instance, might be a manifestation of a colonic diverticular abscess.

Cellulitis infrequently occurs as a result of bacteremia. Uncommonly, pneumococcal cellulitis occurs on the face or limbs in patients with diabetes mellitus, alcohol abuse, systemic lupus erythematosus, the nephrotic syndrome, or a hematologic cancer.[10] Meningococcal cellulitis occurs rarely, although it can affect both children (periorbital cellulitis) and adults (cellulitis on an extremity).[11] Bacteremic cellulitis due to *V. vulnificus* with prominent hemorrhagic bullae may follow the ingestion of raw oysters by patients with cirrhosis, hemochromatosis, or thalassemia.[12,13] Cellulitis caused by other gram-negative organisms (e.g., *E. coli*) usually occurs through a cutaneous source in an immunocompromised patient but can also develop through bacteremia[14]; it sometimes follows

Table 2. Important Processes to Be Distinguished from Cellulitis.

Process	Clinical Clues to Diagnosis
Infectious	
Necrotizing fasciitis	
Type I (mixed infection of anaerobes plus facultative species such as streptococci or Enterobacteriaceae)	Acute, rapidly developing infection of deep fascia; marked pain, tenderness, swelling, and often crepitus; bullae and necrosis of underlying skin
Type II (infection with group A streptococci)	Acute infection, often accompanied by toxic shock syndrome; rapid progression of marked edema to violaceous bullae and necrosis of subcutaneous tissue; absence of crepitus
Anaerobic myonecrosis (gas gangrene, due to *Clostridium perfringens*)	Rapidly progressive toxemic infection of previously injured muscle, producing marked edema, crepitus, and brown bullae (showing large, gram-positive bacilli with scant polymorphonuclear cells); on radiography, extensive gaseous dissection of muscle and fascial planes; bacteremic spread of *C. septicum* from occult colonic cancer can produce myonecrosis without penetrating trauma
Cutaneous anthrax	Gelatinous edema surrounding eschar of anthrax lesion may be mistaken for cellulitis; anthrax lesion is painless or pruritic; epidemiologic factors are of paramount importance
Vaccinia vaccination	Erythema and induration around vaccination site reaches peak at 10–12 days (more slowly than cellulitis); little toxicity; represents cellular response to vaccinia
Inflammatory and neoplastic	
Insect bite (hypersensitivity response)	History of insect bite, local pruritus; absence of fever, toxicity, or leukocytosis
Acute gout	Involvement of foot (podagra); joint pain; repeated attacks; increase in serum uric acid level
Deep venous thrombophlebitis	Involvement of leg; sentinel venous cord and linear extent
Familial Mediterranean fever–associated cellulitis-like erythema[18]	Occurs in Sephardic Jews and persons from the Middle East who have had previous episodes of recurrent fevers with or without episodes of acute abdominal pain
Fixed drug reaction	Skin erythema does not spread as rapidly as cellulitis; fever low, if present; history of medication use
Pyoderma gangrenosa (particularly lesions starting in subcutaneous fat as acute panniculitis)	Lesions become nodular or bullous and ulcerate; occurs particularly in patients with inflammatory bowel disease or collagen vascular syndromes
Sweet's syndrome (acute febrile neutrophilic dermatosis)[19]	Acute, tender erythematous pseudovesiculated plaques, fever, and neutrophilic leukocytosis; often associated with cancer (commonly hematologic); on face, may resemble erysipelas or periorbital cellulitis; corticosteroid-responsive
Kawasaki's disease[20]	Fever, conjunctivitis, acute cervical lymphadenopathy, oropharyngeal erythema; dermatitis of palms and soles; facial appearance may suggest periorbital cellulitis; occurs mainly in infancy and childhood
Wells' syndrome	Urticaria-like lesions with central clearing; lesions progress slowly and persist for weeks or months; histologically, infiltration with eosinophils; peripheral eosinophilia
Carcinoma erysipeloides[21,22]	A form of metastatic carcinoma with lymphatic involvement; occurs most often on anterior chest wall with cancer of the breast but may also occur at sites of distant metastases; absence of fever; slower progression than cellulitis

Pseudomonas aeruginosa bacteremia in patients with neutropenia. In immunocompromised persons, less common opportunistic pathogens (e.g., *Helicobacter cinaedi* in patients with human immunodeficiency virus infection; *Cryptococcus neoformans*; and fusarium, proteus, and pseudomonas species) have also been associated with bloodborne cellulitis.[15-17]

Differential Diagnosis

The differential diagnosis of cellulitis is summarized in Table 2. Soft-tissue infections that resemble cellulitis must be distinguished from it, since the management of necrotizing fasciitis or gas gangrene requires extensive débridement. The diagnosis of necrotizing fasciitis can be established definitively only by direct examination on surgery or by biopsy with frozen section.[23,24]

STRATEGIES AND EVIDENCE

Diagnostic Studies

Cultures of Aspirates and Lesions   The diagnosis of cellulitis is generally based on the morphologic features of the lesion and the clinical setting. Culture of needle aspirates is not indicated in routine care. However, data from five series using needle aspiration have elucidated common pathogens. Among 284 patients, a likely pathogen was identified in 29 percent.[25-30] Of 86 isolates, only 3 represented mixed cultures. Gram-positive microorganisms (mainly *Staphylococcus aureus*, group A or B streptococci, viridans streptococci, and *Enterococcus faecalis*) accounted for 79 percent of cases; the remainder were caused by gram-negative bacilli (Enterobacteriaceae, *H. influenzae*, *Pasteurella multocida*, *P. aeruginosa*, and acinetobacter species). A small study in children demonstrated higher yields when needle aspirates were obtained from the point of maximal inflammation than when they were obtained from the leading edge.[30]

In two small studies, the yield of punch biopsies was slightly better than that of needle aspirates,[27,29] and the biopsies revealed the presence of gram-positive bacteria in all but one case (*S. aureus* alone in 50 percent of cases, and either group A streptococi alone or *S. aureus* with other gram-positive organisms in most of the remainder). Cultures of ulcers and abrasions in areas contiguous to those with cellulitis have similarly revealed the presence of *S. aureus*, group A streptococci, or both in the majority of cases.[28] These data indicate that antimicrobial therapy for cellulitis in immunocompetent hosts should be focused primarily on gram-positive cocci.

Broader coverage is warranted in patients with diabetes. Among 96 leg-threatening foot infections (including cellulitis) in patients with diabetes, the main potential pathogens recovered from deep wounds or débrided tissue were gram-positive aerobes including S. aureus, enterococci, and streptococci (in 56 percent of cases); gram-negative aerobes including proteus, E. coli, klebsiella, enterobacter, acinetobacter, and P. aeruginosa (in 22 percent); and anaerobes including bacteroides and peptococcus (in 22 percent).[31] This broad range of microorganisms should also be considered as potential pathogens in cellulitis that occurs as a complication of decubitus ulcers.

Blood Cultures   Bacteremia is uncommon in cellulitis: among 272 patients, initial blood cultures were positive in 4 percent.[25,26,28-30] Two thirds of the isolates were either group A streptococci or S. aureus, and the remainder were either H. influenzae or P. multocida. A retrospective study of blood cultures in 553 patients with community-acquired celluli-

Table 3. Initial Treatment for Cellulitis at Specific Sites or with Particular Exposures.

Variable	Bacterial Species to Consider*	Standard Antimicrobial Therapy†	Alternative Antimicrobial Agents
Buccal cellulitis	H. influenzae	Ceftriaxone (1–2 g/day intravenously)	Meropenem or imipenem–cilastatin
Limb-threatening diabetic foot ulcer	Aerobic gram-negative bacilli (Enterobacteriaceae, P. aeruginosa, acinetobacter); anaerobes (bacteroides, peptococcus)	Ampicillin–sulbactam (3 g intravenously every 6 hr)	Meropenem or imipenem–cilastatin; clindamycin plus a broad-spectrum fluoroquinolone (ciprofloxacin or levofloxacin); metronidazole plus a fluoroquinolone or ceftriaxone
Human bites	Oral anaerobes (bacteroides species, peptostreptococci); Eikenella corrodens; viridans streptococci; S. aureus	Amoxicillin–clavulanate (500 mg orally every 8 hr)	Penicillin plus a cephalosporin
Dog and cat bites	P. multocida and other pasteurella species; S. aureus, S. intermedius, Neisseria canis, Haemophilus felix, Capnocytophaga canimorsus; anaerobes	Amoxicillin–clavulanate (500 mg orally every 8 hr)	Moxifloxacin plus clindamycin
Exposure to salt water at site of abrasion or laceration	Vibrio vulnificus	Doxycycline (200 mg intravenously initially, followed by 100–200 mg intravenously per day in 2 divided doses)‡	Cefotaxime; ciprofloxacin
Exposure to fresh water at site of abrasion or laceration or after the therapeutic use of leeches	Aeromonas species	Ciprofloxacin (400 mg intravenously every 12 hr) or ceftazidime plus gentamicin‡	Meropenem or imipenem–cilastatin
Working as a butcher, fish or clam handler, veterinarian	Erysipelothrix rhusiopathiae	Amoxicillin (500 mg orally every 8 hr) for mild skin infections; penicillin G (12 million–20 million units intravenously daily) for bacteremic infections or endocarditis	Ciprofloxacin or cefotaxime or imipenem–cilastatin

* These bacterial species should be considered in addition to the common pathogens.
† Doses given are for adults with normal renal function; the duration of treatment should be 7 to 15 days or longer, depending on the clinical response.
‡ Treatment is to be given along with antimicrobial agents targeted to the common pathogens.

tis found a relevant isolate, mainly group A or group G streptococci (but also *S. aureus* and *V. vulnificus*), in only 2 percent,[32] indicating that blood cultures were not likely to be cost effective for most patients with cellulitis.

In contrast, blood cultures are indicated in patients who have cellulitis superimposed on lymphedema. In a study involving 10 such patients, 3 had positive blood cultures (all non–group A streptococci).[9] This high prevalence of bacteremia may be attributable to the preexisting lymphedema and the infecting bacterial species. Blood cultures are also warranted in patients with buccal or periorbital cellulitis, in patients in whom a salt-water or fresh-water source of infection is likely (Table 3), and in patients with chills and high fever, which suggest bacteremia.

Radiology   Radiologic examination is unnecessary in most cases of cellulitis. Plain-film radiography and computed tomography (CT) are of value, however, when the clinical setting suggests a subjacent osteomyelitis. When it is difficult to differentiate cellulitis from necrotizing fasciitis, magnetic resonance imaging (MRI) may be helpful, although surgical exploration for a definitive diagnosis should not be delayed when the latter condition is suspected.[24] In a study involving 17 patients with suspected necrotizing fasciitis, 11 cases were ultimately confirmed to be necrotizing fasciitis (at surgery or, in 1 case, on autopsy), and 6 were confirmed to be cellulitis on the basis of the clinical course[33]; on MRI, all 11 cases of necrotizing fasciitis were identified (100 percent sensitivity), but 1 of the 6 cases of cellulitis was misdiagnosed (for a specificity of 86 percent). The criteria for identifying necrotizing fasciitis on MRI include the involvement of deep fasciae, as evidenced by fluid collection, thickening, and enhancement with contrast material.

Ultrasonography and CT are of less value in distinguishing necrotizing fasciitis from cellulitis, but ultrasonography can be helpful in detecting the subcutaneous accumulation of pus as a complication of cellulitis and can aid in guiding aspiration.[34] Gallium-67 scintillography may aid in the detection of cellulitis superimposed on recently increasing, chronic lymphedema of a limb.[35]

Antimicrobial Treatment

Because most cases of cellulitis are caused by streptococci and *S. aureus*, beta-lactam antibiotics with activity against penicillinase-producing *S. aureus* are the usual drugs of choice. Initial treatment should be given by the intravenous route in the hospital if the lesion is spreading rapidly, if the systemic response is prominent (e.g., chills and a fever, with temperatures of 100.5°F [37.8°C] or higher), or if there are clinically significant coexisting conditions (such as immunocompromise, neutropenia, asplenia, preexisting edema, cirrhosis, cardiac failure, or renal insufficiency) (Table 4). Specially tailored treatment for other bacterial causes is warranted when cellulitis occurs after an unusual exposure (a human or animal bite or exposure to salt or fresh water), in patients with certain underlying conditions (neutropenia, splenectomy, or immunocompromise), or in the presence of bullae (Table 3). Diabetic foot infections involve multiple potential pathogens, and broad antimicrobial coverage is required.[31] Ampicillin–sulbactam and imipenem–cilastatin were shown in a randomized, double-blind trial to have similar cure rates in this setting (81 percent vs. 85 percent), but the former combination was more cost effective.[38]

Several trials have evaluated newer antibiotics. In a multicenter, double-blind trial involving 461 patients, oral ciprofloxacin (750 mg every 12 hours) was as safe and effective as parenteral cefotaxime (overall failure rate, 2 percent vs. 8 percent; P=0.008) in the treatment of various skin and skin-structure infections.[39] The evaluation of these results must be tempered by the facts that most of the skin infections studied were infected ulcers

Table 4. Antimicrobial Treatment for a Usual Case of Cellulitis.*	
Initial Treatment	**Subsequent Treatment**
Cefazolin, 1.0 g intravenously every 6–8 hr	Dicloxacillin, 0.5 g orally every 6 hr or Cephradine, 0.5 g orally every 6 hr or Cephalexin, 0.5 g orally every 6 hr or Cefadroxil, 0.5–1.0 g orally every 12–24 hr
or	
Nafcillin, 1.0 or 1.5 g intravenously every 4–6 hr	Same as above
or	
Ceftriaxone, 1.0 g intravenously every 24 hr†	Same as above
or	
Cefazolin, 2.0 g intravenously once daily, plus probenecid (1.0 g orally once daily)‡	Same as above
If methicillin-resistant *S. aureus* is suspected or patient is highly allergic to penicillin	
Vancomycin, 1.0–2.0 g intravenously daily	Linezolid, 0.6 g orally every 12 hr
or	
Linezolid, 0.6 g intravenously every 12 hr	Same as above

* Doses given are for adults; patients should be switched to oral therapy when they are afebrile and skin findings begin to resolve (after approximately three to five days). The total duration of treatment should be 7 to 14 days or longer, depending on the rate of response. Treatment should last longer in cases with associated abscesses, tissue necrosis, or underlying skin process (e.g., infected ulcer).

† Ceftriaxone has the advantage of allowing early discharge home with intravenous doses of 1.0 g daily.[36]

‡ Cefazolin–probenecid is given as a substitute for a once-daily parenteral third-generation cephalosporin. It has been shown to be similar in efficacy to ceftriaxone (1.0 g intravenously once daily) in home-based therapy for moderate-to-severe cellulitis in adults.[37]

and abscesses rather than cellulitis and that, since the time of the study, the fluoroquinolone resistance of *S. aureus*, the predominant pathogen isolated, has increased. More recently, oral moxifloxacin (400 mg once daily) has been shown to be as effective (84 percent) as oral cephalexin (500 mg three times a day) in the treatment of uncomplicated skin and soft-tissue infections.[40]

In a randomized, open-label trial of treatment of "complicated" skin and skin-structure infections in which high-dose levofloxacin (750 mg intravenously once daily) was compared with ticarcillin–clavulanate (3.1 g intravenously every four to six hours), therapeutic equivalence was demonstrated (success rates of 84 percent and 80 percent, respectively).[41] However, cellulitis (as a complication of preexisting skin lesions, immunosuppression, or vascular insufficiency) accounted for only 7 percent of the 399 skin infections. Linezolid (600 mg intravenously every 12 hours) has been compared with oxacillin (2 g intravenously every 6 hours) in a randomized, double-blind trial of treatment of complicated skin and soft-tissue infections in 819 hospitalized adults,[42] 44 percent of whom had cellulitis. The cure rates were 89 percent for linezolid and 86 percent for oxacillin. Clinically relevant pathogens isolated from contiguous sites included *S. aureus* (in 35 percent), group A streptococci (in 11 percent), and group B streptococci (in 27 percent), but infections due to methicillin-resistant *S. aureus* were excluded. A trial comparing linezolid and vancomycin in the treatment of adults with methicillin-resistant *S. aureus* infections, including 175 skin and soft-tissue infections,[43] found similar cure rates (79 percent with linezolid and 73 percent with vancomycin), but cellulitis accounted for only 13 percent of these infections.

Ancillary Measures

The local care of cellulitis involves the elevation and immobilization of the involved limb to reduce swelling and cool sterile saline dressings to remove purulence from any open lesion. Interdigital dermatophytic infections should be treated with a topical antifungal agent until they have been cleared. Such lesions may provide ingress for infecting bacteria. Several classes of topical antifungal agents are effective in clearing up fungal infection when applied one to two times daily; these include imidazoles (clotrimazole and miconazole), allylamines (terbinafine), and substituted pyridones (ciclopirox olamine).[44] Observational data suggest that after the successful treatment of such dermatophytic infections, the subsequent prompt use of topical antifungal agents at the earliest evidence of recurrence (or prophylactic application once or twice per week) will reduce the risk of recurrences of cellulitis.

Patients with peripheral edema are predisposed to recurrent cellulitis. Support stockings, good skin hygiene, and prompt treatment of tinea pedis can prevent recurrences.

In patients who, despite these measures, continue to have frequent episodes of cellulitis or erysipelas, the prophylactic use of penicillin G (250 to 500 mg orally twice daily) may prevent additional episodes; if the patient is allergic to penicillin, erythromycin (250 mg orally once or twice daily) may be used.

AREAS OF UNCERTAINTY

A variety of antimicrobial agents have been used to treat cellulitis because of their spectrum of action against likely causative organisms and have been approved by the Food and Drug Administration for use in skin and soft-tissue infections. However, such approval is often based on clinical studies of heterogeneous collections of cutaneous infections (including infected ulcers, abscesses, and wound infections); in some studies, cellulitis accounts for a minority of the infections.[39,43]

Most studies of cellulitis have involved patients with serious infections. Studies are needed to determine specific criteria that define the types of mild cases that are highly likely to respond to oral antibiotics administered at home. Penicillinase-resistant penicillins and cephalosporins have been used because most community-acquired pathogens causing cellulitis (streptococci and *S. aureus*) are susceptible to methicillin. However, the rate of community-acquired methicillin-resistant *S. aureus* infections in patients without identified risk factors appears to be increasing. In a rural Native American community, 55 percent of 112 isolates of *S. aureus* were methicillin-resistant, and 74 percent of these cases were community-acquired; the risk factors did not differ from those in patients with community-acquired methicillin-susceptible strains.[45] It remains uncertain how this change in resistance patterns will affect the management of cellulitis.[46]

Although there is a rationale for the empirical prophylactic use of penicillin to prevent recurrences of cellulitis in patients with multiple previous episodes, the results of efficacy studies have been conflicting. In a study of prophylaxis with monthly intramuscular doses of penicillin G benzathine (1.2 million units) after treatment for an acute episode of streptococcal cellulitis in the lower leg, such prophylaxis reduced the rate of recurrence from 17 percent to 0 (0 of 11) among patients who did not have predisposing factors, but it failed to prevent recurrence in those who had such predisposing factors as lymphedema (4 of 20 cases).[47] Whether it would be more effective to shorten the interval between doses to two or three weeks or to increase the dose is not known. Long-term erythromycin therapy (250 mg orally twice daily for 18 months) has been used to prevent recurrences in patients with a history of two or more episodes of cellulitis or erysipelas.[48] Episodes did not occur in 16 treated patients, whereas 8 of 16 controls had one or more recurrences.

GUIDELINES

Guidelines for the treatment of skin and soft-tissue infections (including cellulitis) are being prepared by the Infectious Diseases Society of America.

SUMMARY AND RECOMMENDATIONS

Cellulitis is a clinical diagnosis based on the spreading involvement of skin and subcutaneous tissues with erythema, swelling, and local tenderness, accompanied by fever and malaise. The approach to therapy involves the identification of the likely source as either local (secondary to abrasion or ulcer or due to another exposure, such as an animal bite or seawater, which implicates particular bacterial species — *P. multocida* and *V. vulnificus*, respectively) or an uncommon bacteremic spread of infection. Distinctive features of the patient (such as the presence of diabetes or immunocompromise) or anatomical sites should also be considered in treatment decisions. Streptococci (groups A, G, and B) and *S. aureus* are the most frequently isolated bacterial species.

Initial empirical antimicrobial treatment for moderate or severe cellulitis in a patient such as the one described in the vignette would thus consist of an intravenous cephalosporin (cefazolin or ceftriaxone) or nafcillin (vancomycin in patients with an allergy to penicillin), followed by dicloxacillin or an oral cephalosporin, generally for a course of 7 to 14 days. In patients with recurrent cellulitis of the leg, any fissures in the interdigital spaces caused by epidermophytosis should be treated with topical antifungal agents in order to prevent recurrences. Daily prophylaxis with oral penicillin G (or amoxicillin) should be considered for patients who have had more than two episodes of cellulitis at the same site.

This article first appeared in the February 26, 2004, issue of the New England Journal of Medicine.

REFERENCES

1.
Barzilai A, Choen HA. Isolation of group A streptococci from children with perianal cellulitis and from their siblings. Pediatr Infect Dis J 1998;17:358-60.

2.
Binswanger IA, Kral AH, Blumenthal RN, Rybold DJ, Edlin BR. High prevalence of abscesses and cellulitis among community-recruited injection drug users in San Francisco. Clin Infect Dis 2000;30:579-81.

3.
Dancer SJ, McNair D, Finn P, Kolsto AB. Bacillus cereus cellulitis from contaminated heroin. J Med Microbiol 2002;51:278-81.

4.
Simon MS, Cody RL. Cellulitis after axillary lymph node dissection for carcinoma of the breast. Am J Med 1992;93:543-8.

5.
Mertz KR, Baddour LM, Bell JL, Gwin JL. Breast cellulitis following breast conservation therapy: a novel complication of medical progress. Clin Infect Dis 1998;26:481-6.

6.
Miller SR, Mondry T, Reed JS, Findley A, Johnstone PA. Delayed cellulitis associated with conservative therapy for breast cancer. J Surg Oncol 1998;67:242-5.

7.
Baddour LM, Bisno AL. Non-group A beta-hemolytic streptococcal cellulitis: association with venous and lymphatic compromise. Am J Med 1985;79:155-9.

8.
Dupuy A, Benchikhi H, Roujeau JC, et al. Risk factors for erysipelas of the leg (cellulitis): case-control study. BMJ 1999;318:1591-4.

9.
Woo PCY, Lum PNL, Wong SSY, Cheng VC, Yuen KY. Cellulitis complicating lymphoedema. Eur J Clin Microbiol Infect Dis 2000;19:294-7.

10.
Parada JP, Maslow JN. Clinical syndromes associated with adult pneumococcal cellulitis. Scand J Infect Dis 2000;32:133-6.

11.
Porras MC, Martínez VC, Ruiz IM, et al. Acute cellulitis: an unusual manifestation of meningococcal disease. Scand J Infect Dis 2001;33:56-9.

12.
Chuang Y-C, Yuan C-Y, Liu C-Y, Lan CK, Huang AH. Vibrio vulnificus infection in Taiwan: report of 28 cases and review of clinical manifestations and treatment. Clin Infect Dis 1992;15:271-6.

13.
Fernandez JM, Serrano M, De Arriba JJ, Sanchez MV, Escribano E, Ferreras P. Bacteremic cellulitis caused by non-01, non-0139 Vibrio cholerae: report of a case in a patient with hemochromatosis. Diagn Microbiol Infect Dis 2000;37:77-80.

14.
Gach JE, Charles-Holmes R, Ghose A. E. coli cellulitis. Clin Exp Dermatol 2002;27:523-5.

15.
Kiehlbauch JA, Tauxe RV, Baker CN, Wachsmuth IK. Helicobacter cinaedi-associated bacteremia and cellulitis in immunocompromised patients. Ann Intern Med 1994;121:90-3.

16.
Horrevorts AM, Huysmans FTM, Koopman RJJ, Meis JFG. Cellulitis as first clinical presentation of disseminated cryptococcosis in renal transplant recipients. Scand J Infect Dis 1994;26:623-6.

17.
Nucci M, Anaissie E. Cutaneous infection by Fusarium species in healthy and immunocompromised hosts: implications for diagnosis and management. Clin Infect Dis 2002;35:909-20.

18.
Majeed HA, Quabazard Z, Hijazi Z, Farwana S, Harshani F. The cutaneous manifestations in children with familial Mediterranean fever (recurrent hereditary polyserositis): a six-year study. Q J Med 1990;75:607-16.

19.
Morgan KW, Callen JP. Sweet's syndrome in acute myelogenous leukemia presenting as periorbital cellulitis with an infiltrate of leukemic cells. J Am Acad Dermatol 2001;45:590-5.

20.
Sheard RM, Pandey KR, Barnes ND, Vivian AJ. Kawasaki disease presenting as orbital cellulitis. J Pediatr Ophthalmol Strabismus 2000;37:123-5.

21.
Taylor GW, Meltzer A. "Inflammatory carcinoma" of the breast. Am J Cancer 1938;33:33-49.

22.
Faber J, Shroeder L, Thill M-P, Jacob F. Carcinoma erysipeloides of the neck. Lancet 2002;359:1025.

23.
Stevens DL, Tanner MH, Winship J, et al. Severe group A streptococcal infections associated with a toxic shock–like syndrome and scarlet fever toxin A. N Engl J Med 1989;321:1-7.

24.
Stamenkovic I, Lew PD. Early recognition of potentially fatal necrotizing fasciitis: the use of frozen-section biopsy. N Engl J Med 1984;310:1689-93.

25.
Kielhofner MA, Brown B, Dall L. Influence of underlying disease process on the utility of cellulitis needle aspirates. Arch Intern Med 1988;148:2451-2.

26.
Sachs MK. The optimum use of needle aspiration in the bacteriologic diagnosis of cellulitis in adults. Arch Intern Med 1990;150:1907-12. [Erratum, Arch Intern Med 1991;151:244.]

27.
Duvanel T, Auckenthaler R, Rohner P, Harms M, Saurat JH. Quantitative cultures of biopsy specimens from cutaneous cellulitis. Arch Intern Med 1989;149:293-6.

28.
Sigurdsson AF, Gudmundsson S. The etiology of bacterial cellulitis as determined by fine-needle aspiration. Scand J Infect Dis 1989;21:537-42.

29.
Hook EW III, Hooton TM, Horton CA, Coyle MB, Ramsey PG, Turck M. Microbiologic evaluation of cutaneous cellulitis in adults. Arch Intern Med 1986;146:295-7.

30.
Howe PM, Eduardo Fajardo J, Orcutt MA. Etiologic diagnosis of cellulitis: comparison of aspirates obtained from the leading edge and the point of maximal inflammation. Pediatr Infect Dis J 1987;6:685-6.

31.
Grayson ML, Gibbons GW, Habershaw GW, et al. Use of ampicillin/sulbactam versus imipenem/cilastatin in the treatment of limb-threatening foot infections in diabetic patients. Clin Infect Dis 1994;18:683-93. [Erratum, Clin Infect Dis 1994;19:820.]

32.
Perl B, Gottehrer NP, Ravek D, Schlesinger Y, Rudensky B, Yinnon AM. Cost-effectiveness of blood cultures for adult patients with cellulitis. Clin Infect Dis 1999;29:1483-8.

33.
Schmid MR, Kossmann T, Duewell S. Differentiation of necrotizing fasciitis and cellulitis using MR imaging. AJR Am J Roentgenol 1998;170:615-20.

34.
Chao H-C, Lin S-J, Huang Y-C, Lin TY. Sonographic evaluation of cellulitis in children. J Ultrasound Med 2000;19:743-9.

35.
Suga K, Ariga M, Motoyama K, Hara A, Kume N, Matsunaga N. Ga-67-avid massive cellulitis within a chronic lymphedematous limb in a survivor of Hodgkin's disease. Clin Nucl Med 2001;26:791-2.

36.
Bradsher RW Jr, Snow RM. Ceftriaxone treatment of skin and soft tissue infections in a once daily regimen. Am J Med 1984;77:63-7.

37.
Grayson ML, McDonald M, Gibson K, et al. Once-daily intravenous cefazolin plus oral probenecid is equivalent to once-daily intravenous ceftriaxone plus oral placebo for the treatment of moderate-to-severe cellulitis in adults. Clin Infect Dis 2002;34:1440-8.

38.
McKinnon PS, Paladino JA, Grayson ML, Gibbons GW, Karchmer AW. Cost-effectiveness of ampicillin/sulbactam versus imipenem/cilastatin in the treatment of limb-threatening foot infections in diabetic patients. Clin Infect Dis 1997;24:57-63.

39.
Gentry LO, Ramirez-Ronda CH, Rodriguez-Noriega E, Thadepalli H, del Rosal PL, Ramirez C. Oral ciprofloxacin vs parenteral cefotaxime in the treatment of difficult skin and skin structure infections: a multicenter trial. Arch Intern Med 1989;149:2579-83.

40.
Muijsers RB, Jarvis B. Moxifloxacin in uncomplicated skin and skin structure infections. Drugs 2002;62:967-73.

41.
Graham DR, Talan DA, Nichols RL, et al. Once-daily, high-dose levofloxacin versus ticarcillin-clavulanate alone or followed by amoxicillin-clavulanate for complicated skin and skin-structure infections: a randomized, open-label trial. Clin Infect Dis 2002;35:381-9.

42.
Stevens DL, Smith LG, Bruss JB, et al. Randomized comparison of linezolid (PNU-100766) versus oxacillin-dicloxacillin for treatment of complicated skin and soft tissue infections. Antimicrob Agents Chemother 2000;44:3408-13.

43.
Stevens DL, Herr D, Lamperis H, Hunt JL, Batts DH, Hafkin B. Linezolid versus vancomycin for the treatment of methicillin-resistant Staphylococcus aureus infections. Clin Infect Dis 2002;34:1481-90.

44.
Liu V, Mackool BT. Current diagnosis and management of chronic fungal infection of the feet and nails. In: Remington JS, Swartz MN, eds. Current clinical topics in infectious diseases. Vol. 19. Malden, Mass.: Blackwell Science, 1999:305-26.

45.
Groom AV, Wolsey DH, Naimi TS, et al. Community-acquired methicillin-resistant Staphylococcus aureus in a rural American Indian community. JAMA 2001;286:1201-5.

46.
Eady EA, Cove JH. Staphylococcal resistance revisited: community-acquired methicillin resistant Staphylococcus aureus — an emerging problem for the management of skin and soft tissue infections. Curr Opin Infect Dis 2003;16:103-24.

47.
Wang J-H, Liu Y-C, Cheng DL, et al. Role of benzathine penicillin G in prophylaxis for recurrent streptococcal cellulitis of the lower legs. Clin Infect Dis 1997;25:685-9.

48.
Kremer M, Zuckerman R, Avraham Z, Raz R. Long-term antimicrobial therapy in the prevention of recurrent soft-tissue infections. J Infect 1991;22:37-40.

ADDENDUM

Since publication of this article, the role of community-acquired methicillin-resistant *Staphylococcus aureus* (CA-MRSA) in skin and soft tissue infections, noted in the section entitled "Areas of Uncertainty," has increased in prominence. Outbreaks of skin infections due to CA-MRSA have occurred among prison inmates, members of football teams, children in daycare centers, users of parenteral illicit drugs, and the homeless.[1-3] In addition, CA-MRSA has been recognized as a cause of necrotizing fasciitis in Los Angeles.[4] In surveillance in three areas (Baltimore, Atlanta, and 12 hospitals in Minnesota), 8 to 20 percent of all MRSA isolates from infections were CA-MRSA, and 77 percent of those were from skin and soft-tissue infections.[5] Antimicrobial susceptibilities of these isolates differed from those of hospital-associated methicillin-resistant *S. aureus* (HA-MRSA) that had been carried into the community; community-acquired isolates were more often susceptible to commonly used antimicrobials than HA-MRSA isolates: community-acquired isolates were susceptible to clindamycin (87 percent), rifampin (98 percent), trimethoprim–sulfamethoxazole (97 percent), tetracycline (88 percent), ciprofloxacin (65 percent), vancomycin (100 percent), and linezolid (96 percent).

Initial antimicrobial treatment for the usual case of community-acquired cellulitis typically remains a drug like cefazolin since the microbial etiology still is likely to be streptococcal or a methicillin-susceptible *S. aureus* strain. However, the presence of CA-MRSA in an associated skin lesion (infected ulcer, abscess) might furnish a rationale for use of an antimicrobial such as clindamycin or trimethoprim–sulfamethoxazole, provided the severity of the process does not warrant use of vancomycin or linezolid. If clindamycin is used, the *S. aureus* strain should be tested for inducible clindamycin resistance.

1. Kazakova SV, Hageman JC, Matava M, et al. A clone of methicillin-resistant *Staphylococcus aureus* among professional football players. N Engl J Med 2005;352:468-75.

2. Chambers HF. Community-associated MRSA: resistance and virulence converge. N Engl J Med 2005;352: 1485-7.

3. Rybak MJ, LaPlante KL. Community-associated methicillin-resistant Staphylococcus aureus: a review. Pharmacotherapy 2005;25:74-85.

4. Miller LG, Perdreau-Remington F, Rieg G, et al. Necrotizing fasciitis caused by community-associated methicillin-resistant *Staphylococcus aureus* in Los Angeles. N Engl J Med 2005;352:1445-53.

5. Fridkin SK, Hageman JC, Morrison M, et al. Methicillin-resistant *Staphylococcus aureus* disease in three communities. N Engl J Med 2005;352:1436-44.

Asymptomatic Primary Hyperparathyroidism

JOHN P. BILEZIKIAN, M.D., AND SHONNI J. SILVERBERG, M.D.

A 60-year-old woman is noted incidentally to have a calcium level of 10.8 mg per deciliter (2.70 mmol per liter; normal range, 8.4 to 10.2 mg per deciliter [2.10 to 2.55 mmol per liter]). The parathyroid hormone level, as measured on immunoradiometric assay, is 84 pg per milliliter (normal range, 10 to 65). She has never had a kidney stone or a fracture, and she feels well. Her urinary calcium excretion is normal. Her bone density is within 0.5 SD of the peak bone mass at the lumbar spine and the hip and is 1.0 SD below the peak bone mass at the forearm. How should her case be managed?

THE CLINICAL PROBLEM

For the first 40 years after its recognition as a clinical entity, primary hyperparathyroidism was a symptomatic disorder in which kidney stones and bone disease were common.[1,2] Management was straightforward, since parathyroidectomy was always indicated. The advent of a multichannel biochemical screening test in the early 1970s ushered in the era of asymptomatic primary hyperparathyroidism, and the incidence of this disorder increased by a factor of four to five.[3,4]

In patients with asymptomatic primary hyperparathyroidism, the serum calcium concentration is elevated, but usually only to within 1 mg per deciliter above the upper limit of normal (10.2 mg per deciliter). The parathyroid hormone level, measured by means of immunoradiometric assay, is usually 1.5 to 2.0 times the upper limit of normal (65 pg per milliliter), although it may be inappropriately "normal." Hypophosphatemia and hyperchloremia, which were common among patients with symptomatic disease, are uncommon among patients with asymptomatic disease. The 24-hour urinary calcium excretion tends to be near the upper limit of normal.

Although radiography almost never shows skeletal involvement, bone densitometry typically does. As measured on dual-energy x-ray absorptiometry, the greatest reduction in bone density is at the distal third of the radius, a site composed predominantly of cortical bone that is vulnerable to the catabolic actions of parathyroid hormone. The hip and the lumbar spine, sites where bone becomes progressively more cancellous, show smaller reductions.[5] This pattern of bone loss differs from the usual pattern of the early postmenopausal years, when cancellous bone of the lumbar spine is lost preferentially. But in estrogen-deficient postmenopausal women with primary hyperparathyroidism, bone density at the lumbar spine is generally well preserved, emphasizing a protective effect of parathyroid hormone against the loss of cancellous bone. Recent trials showing improved bone density at the lumbar spine in postmenopausal women with osteoporosis who were treated with intermittent low-dose parathyroid hormone have confirmed its anabolic potential.[6] However, occasionally, patients with primary hyperparathyroidism do have bone loss at the lumbar spine.[7-9]

Approximately 20 percent of patients are symptomatic, with kidney stones, overt bone disease, or proximal neuromuscular weakness.[10,11] Some patients do report weakness, easy fatigability, intellectual weariness, and even depression.[12,13] Since these symptoms are nonspecific and are hard to attribute to primary hyperparathyroidism in particular, they do not enter prominently into decisions regarding surgery, nor do they necessarily define patients as symptomatic. When the calcium level exceeds 12 mg per deciliter (3.0 mmol per liter), such nonspecific problems are more likely to be related to primary hyperparathyroidism.

A less common presentation of asymptomatic primary hyperparathyroidism is characterized by a normal serum calcium level but an elevated parathyroid hormone level. This condition is typically identified during an evaluation of skeletal health. The diagnosis is made when there is no apparent cause of secondary elevations of the parathyroid hormone level and the serum 25-hydroxyvitamin D level is not below the lower limit of the physiologically normal range (i.e., is above 20 ng per milliliter). This normocalcemic variant may represent the earliest manifestation of primary hyperparathyroidism.[14]

Although asymptomatic primary hyperparathyroidism commonly occurs in countries that use multichannel screening tests, symptomatic disease is common in other geographic areas, such as India, northeastern Brazil, and China, where access to multichannel screening is limited.[15] In addition, the high prevalence of vitamin D deficiency in these countries may fuel the processes associated with overactivity of the parathyroid glands, leading to more cases of symptomatic disease.

Diagnosis

Although there are clear advantages to measuring the concentration of ionized calcium rather than the total calcium concentration, most experts in the United States use the total serum calcium concentration, corrected for the patient's albumin concentration (by adding 0.8 mg per deciliter to the total serum calcium value for every 1 g per deciliter below a serum albumin concentration of 4 g per deciliter). The corrected total serum calcium concentration is used because of the technical challenges involved in the accurate measurement of ionized calcium. The diagnosis of primary hyperparathyroidism is made on the basis of the combination of an elevated total serum calcium concentration and an elevated or inappropriately normal parathyroid hormone level.[16]

There are many causes of hypercalcemia, but few are associated with elevated levels of parathyroid hormone, and thus the differential diagnosis of hypercalcemia does not usually present difficulties. A newly introduced immunoradiometric assay for parathyroid hormone detects only the intact, full-length 84-amino-acid molecule.[17] This more specific assay has the potential to be more clinically useful than the established immunoradiometric assay for parathyroid hormone, in which large fragments truncated at the N-terminal end are measured along with the full-length molecule.[18]

When the parathyroid hormone level is elevated in a patient with hypercalcemia, the differential diagnosis includes hyperparathyroidism due to thiazide diuretics or lithium, familial hypocalciuric hypercalcemia, and the tertiary hyperparathyroidism associated with end-stage renal disease. If the patient is taking a thiazide diuretic or lithium and it is considered to be safe to discontinue the use of the medication, then it should be withdrawn and the patient retested three months later. If the serum calcium concentration continues to be elevated, it can be concluded that the hypercalcemia is due to primary hyperparathyroidism. Familial hypocalciuric hypercalcemia is distinguished from primary hyperparathyroidism by a family history of mild hypercalcemia, a usual onset in young adulthood, and a ratio of urinary calcium to urinary creatinine of less than 0.01.[19] Humoral hypercalcemia of malignancy should not be a consideration when the parathyroid hormone level is high, because the hypercalcemic agent in this condition, parathyroid hormone–related protein, is not detected by the immunoradiometric assay for parathyroid hormone. If the parathyroid hormone level is high in a patient with humoral hypercalcemia of malignancy, he or she is more likely to have concomitant primary hyperparathyroidism and cancer than to have a cancer that has produced authentic parathyroid hormone (a situation that is reported rarely).

Natural History of Asymptomatic Primary Hyperparathyroidism without Surgery

Management decisions about asymptomatic primary hyperparathyroidism require knowledge of its natural history. Most patients who do not meet the criteria for surgery (listed below) do well, with no evidence of progressive disease.[20] In most patients who are followed without surgery, the average serum levels of calcium and parathyroid hormone do not change over a 10-year period. Average bone mass as measured by dual-energy x-ray absorptiometry is typically stable, and hypercalciuria does not worsen. The microarchitecture of cancellous bone appears to be maintained. However, approximately 25 percent of patients have evidence of progressive disease, including worsening hypercalcemia, hypercalciuria, and reductions in bone mass. Only age appears to be predictive of progression; younger patients (younger than 50 years of age) are approximately three times as likely to have worsening disease.[21] Therefore, despite the generally benign natural history of primary hyperparathyroidism, patients who are not candidates for surgery should be monitored.

Surgery is routinely warranted in patients with a history of nephrolithiasis. Over a 10-year follow-up period, all patients with such a history who did not undergo parathyroidectomy had progressive disease.

Outcomes after Parathyroid Surgery

Most adults with primary hyperparathyroidism (80 to 85 percent) have a single benign adenoma, whereas 15 to 20 percent have hyperplasia of all four parathyroid glands. Parathyroid cancer is exceedingly rare (found in less than 0.5 percent of patients with hyperparathyroidism).

Although the standard surgical approach is the exploration of all four parathyroid glands with the use of general anesthesia,[22] an alternative approach is to perform the same four-gland operation with the use of local anesthesia. Another strategy is a unilateral operation in which the other gland on the side that harbors the adenoma is ascertained to be normal. Since multiple parathyroid adenomas are unusual, the presence of one normal parathyroid gland is considered by some to be sufficient evidence of single-gland disease.

When performed by an expert parathyroid surgeon, these approaches are successful more than 90 percent of the time. However, since not all surgeons are experts and the parathyroid glands are notoriously variable in their location, preoperative localization has become popular in recent years.[23,24] Imaging with technetium-labeled sestamibi, with or without single-photon-emission computed tomography, is a preferred method, although there are other approaches to localization (ultrasonography, computed tomography, and magnetic resonance imaging). Most experts consider preoperative imaging to be mandatory for patients who have had previous neck surgery, but its use in patients without such a history remains controversial.

Preoperative parathyroid imaging is required for all patients who are to undergo minimally invasive parathyroidectomy, a procedure that is directed only at the site where the abnormal parathyroid gland has been visualized.[25] After the removal of the parathyroid gland that is presumed to be abnormal, a sample of peripheral blood is obtained intraoperatively for a rapid parathyroid hormone assay. If the level decreases by more than 50 percent after resection, the gland that has been removed is considered to be the sole source of overactive parathyroid tissue, and the operation is terminated. If the parathyroid hormone level does not decrease by more than 50 percent, the operation is extended to a more traditional one in a search for other overactive parathyroid tissue. There is controversy over the use of minimally invasive parathyroidectomy, since it may miss another overactive gland (a second adenoma or four-gland hyperplasia) whose activity is relatively suppressed when a larger, more dominant gland is present.[26,27]

Complications of parathyroidectomy include injury to the recurrent laryngeal nerve or hypoparathyroidism, both of which are very uncommon if the procedure is performed by an expert parathyroid surgeon. Symptomatic hypocalcemia may occur in the postoperative period in patients with more severe primary hyperparathyroidism (termed "hungry bone syndrome"), but it is rare in patients with mild disease.

After the removal of the parathyroid adenoma or multiple overactive glands, the serum and urinary calcium concentrations return to normal. The rate of recurrence of kidney stones has been reduced by more than 90 percent after parathyroid surgery in some series.[10] Over a period of three to four years, bone density improves, with the lumbar spine and hip regions typically showing increases of 12 to 14 percent without the need to resort to antiresorptive therapy.[20] In patients with vertebral osteopenia, increases in bone density at these sites can approach 20 percent.[7] The density of the distal third of the radius changes little, if at all. Although some reports have suggested that patients feel better in terms of a number of subjective variables after surgery,[13,28] more rigorous quantitative assessment of quality-of-life measures after surgery is still needed.

AREAS OF UNCERTAINTY

Long-Term Risks

The long-term risks associated with living with chronic hypercalcemia are unknown. In a population-based study from the United States, mild, asymptomatic primary hyperparathyroidism was not associated with increased overall mortality, although mortality was increased among patients in the highest quartile of serum calcium concentrations.[29] Whereas classic primary hyperparathyroidism has been linked to cardiovascular disorders (hypertension), gastrointestinal disorders (peptic ulcer disease), and metabolic disorders (diabetes mellitus), it is not clear whether these individual associations are causal.[13] Studies from Europe, however, indicate that patients with primary hyperparathyroidism may have increased cardiovascular risk, rates of lipid disorders, rates of glucose intolerance, and mortality.[30-34]

The incidence of fracture among patients with primary hyperparathyroidism is unknown. Although the risk of fracture has been reported to be increased at all sites,[35] an increased risk of vertebral fracture is a surprising finding, since most patients have relatively well preserved vertebral bone density. An increased incidence of forearm fractures is more consistent with the finding of reduced bone density at that site. However, even this risk is uncertain, because it is now known that parathyroid hormone may increase the cross-sectional area of bone and therefore strengthen it, even if the bone density appears to be reduced.[36]

Medical Therapy

There is considerable interest in the development of a safe, medical approach to asymptomatic primary hyperparathyroidism. The use of estrogen therapy in postmenopausal women with primary hyperparathyroidism is associated with small reductions (of 0.5 to 1 mg per deciliter) in the serum calcium concentration and increases in bone density, along with stable parathyroid hormone levels.[37] However, risks associated with estrogen use have been well publicized recently.[38] In addition, doses higher than the current standard have been most consistently associated with beneficial effects in primary hyperparathyroidism, although some positive studies have used lower doses.[39] Raloxifene, a selective estrogen-receptor modulator, is a potential alternative. In a short-term (eight-week) trial involving 18 postmenopausal women, raloxifene was associated with a statistically significant, although small (0.5 mg per deciliter), reduction in the serum calcium concentration and in the levels of markers of bone turnover.[40]

Since primary hyperparathyroidism is characterized by high bone turnover, potent bisphosphonates are another therapeutic option. In recent clinical trials involving small numbers of patients with primary hyperparathyroidism, the use of alendronate has resulted in significant increases (of 4 to 6 percent) in vertebral bone density.[41,42] Serum calcium and parathyroid hormone levels do not change significantly.

The calcimimetic drug cinacalcet has been investigated in patients with primary hyperparathyroidism.[43] By increasing the affinity of the parathyroid-cell calcium receptor for

Table 1. Comparison of Old and New Criteria for Parathyroid Surgery in Patients with Asymptomatic Primary Hyperparathyroidism.*

Variable	1990 Guidelines	2002 Guidelines
Serum calcium concentration	1.0–1.6 mg/dl above upper limit of normal	1.0 mg/dl above upper limit of normal
24-Hr urinary calcium excretion	>400 mg	>400 mg
Reduction in creatinine clearance	30%	30%
Bone mineral density	Z score below −2.0 in the forearm	T score below −2.5 at any site
Age	<50 Yr	<50 Yr

* Data are from Bilezikian et al.[46]

Table 2. Comparison of Old and New Management Guidelines for Monitoring Patients with Asymptomatic Primary Hyperparathyroidism Who Do Not Undergo Parathyroid Surgery.*

Variable	Recommended Monitoring	
	1990 Guidelines	2002 Guidelines
Serum calcium level	Every 6 mo	Every 6 mo
24-Hr urinary calcium excretion	Annual	Not recommended
Creatinine clearance	Annual	Not recommended
Serum creatinine concentration	Annual	Annual
Bone density	Annual	Annual, at all 3 sites
Abdominal radiography	Annual	Not recommended

* Data are from Bilezikian et al.[46]

extracellular calcium, this agent leads to an increase in intracellular calcium and a subsequent reduction in parathyroid hormone secretion. This action, in turn, reduces the serum calcium level. Clinical trials have demonstrated prolonged normalization (lasting up to three years) of the serum calcium level[44] but no change in bone density as measured on dual-energy x-ray absorptiometry. There are no data regarding the incidence of fractures with this agent or any other medical therapy in patients with primary hyperparathyroidism. More information is required about all these potential medical approaches to asymptomatic primary hyperparathyroidism before evidence-based recommendations can be made regarding their use in this disorder.

Calcium and Vitamin D Intake

Although it is prudent for patients to refrain from the ingestion of more calcium than is recommended for adults (1200 to 1500 mg per day), it is also important not to restrict calcium intake too much (to less than 750 mg per day). Calcium-poor diets may fuel processes associated with excessive secretion of parathyroid hormone. Many patients with asymptomatic primary hyperparathyroidism have levels of 25-hydroxyvitamin D that are at the lower end of the normal range or frankly low,[45] and a low level of supplementation, achievable with a multivitamin (400 IU of vitamin D daily), is reasonable. Patients should be advised to be cautious about using higher doses of vitamin D, because hypercalcemia and hypercalciuria can develop and worsen quickly. They should also be advised to maintain adequate fluid intake, because dehydration can exacerbate hypercalcemia.

Other Uncertainties

Data are lacking regarding the natural history of the recently recognized normocalcemic variant of primary hyperparathyroidism. In addition, more research is needed on possible neuropsychological, cardiovascular, and metabolic manifestations of mild hyperparathyroidism. The roles of newer assays for parathyroid hormone, newer imaging methods, and different surgical approaches require further study.

GUIDELINES

In 2002, the National Institutes of Health (NIH) Workshop on Asymptomatic Primary Hyperparathyroidism[46] revisited key issues related to the management of this condition that had previously been addressed in the 1990 NIH Consensus Development Conference.[4] A panel convened after the workshop recommended new management guidelines that relate specifically to the asymptomatic form of the disease. The current guidelines for surgery are compared with the 1990 guidelines in Table 1. In the new guidelines, the serum calcium concentration above which surgery is recommended has been lowered to 1 mg per deciliter above the upper limit of normal, because the panel judged that levels that are consistently higher than this are associated with greater risks of complications. The recommendation that bone densitometry be performed at three sites (the lumbar spine, the hip, and the distal third of the radius) reflects the fact that this disease can affect all bones and that the radius is particularly vulnerable. The use of the T score for bone mineral density and the guideline recommending surgery if the T score is less than −2.5 are consistent with the definition of osteoporosis established by the World Health Organization.

Some patients with asymptomatic primary hyperparathyroidism do not meet any of these criteria for surgery. For these patients, a conservative approach including monitoring (as outlined in Table 2) is considered to be an appropriate and safe alternative.

CONCLUSIONS AND RECOMMENDATIONS

Many patients with asymptomatic primary hyperparathyroidism will not require surgery. On the basis of long-term follow-up in patients as well as expert opinion, accepted indications for surgery include a serum calcium concentration that is at least 1 mg per deciliter above the upper limit of normal, marked hypercalciuria (urinary calcium excretion of more than 400 mg per day), reduced bone density (a T score of less than −2.5 at any site), and an age of less than 50 years. For patients who do not meet any of these criteria, such as the patient described in the vignette, monitoring with semiannual measurement of serum calcium and annual measurement of bone mass is recommended. Patients should be encouraged to maintain an active lifestyle, with normal intakes of calcium and vitamin D.

Supported by a grant (NIDDK 32333) from the National Institute of Diabetes and Digestive and Kidney Diseases.

This article first appeared in the April 22, 2004, issue of the New England Journal of Medicine.

REFERENCES

1.
Albright F, Reifenstein EC. The parathyroid glands and metabolic bone disease. Baltimore: Williams & Wilkins, 1948.

2.
Cope O. The story of hyperparathyroidism at the Massachusetts General Hospital. N Engl J Med 1966;21:1174-82.

3.
Heath H III, Hodgson SF, Kennedy MA. Primary hyperparathyroidism: incidence, morbidity, and potential economic impact in a community. N Engl J Med 1980;302:189-93.

4.
Potts JT Jr, Fradkin JE, Aurbach GD, Bilezikian JP, Raisz LG, eds. Proceedings of the NIH consensus development conference on diagnosis and management of asymptomatic primary hyperparathyroidism. J Bone Miner Res 1991;6:Suppl 2.

5.
Silverberg SJ, Shane E, De La Cruz L, et al. Skeletal disease in primary hyperparathyroidism. J Bone Miner Res 1989;4:283-91.

6.
Neer RM, Arnaud CD, Zanchetta JR, et al. Effect of parathyroid hormone (1-34) on fractures and bone mineral density in postmenopausal women with osteoporosis. N Engl J Med 2001;344:1434-41.

7.
Silverberg SJ, Locker F, Bilezikian JP. Vertebral osteopenia: a new indication for surgery in primary hyperparathyroidism. J Clin Endocrinol Metab 1996;81:4007-12.

8.
Fuleihan GE, Moore F Jr, LeBoff MS, et al. Longitudinal changes in bone density in hyperparathyroidism. J Clin Densitom 1999;2:153-62.

9.
Guo C-Y, Thomas WEG, al-Dehaimi AW, Assiri AMA, Eastell R. Longitudinal changes in bone mineral density and bone turnover in postmenopausal women with primary hyperparathyroidism. J Clin Endocrinol Metab 1996;81:3487-91.

10.
Bilezikian JP. Nephrolithiasis in primary hyperparathyroidism. In: Coe FL, Favus MJ, Pak CYC, Parks JH, Preminger GM, eds. Kidney stones: medical and surgical treatment. Philadelphia: Lippincott-Raven, 1996:783-802.

11.
Turken SA, Cafferty M, Silverberg SJ, et al. Neuromuscular involvement in mild, asymptomatic primary hyperparathyroidism. Am J Med 1989;87:553-7.

12.
Solomon BL, Schaaf M, Smallridge RC. Psychologic symptoms before and after parathyroid surgery. Am J Med 1994;96:101-6.

13.
Silverberg SJ. Non-classical target organs in hyperparathyroidism. J Bone Miner Res 2002;17:Suppl 2:N117-N125.

14.
Silverberg SJ, Bilezikian JP. "Incipient" primary hyperparathyroidism: a "forme fruste" of an old disease. J Clin Endocrinol Metab 2003;88:5348-52.

15.
Mithal A, Bandeira F, Meng X, et al. Clinical presentation of primary hyperparathyroidism in India, Brazil and China. In: Bilezikian JP, ed. The parathyroids: basic and clinical concepts. 2nd ed. San Diego, Calif.: Academic Press, 2001:375-86.

16.
Jüppner H, Potts JT Jr. Immunoassays for the detection of parathyroid hormone. J Bone Miner Res 2002;17:Suppl 2:N81-N86.

17.
Gao P, Scheibel S, D'Amour P, et al. Development of a novel immunoradiometric assay exclusively for biologically active whole parathyroid hormone 1-84: implications for improvement of accurate assessment of parathyroid function. J Bone Miner Res 2001;16:605-14.

18.
Silverberg SJ, Brown I, LoGerfo P, Gao P, Cantor TL, Bilezikian JP. Clinical utility of an immunoradiometric assay for parathyroid hormone (1-84) in primary hyperparathyroidism. J Clin Endocrinol Metab 2003;88:4725-30.

19.
El-Hajj Fuleihan G, Brown EM, Heath H III. Familial benign hypocalciuric hypercalcemia and neonatal primary hyperparathyroidism. In: Bilezikian JP, Raisz LG, Rodan GA, eds. Principles of bone biology. 2nd ed. San Diego Calif.: Academic Press, 2001:1031-45.

20.
Silverberg SJ, Shane E, Jacobs TP, Siris E, Bilezikian JP. A 10-year prospective study of primary hyperparathyroidism with or without parathyroid surgery. N Engl J Med 1999;341:1249-55.

21.
Silverberg SJ, Brown I, Bilezikian JP. Age as a criterion for surgery in primary hyperparathyroidism. Am J Med 2002;113:681-4.

22.
Clark OH. How should patients with primary hyperparathyroidism be treated? J Clin Endocrinol Metab 2003;88:3011-4.

23.
Allendorf J, Kim L, Chabot J, DiGiorgi M, Spanknebel K, LoGerfo P. The impact of sestamibi scanning on the outcome of parathyroid surgery. J Clin Endocrinol Metab 2003;88:3015-8.

24.
Alexander HR Jr, Chen CC, Shawker T, et al. Role of preoperative localization and intraoperative localization maneuvers including intraoperative PTH assay determination for patients with persistent or recurrent hyperparathyroidism. J Bone Miner Res 2002;17:Suppl 2:N133-N140.

25.
Udelsman R, Donovan POI, Sokoll LT. One hundred consecutive minimally invasive parathyroid explorations. Ann Surg 2000;232:331-9.

26.
Lee NC, Norton JA. Multiple-gland disease in primary hyperparathyroidism: a function of operative approach? Arch Surg 2002;137:896-9.

27.
Genc H, Morita E, Perrier ND, et al. Differing histologic findings after bilateral and focused parathyroidectomy. J Am Coll Surg 2003;196:535-40.

28.
Chan AK, Duh QY, Katz MH, Siperstein AE, Clark OH. Clinical manifestations of primary hyperparathyroidism before and after parathyroidectomy: a case-control study. Ann Surg 1995;22:402-12.

29.
Wermers RA, Khosla S, Atkinson EJ, et al. Survival after the diagnosis of primary hyperparathyroidism: a population-based study. Am J Med 1998;104:115-22.

30.
Stefenelli T, Abela C, Frank H, et al. Cardiac abnormalities in patients with primary hyperparathyroidism: implications for follow-up. J Clin Endocrinol Metab 1997;82:106-12.

31.
Piovesan A, Molineri N, Casasso F, et al. Left ventricular hypertrophy in primary hyperparathyroidism: effects of successful parathyroidectomy. Clin Endocrinol 1999;50:321-8.

32.
Palmer M, Adami HO, Bergstrom R, Akerstrom G. Mortality after surgery for primary hyperparathyroidism: a follow-up of 441 patients operated on from 1956 to 1979. Surgery 1987;102:1-7.

33.
Hedback G, Oden A. Increased risk of death from primary hyperparathyroidism — an update. Eur J Clin Invest 1998;28:271-6.

34.
Nilsson IL, Yin L, Lundgren E, Rastad J, Ekbom A. Clinical presentation of primary hyperparathyroidism in Europe — nationwide cohort analysis on mortality from non-malignant causes. J Bone Miner Res 2002;17:Suppl 2:N68-N74.

35.
Khosla S, Melton LJ III, Wermers RA, Crowson CS, O'Fallon WM, Riggs BL. Primary hyperparathyroidism and the risk of fracture: a population-based study. J Bone Miner Res 1999;14:1700-7.

36.
Zanchetta JR, Bogado CE, Ferretti JL, et al. Effects of teriparatide [recombinant human parathyroid hormone(1-34)] on cortical bone in postmenopausal women with osteoporosis. J Bone Miner Res 2003;18:539-43.

37.
Marcus R. The role of estrogens and related compounds in the management of primary hyperparathyroidism. J Bone Miner Res 2002;17: Suppl 2:N146-N149.

38.
Roussow JE, Anderson GL, Prentice RL, et al. Risks and benefits of estrogen plus progestin in healthy postmenopausal women: principal results from the Women's Health Initiative randomized controlled trial. JAMA 2002;228:321-33.

39.
Grey AB, Stapleton JP, Evans MC, Tatnell MA, Reid IR. Effect of hormone replacement therapy on bone mineral density in postmenopausal women with mild primary hyperparathyroidism. Ann Intern Med 1996;125:360-8.

40.
Rubin MA, Lee KH, McMahon DJ, Silverberg SJ. Raloxifene lowers serum calcium and markers of bone turnover in postmenopausal women with primary hyperparathyroidism. J Clin Endocrinol Metab 2003;88:1174-8.

41.
Parker CR, Blackwell PJ, Fairbairn KJ, Hosking DJ. Alendronate in the treatment of primary hyperparathyroidism-related osteoporosis: a 2-year study. J Clin Endocrinol Metab 2002;87:4482-9.

42.
Chow CC, Chan WB, Li JKY, et al. Oral alendronate increases bone mineral density in postmenopausal women with primary hyperparathyroidism. J Clin Endocrinol Metab 2003;88:581-7.

43.
Shoback DM, Bilezikian JP, Turner SA, McCary LC, Guo MD, Peacock M. The calcimimetic cinacalcet normalizes serum calcium in patients with primary hyperparathyroidism. J Clin Endocrinol Metab 2003;88:5644-9.

44.
Peacock M, Scumpia S, Bolognese MA, et al. Long term control of primary hyperparathyroidism with cinacalcet HCl. J Bone Miner Res 2003;18:Suppl 2:S17. abstract.

45.
Silverberg SJ, Shane E, Dempster DW, Bilezikian JP. The effects of vitamin D insufficiency in primary hyperparathyroidism. Am J Med 1999;107:561-7.

46.
Bilezikian JP, Potts JT Jr, Fuleihan Gel-H, et al. Summary statement from a workshop on asymptomatic primary hyperparathyroidism: a perspective for the 21st century. J Bone Miner Res 2002;17:Suppl 2:N2-N11.

Treatment of Deep-Vein Thrombosis

SHANNON M. BATES, M.D.C.M.,

AND JEFFREY S. GINSBERG, M.D.

A 52-year-old-woman with no history of venous thromboembolism presents with a four-day history of discomfort in her left calf. Proximal deep-vein thrombosis is diagnosed by compression ultrasonography. How should her case be managed?

THE CLINICAL PROBLEM

The annual incidence of venous thromboembolism is approximately 0.1 percent; the rate increases from 0.01 percent among persons in early adulthood to nearly 1 percent among those who are at least 60 years old.[1,2] More than half of these events involve deep-vein thrombosis. To minimize the risk of fatal pulmonary embolism, accurate diagnosis and prompt therapy are crucial.[3] Long-term complications include the post-thrombotic syndrome[4-6] and recurrent thromboembolism.[4,7-13]

The pathogenesis of venous thrombosis involves three factors, which are referred to as Virchow's triad. Those factors are damage to the vessel wall, venous stasis, and hypercoagulability. Damage to the vessel wall prevents the endothelium from inhibiting coagulation and initiating local fibrinolysis. Venous stasis due to immobilization or venous obstruction inhibits the clearance and dilution of activated coagulation factors. Finally, congenital or acquired thrombophilia promotes coagulation. Venous thromboembolism is multifactorial and often results from a combination of risk factors (Table 1).[14,15]

Deep-vein thrombosis typically originates in the venous sinuses of the calf muscles[16] but occasionally originates in the proximal veins, usually in response to trauma or surgery.[17] Signs and symptoms result from venous outflow obstruction and from inflammation of the vessel wall and perivascular tissue. Calf-vein thrombi often spontaneously lyse and rarely lead to symptomatic pulmonary embolism.[16,18] Approximately 25 percent of untreated calf thrombi extend into the proximal veins, usually within a week after presentation.[19] The risk of pulmonary embolism (either symptomatic or asymptomatic) with

Table 1. Risk Factors for Venous Thromboembolism.*

Risk Factor	Estimated Relative Risk
Inherited conditions†	
Antithrombin deficiency	25
Protein C deficiency	10
Protein S deficiency	10
Factor V Leiden mutation	
Heterozygous	5
Homozygous	50
G20210A prothrombin-gene mutation (heterozygous)	2.5
Dysfibrinogenemia	18
Acquired conditions	
Major surgery or major trauma	5–200‡
History of venous thromboembolism	50
Antiphospholipid antibodies	
Elevated anticardiolipin antibody level	2
Nonspecific inhibitor (e.g., lupus anticoagulant)	10
Cancer	5
Major medical illness with hospitalization	5
Age	
>50 years	5
>70 years	10
Pregnancy	7
Estrogen therapy	
Oral contraceptives	5
Hormone-replacement therapy	2
Selective estrogen-receptor modulators	
Tamoxifen	5
Raloxifene	3
Obesity	1–3
Hereditary, environmental, or idiopathic conditions	
Hyperhomocysteinemia§	3
Elevated levels of factor VIII (>90th percentile)	3
Elevated levels of factor IX (>90th percentile)	2.3
Elevated levels of factor XI (>90th percentile)	2.2

* Data are from Rosendaal[14] and Kearon.[15] Relative risks are for patients with the specified risk factor, as compared with those without the risk factor.

† The definition of deficiency of antithrombin, protein C, or protein S varies among studies; it is usually defined as a functional or immunologic value that is less than the 5th percentile of values in the control population.

‡ The risk varies greatly, depending on the type of surgery, the use and type of prophylaxis, and the method of diagnosis.

§ The definition of hyperhomocysteinemia varies among studies; it is usually defined as a persistent elevation of fasting plasma homocysteine levels or plasma homocysteine levels after methionine loading that are greater than the 95th percentile of the control population or more than 2 SD above the mean for the control population.

Table 2. Contraindications to Anticoagulant Therapy.*
Absolute contraindications
Active bleeding
Severe bleeding diathesis or platelet count ≤20,000/mm³
Neurosurgery, ocular surgery, or intracranial bleeding within the past 10 days
Relative contraindications
Mild-to-moderate bleeding diathesis or thrombocytopenia†
Brain metastases
Recent major trauma
Major abdominal surgery within the past 2 days
Gastrointestinal or genitourinary bleeding within the past 14 days
Endocarditis
Severe hypertension (i.e., systolic blood pressure >200 mm Hg, diastolic blood pressure >120 mm Hg, or both) at presentation

* Data are from Abrams et al.[25]
† Mild-to-moderate thrombocytopenia is defined as a platelet count that is less than normal but greater than 20,000 per cubic millimeter.

proximal-vein thrombosis is approximately 50 percent,[20] and most fatal emboli probably arise from proximal thrombi.[21] Rarely, thrombosis is massive, causing vascular compromise of the leg (i.e., phlegmasia cerulea dolens).

STRATEGIES AND EVIDENCE

Diagnosis

Because clinical diagnosis is unreliable, accurate diagnostic tests are required when deep-vein thrombosis is suspected. The failure of a proximal deep vein to flatten when compressed with an ultrasound probe or the finding of a persistent intraluminal filling defect in any deep vein on venography provides a definitive diagnosis.[22] Venography is often not used clinically because of its invasive nature, its technical demands, its costs, and its potential risks, such as allergic reactions and renal dysfunction. Therefore, compression ultrasonography is the diagnostic test of choice when deep-vein thrombosis is suspected. The sensitivity and specificity of compression ultrasonography for proximal deep-vein thrombosis are more than 95 percent.[23] However, for isolated deep-vein thrombosis in the calf, the sensitivity of ultrasonography is lower (approximately 70 percent), and its positive predictive value is only 80 percent.[23] Therefore, imaging of the calf veins is not routinely performed. Consequently, follow-up ultrasonography one week after a normal test result has been obtained is recommended to detect the possible extension of a deep-vein thrombosis from the calf into the proximal veins; if the test is negative at this time, subsequent extension is unlikely. Venography may be useful to confirm the diagnosis when ultrasonography suggests isolated distal thrombosis[23] and when patients are unable to return for serial ultrasonography or have highly suggestive clinical signs or symptoms but negative results on ultrasonography.

Initial Therapy

Once deep-vein thrombosis is diagnosed, the goals of treatment are relief of symptoms and prevention of embolization and recurrence. The cornerstone of initial therapy is either unfractionated or low-molecular-weight heparin, followed by an oral anticoagulant drug.[3,19,22,24] Table 2 lists the contraindications to anticoagulant therapy.[25]

Table 3. Options for the Initial Treatment of Deep-Vein Thrombosis with Anticoagulant Agents.

Drug	Method of Administration	Dose*	Reported Risks	
			Risk of Heparin-Induced Thrombocytopenia†	Risk of Major Bleeding‡
			no./total no. (%)	
Unfractionated heparin	Intravenous	Loading dose, 5000 U or 80 U/kg of body weight with infusion adjusted to maintain activated partial-thromboplastin time within the therapeutic range§	9/332 (2.7)	35/1853 (1.9)
Low-molecular-weight heparin			0/333 (0)	20/1821 (1.1)
Dalteparin	Subcutaneous	100 U/kg every 12 hr or 200 U/kg daily; maximum, 18,000 U/day		
Enoxaparin	Subcutaneous	1 mg/kg every 12 hr or 1.5 mg/kg daily; maximum, 180 mg/day		
Tinzaparin	Subcutaneous	175 U/kg daily; maximum, 18,000 U/day		
Nadroparin	Subcutaneous	86 U/kg every 12 hr or 171 U/kg daily; maximum, 17,100 U/day		

* Doses vary in patients who are obese or who have renal dysfunction. Monitoring of anti–factor Xa levels has been suggested for these patients, with dose adjustment to a target range of 0.6 to 1.0 U per milliliter four hours after injection for twice-daily administration or 1.0 to 2.0 U per milliliter for once-daily administration. Even though there are few supporting data, most manufacturers recommend capping the dose for obese patients at that for a 90-kg patient.
† Data are from Warkentin et al.[29] and are based on the incidence in patients who had undergone orthopedic surgery and were receiving prophylactic doses of unfractionated heparin or low-molecular-weight heparin (i.e., enoxaparin).
‡ Data are from Gould et al.[30]
§ The therapeutic range of activated partial-thromboplastin time corresponds to heparin levels of 0.3 to 0.7 U per milliliter, as determined by anti–factor Xa assay. High levels of heparin-binding proteins and factor VIII may result in so-called heparin resistance. In patients requiring more than 40,000 U per day to attain a therapeutic activated partial-thromboplastin time, the dosage can be adjusted on the basis of plasma heparin levels.[31]

Unfractionated Heparin   Unfractionated heparin is usually given intravenously by continuous infusion after a loading dose has been administered.[26] The anticoagulant response varies among patients, because this drug binds nonspecifically to plasma and cellular proteins. Laboratory monitoring, with assessment of the activated partial-thromboplastin time, is required, with adjustment of the dose to achieve the target therapeutic range. This range depends on which reagent and coagulometer are used to measure the activated partial-thromboplastin time. Although the use of a fixed ratio of 1.5 to 2.5 between the patient's value and the control value is commonly suggested, this strategy results in variable (and usually subtherapeutic) degrees of anticoagulation, because of the differing degrees of responsiveness among the available reagents. Ideally, the therapeutic range of activated partial-thromboplastin times for each reagent should correspond to ex vivo plasma levels of activity against activated factor X (anti–factor Xa) of 0.3 to 0.7 U per milliliter.[26] Weight-based heparin nomograms facilitate the achievement of a therapeutic anticoagulant effect.

Hemorrhage occurs in up to 7 percent of patients during initial treatment; the risk is affected by the heparin dose, the patient's age, and concomitant use or nonuse of thrombolytic and antiplatelet agents. Long-term use of heparin (i.e., longer than one month) can cause osteoporosis.[26-28] Heparin-induced thrombocytopenia is immune-mediated and in 30 to 50 percent of cases is associated with venous or arterial thrombosis.[26] Patients with previous heparin-induced thrombocytopenia should receive alternative anticoagulant agents, such as danaparoid, lepirudin, or argatroban.[26]

Low-Molecular-Weight Heparins   Meta-analyses suggest that low-molecular-weight heparins are as effective as unfractionated heparin in preventing recurrent venous thromboembolism, and they cause less bleeding (Table 3).[30] These heparin products — which show less nonspecific binding, have improved bioavailability, and elicit more predictable dose responses than unfractionated heparin — are administered subcutaneously once or twice daily in weight-adjusted doses,[26] generally without monitoring.

Although heparin-induced thrombocytopenia develops less frequently with low-molecular-weight heparins than it does with unfractionated heparin,[26,29] these agents often cross-react with the antibody that causes heparin-induced thrombocytopenia and are therefore contraindicated in patients with a history of this condition. Low-molecular-weight heparins also cause less osteoporosis than does unfractionated heparin.[27,28] In a randomized study comparing prophylactic regimens during pregnancy and the puerperium, 2 of 23 women who received unfractionated heparin were given a diagnosis of osteoporosis on the basis of postpartum studies of bone mineral density, whereas none of the 21 women who received low-molecular-weight heparin (dalteparin) had osteoporosis.[27] In another study, symptomatic vertebral fractures occurred in 6 of 40 patients with contraindications to warfarin therapy who received three to six months of unfractionated heparin (10,000 U subcutaneously twice daily), as compared with 1 of 40 patients who received dalteparin (5000 U subcutaneously twice daily) for the same length of time.[28]

Outpatient therapy with low-molecular-weight heparins is safe and effective.[32,33] If there is a system in place for administering the medication (or for teaching patients or caregivers to administer it) and for monitoring, more than 80 percent of patients can be treated without hospitalization.[26] However, outpatient treatment is unsuitable for patients with massive thrombosis, serious coexisting illnesses, or a high risk of hemorrhage (e.g., patients who are very old, have recently undergone surgery, or have a history of bleeding or renal or liver disease). Low-molecular-weight heparins are more expensive than is unfractionated heparin, but they cut costs by reducing the frequency of hospital admissions and the need for laboratory monitoring.[34] Reductions in nursing time also make low-molecular-weight heparins cost effective for inpatients.

Thrombolytic Therapy   Thrombolytic agents dissolve fresh clots and restore venous patency more rapidly than do anticoagulants.[35] They are given systemically or by regional catheter-directed infusion, which results in a higher local concentration of the drug than does systemic administration. Theoretically, catheter-directed infusion should result in improved efficacy, but this hypothesis remains untested. Both routes of administration cause substantially more bleeding than does heparin,[35] and it is unclear whether either agent reduces the incidence of the post-thrombotic syndrome. Consequently, thrombolytic therapy is generally reserved for patients who have limb-threatening thrombosis, who have had symptoms for less than one week, and who have a low risk of bleeding.[36]

Long-Term Therapy

Warfarin (or another coumarin) at a dose that is titrated to achieve an international normalized ratio (INR) of 2.0 to 3.0 is used for secondary prophylaxis and, as compared with placebo, reduces the risk of recurrence by 90 percent among patients who have received four weeks to three months of therapy.[36,37] Because the antithrombotic effect of warfarin is delayed for 72 to 96 hours, heparin therapy is overlapped with initiation of warfarin. When therapy with the two drugs is started on the same day, heparin can be discontinued after five days, provided the INR has been at a therapeutic level for two consecutive days. Patients with massive thrombosis often receive an extended course (i.e., 7 to 14 days) of heparin. The use of oral anticoagulant therapy was reviewed recently in the *Journal*.[38]

Patients with cancer who have venous thromboembolism have a substantial risk of a recurrent event when they are treated with warfarin. A randomized study involving such patients showed that after standard initial therapy with low-molecular-weight heparin, patients who were taking the drug on a long-term basis had half as many recurrent events as those who were taking coumarin derivatives.[39] Bleeding rates were similar with both medications, and daily injections were acceptable to the patients. Therefore, this therapy should be considered for all patients with cancer who also have deep-vein thrombosis.

For other patients, the role of long-term therapy with low-molecular-weight heparin is less clear. In a systematic review of randomized, controlled trials in which low-molecular-weight heparin was compared with warfarin for secondary prophylaxis, the rates of recurrent thrombosis and major bleeding were similar with the two regimens.[40] Although low-molecular-weight heparin has advantages over warfarin, its cost, the need for daily injections, and the risk of osteoporosis with long-term therapy make it unsuitable for routine secondary prophylaxis.

Inferior vena cava filters are useful in patients who have a contraindication to anticoagulation or those in whom treatment has failed (Table 2).[36] In a randomized trial of 400 patients with proximal-vein thrombosis who received anticoagulants either alone or with a filter, the incidence of early pulmonary embolism by day 12 was significantly lower among patients treated with filters.[41] However, this difference did not persist; at two years, the reduction in symptomatic pulmonary embolism in the filter-treated patients was not significant, and mortality was similar in the two groups. The approximate doubling of the risk of recurrent deep-vein thrombosis in patients treated with filters suggests that anticoagulant therapy should be started if it is safe to do so. It remains a matter of controversy whether filters can be used to prevent embolization of "free-floating" iliofemoral thrombi to avert pulmonary embolism in patients who have deep-vein thrombosis and a reduced cardiopulmonary reserve and to treat venous thromboembolism in patients with cancer.[36]

Duration of Anticoagulation

Patients should receive anticoagulant therapy for at least three months. The optimal duration of treatment should be determined so as to balance the risks of recurrence and bleeding. When anticoagulation is adjusted to achieve an INR of 2.0 to 3.0, the annual risk of major bleeding is approximately 3 percent.[42] In patients whose thrombosis is associated with a major transient risk factor, the risk of recurrence after three months of anticoagulation is also approximately 3 percent per year.[36] Case fatality rates of 5 percent for recurrence[43] and 10 percent for major bleeding[42] have been reported. After three months, the risk of a fatal recurrence among patients who are not receiving treatment is lower than the

Table 4. Recommendations for the Duration of Anticoagulant Therapy for Patients with Deep-Vein Thrombosis.*

Characteristics of Patient†	Risk of Recurrence in the Year after Discontinuation (%)	Duration of Therapy
Major transient risk factor	3	3 mo
Minor risk factor; no thrombophilia	<10 if risk factor avoided >10 if risk factor persistent	6 mo Until factor resolves
Idiopathic event; no thrombophilia or low-risk thrombophilia	<10	6 mo‡
Idiopathic event; high-risk thrombophilia	>10	Indefinite
More than one idiopathic event	>10	Indefinite
Cancer; other ongoing risk factor	>10	Indefinite

* Data are from Hirsh and Hoak,[22] Hyers et al.,[36] and Kearon.[44]
† Examples of major transient risk factors are major surgery, a major medical illness, and leg casting. Examples of minor transient risk factors are the use of an oral contraceptive and hormone-replacement therapy. Examples of low-risk thrombophilias are heterozygosity for the factor V Leiden and G20210A prothrombin-gene mutations. Examples of high-risk thrombophilia are antithrombin, protein C, and protein S deficiencies; homozygosity for the factor V Leiden or prothrombin-gene mutation or heterozygosity for both; and the presence of antiphospholipid antibodies.
‡ Therapy may be prolonged if the patient prefers to prolong it or if the risk of bleeding is low.

risk of fatal hemorrhage among patients taking warfarin (i.e., approximately 0.15 percent vs. 0.3 percent per year); therefore, therapy of three months' duration is generally sufficient for patients whose thrombosis is associated with a major transient risk factor.[36]

The optimal duration of therapy for patients who have had idiopathic events or who have continuing risk factors remains controversial.[7-13,36,44] Patients with idiopathic deep-vein thrombosis who are treated for approximately three months have a 10 to 27 percent risk of recurrence during the year after they discontinue anticoagulants.[8-12] With six months of treatment, the risk of recurrence is approximately 10 percent in the year after anticoagulation is stopped[12,13]; patients whose initial events occur in association with a minor transient risk factor probably have a lower risk of recurrence. Extending therapy beyond six months does not substantially reduce the risk of recurrence after discontinuation of treatment.[11] Although continuing treatment prevents recurrences, it also exposes the patient to the risk of anticoagulant-induced bleeding. On the basis of the rates of recurrent venous thromboembolism and major bleeding that are cited above, extended anticoagulant therapy should be considered for patients with idiopathic deep-vein thrombosis whose estimated risk of major bleeding is less than 5 percent per year. However, therapy for six months or less may be more appropriate for patients at higher risk of bleeding or those in whom thrombosis occurred in association with a minor transient risk factor (Table 4).

Table 5. Prevalence of Thrombophilic Abnormalities and the Associated Risk of Recurrent Venous Thromboembolism after the Cessation of Anticoagulant Therapy.*

Risk Factor†	Estimated Prevalence (%)‡	Estimated Relative Risk of Recurrence
Antithrombin deficiency	1	1.5–3
Protein C deficiency	3	1.5–3
Protein S deficiency	3	1.5–3
Factor V Leiden mutation		
Heterozygous	20	1–4
Homozygous	2	About 4
G20210A prothrombin-gene mutation (heterozygous)	5	1–5
Dysfibrinogenemia	<1	NA
Factor V Leiden and G20210A prothrombin-gene mutations	2	2–5
Antiphospholipid antibodies	5	2–4
Elevated factor VIII levels	10–50	1–7
Elevated factor IX levels	10–50	1–5
Hyperhomocysteinemia	10–25	1–3

* Data are from Kearon,[44] Christiansen et al.,[50] Baglin et al.,[51] Margaglinone et al.,[52] and Kyrle et al.[53] Relative risks are for patients with the risk factor in question, as compared with those without the risk factor.
† The definition of deficiency of antithrombin, protein C, or protein S varies; it is usually defined as a functional or immunologic value that is less than the 5th percentile of values in the control population.
‡ Prevalence and relative risk depend on the definitions of hyperhomocysteinemia and elevations in levels of factor VIII and factor IX and on the reference group.

AREAS OF UNCERTAINTY

The Role of Reduced-Intensity Anticoagulation

The role of reduced-intensity anticoagulation (that is, anticoagulant therapy targeted to achieve an INR of 1.5 to 1.9) after three months of conventional therapy has been examined in two randomized, controlled trials. One of the studies suggested that, as compared with placebo, low-intensity warfarin is highly effective and safe when used to prevent recurrences.[45] The other study suggested that low-intensity warfarin was less effective and not safer than conventional-intensity warfarin for extended treatment after idiopathic venous thromboembolism.[46] In both studies, the small number of major bleeding events probably precludes an accurate assessment of the true risk of major hemorrhage with either regimen.

New Anticoagulants

The limitations of traditional anticoagulants have prompted the development of new agents. Drugs that are in an advanced stage of development but have not yet received approval from the Food and Drug Administration include parenteral synthetic pentasaccharide analogues (e.g., fondaparinux and idraparinux) and oral direct thrombin inhibitors (e.g., ximelagatran). In a large randomized trial comparing fondaparinux with enoxaparin for the initial treatment of deep-vein thrombosis, rates of symptomatic, recurrent venous thromboembolism and major bleeding were not statistically different between the two groups.[47] Similar results were obtained in a randomized trial involving 2489 patients with acute deep-vein thrombosis (with or without pulmonary embolism) that compared six months of ximelagatran monotherapy with six months of therapy consisting of enoxaparin followed by warfarin.[48]

A placebo-controlled trial showed that ximelagatran reduced the risk of recurrent venous thromboembolism without increasing the risk of major hemorrhage in patients who had already completed six months of standard treatment.[49] In contrast to warfarin, ximelagatran does not require monitoring of the degree of anticoagulation. However, ximelagatran has potential limitations, including the occurrence of elevations in liver enzyme levels (specifically, alanine aminotransferase) in 5 to 10 percent of patients receiving long-term therapy. To date, such elevations are not usually associated with symptoms and are reversible, even if the medication is continued. Further studies are required to define the appropriate role of these new agents.

Testing for Thrombophilia

At least one third of patients with idiopathic venous thromboembolism have an identifiable thrombophilia on laboratory testing.[15,44] Although testing for hypercoagulable states is costly, the procedure is routine in many centers for patients who have had a single episode of thrombosis. However, there is no clear evidence that modifying treatment because a hypercoagulable state has been found improves outcome or that more intensive therapy is required in patients with laboratory evidence of thrombophilia. Although it is assumed that the presence of a thrombophilic abnormality increases the risk of recurrence and, consequently, justifies prolonged therapy, the available data are inconsistent, and these assumptions remain unproved (Table 5).[15,44,50-52] The effectiveness of testing asymptomatic relatives and its potential consequences — including anxiety, avoidance of effective hormonal contraception, unnecessary exposure to anticoagulants in patients with a positive test, and possibly false reassurance from a negative test — have not been formally assessed. Thus, there are no unequivocal indications for testing for the presence of thrombophilic abnormalities in either patients or their relatives.

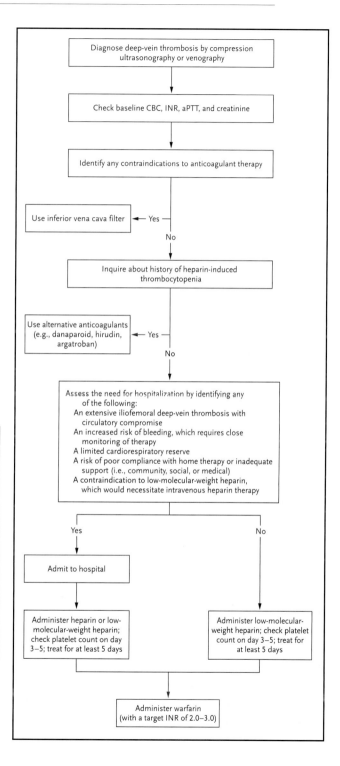

Figure 1. Management of Uncomplicated Deep-Vein Thrombosis.

For patients with limb-threatening iliofemoral thrombosis, symptoms for less than one week, and a low risk of bleeding, thrombolysis should be considered. Absolute contraindications to thrombolysis include suspected aortic dissection, acute pericarditis, active bleeding, cerebral neoplasm, intracranial vascular lesion, and previous central nervous system hemorrhage. The following are relative contraindications to thrombolysis: head trauma, major surgery, organ biopsy, major trauma, prolonged cardiopulmonary resuscitation with resultant chest trauma, or puncture of a noncompressible vessel within the past two to four weeks; severe hypertension at presentation (i.e., systolic blood pressure above 200 mm Hg, diastolic blood pressure above 120 mm Hg, or both); nonhemorrhagic stroke within the past six months; endocarditis; pregnancy; cancer; bleeding diathesis; and hepatic dysfunction.[25] For patients with cancer, long-term therapy with low-molecular-weight heparin should be considered. CBC denotes complete blood count, INR international normalized ratio, and aPTT activated partial-thromboplastin time.

Prevention of the Post-Thrombotic Syndrome

In an unblinded, randomized trial, daytime use of knee-length, graduated compression stockings for at least two years starting two to three weeks after the diagnosis of proximal deep-vein thrombosis reduced the frequency of the post-thrombotic syndrome by 50 percent.[5] However, in a placebo-controlled trial in which the definition of the post-thrombotic syndrome focused on the quality of life (i.e., the presence of chronic pain and swelling six months or more after deep-vein thrombosis), compression stockings worn "as much as possible" during waking hours did not prevent the condition.[6] Although the role of compression stockings in preventing the post-thrombotic syndrome remains uncertain, they are widely used to control symptoms in patients with established disease. Thrombolytic therapy has the potential to prevent the post-thrombotic syndrome by preventing damage to venous valves and subsequent venous hypertension, but outcome data supporting such an effect are lacking.

GUIDELINES

Guidelines for the treatment of deep-vein thrombosis have been published by the American College of Chest Physicians[36] and the American Heart Association[22] and are consistent with the approach outlined in this article.

RECOMMENDATIONS

For most patients with deep-vein thrombosis, such as the patient described in the vignette, low-molecular-weight heparin administered on an outpatient basis is appropriate as initial therapy. If patients or family members cannot administer injections, home care should be arranged. Hospital admission is still warranted for some patients (Figure 1). Thrombolytic therapy should be considered for patients less than 60 years of age who have limb-threatening circulatory compromise. Inferior vena cava filters should be inserted in patients with contraindications to anticoagulation (Table 2) and in those who require urgent surgery that precludes anticoagulation. Temporary filters should be used if anticoagulation is likely to be safe within 14 days after the bleeding event.

Oral anticoagulation should generally be started on the first day of treatment. Heparin should be given for a minimum of five days and not stopped until the patient's INR has been 2.0 or higher for two consecutive days. A platelet count should be obtained three to five days after initiating heparin administration. The INR should be measured after three to four days of warfarin treatment and the dose adjusted to maintain a target INR of 2.5. Twice-weekly monitoring of the INR is usually required for the first one to two weeks, followed by weekly monitoring until the INR is stable. Thereafter, the INR can be measured every two to four weeks, or more frequently if there are changes in medications or health status. Patients with cancer should receive long-term maintenance therapy with low-molecular-weight heparin, if that is practical.

Although the indications for testing for thrombophilia remain controversial, we test for the presence of thrombophilic states — the factor V Leiden mutation, the G20210A prothrombin-gene mutation, hyperhomocysteinemia, antiphospholipid antibodies, and deficiencies of antithrombin, protein C, and protein S — if patients have clinical features suggestive of these abnormalities. These features include a family history of venous thromboembolism, venous thromboembolism before the age of 45 years, recurrent venous thromboembolism, thrombosis in an unusual site (e.g., in mesenteric, renal, hepatic, or cerebral veins), idiopathic venous thromboembolism or thromboembolism after minimal provocation, heparin resistance (in the case of antithrombin deficiency), warfarin-induced skin necrosis (in the case of protein C or protein S deficiency), and neonatal purpura fulminans (in the case of homozygous protein C or protein S deficiency). We also offer the test if identifying a thrombophilic mutation will alter the care of patients or their relatives or if a patient requests it. Testing for dysfibrinogenemia is often not undertaken, given its low yield. We do not routinely test for elevated levels of factor VIII or IX, given the concern about the variability of this assay, the variation in factor levels among patients, and the most appropriate cutoff values.

We treat patients with a major transient risk factor for three months and those with a first episode of idiopathic thrombosis for at least six months. We recommend indefinite therapy for patients with a high-risk thrombophilia (e.g., a deficiency of antithrombin, protein C, or protein S; persistent antiphospholipid antibodies; or homozygosity for factor V Leiden or the prothrombin-gene mutation or heterozygosity for both), a continuing risk factor (e.g., advanced cancer), or recurrent episodes of idiopathic venous thrombosis, provided the risk of bleeding is not high. Although it has recently been suggested that the risk of recurrent venous thromboembolism is significantly higher in men than it is in women,[53] more data are required before these findings can be incorporated into routine recommendations regarding the duration of treatment.

Dr. Bates is the recipient of a New Investigator Award from the University Industry (bioMérieux) program of the Canadian Institutes of Health Research. Dr. Ginsberg is the recipient of a Career Investigator Award from the Heart and Stroke Foundation of Ontario and reports consulting fees from AstraZeneca.

This article first appeared in the July 15, 2004, issue of the New England Journal of Medicine.

REFERENCES

1.
Nordstom M, Lindblad B, Bergqvist D, Kjellstrom T. A prospective study of the incidence of deep-vein thrombosis within a defined urban population. J Intern Med 1992;232:155-60.
2.
Silverstein MD, Heit JA, Mohr DN, Petterson TM, O'Fallon WM, Melton LJ III. Trends in the incidence of deep vein thrombosis and pulmonary embolism: a 25-year population-based study. Arch Intern Med 1998;158:585-93.
3.
Barritt DW, Jordan SC. Anticoagulant drugs in the treatment of pulmonary embolism: a controlled trial. Lancet 1960;1:1309-12.
4.
Prandoni P, Lensing AWA, Cogo A, et al. The long-term clinical course of acute deep venous thrombosis. Ann Intern Med 1996;125:1-7.
5.
Brandjes DPM, Buller HR, Heijboer H, et al. Randomized trial of effect of compression stockings in patients with symptomatic proximal-vein thrombosis. Lancet 1997;349:759-62.
6.
Ginsberg JS, Hirsh J, Julian J, et al. Prevention and treatment of postphlebitic syndrome: results of a 3-part study. Arch Intern Med 2001;161:2105-9.

7.
Prandoni P, Lensing AW, Buller HR, et al. Deep-vein thrombosis and the incidence of subsequent symptomatic cancer. N Engl J Med 1992;327:1128-33.
8.
Shulman S, Rhedin AS, Lindmarker P, et al. A comparison of six weeks with six months of oral anticoagulant therapy after a first episode of venous thromboembolism. N Engl J Med 1995;332:1661-5.
9.
Kearon C, Gent M, Hirsh J, et al. A comparison of three months of anticoagulation with extended anticoagulation for a first episode of idiopathic venous thromboembolism. N Engl J Med 1999;340:901-7. [Erratum, N Engl J Med 1999;341:298.]
10.
Agnelli G, Prandoni P, Santamaria MG, et al. Three months versus one year of oral anticoagulant therapy for idiopathic deep venous thrombosis. N Engl J Med 2001;345:165-9.
11.
Kearon C. Rate of recurrent venous thromboembolism (VTE) after completing two years of anticoagulation for a first episode of idiopathic VTE. In: Program and abstracts of the XVIII Congress of the International Society on Thrombosis and Haemostasis, Paris, July 6–12, 2001. Stuttgart, Germany: Schattauer, 2001. abstract (computer disk).

12.
Pinede L, Ninet J, Duhaut P, et al. Comparison of 3 and 6 months of oral anticoagulant therapy after a first episode of proximal deep vein thrombosis or pulmonary embolism and comparison of 6 and 12 weeks of therapy after isolated calf deep vein thrombosis. Circulation 2001;103:2453-60.
13.
Baglin T, Luddington R, Brown K, Baglin C. Incidence of recurrent venous thromboembolism in relation to clinical and thrombophilic risk factors: prospective cohort study. Lancet 2003;362:523-6.
14.
Rosendaal FR. Venous thrombosis: a multicausal disease. Lancet 1999;353:1167-73.
15.
Kearon C. Epidemiology of venous thromboembolism. Semin Vasc Med 2001;1:7-26.
16.
Kakkar VV, Howe CT, Flanc C, Clarke MB. Natural history of postoperative deep-vein thrombosis. Lancet 1969;2:230-2.
17.
Stamatakis JD, Kakkar VV, Sagar S, Lawrence D, Nairn D, Bentley PG. Femoral vein thrombosis and total hip -replacement. Br Med J 1977;2:223-5.
18.
Moser KM, LeMoine JR. Is embolic risk conditioned by location of deep venous thrombosis? Ann Intern Med 1981;94:439-44.
19.
Lagerstedt CI, Olsson CB, Fagher BO, Oqvist BW, Albrechtsson U. Need for long-term anticoagulant treatment in patients with symptomatic calf-vein thrombosis. Lancet 1985;2:515-8.

20.
Moser KM, Fedullo PF, LittleJohn JK, Crawford R. Frequent asymptomatic pulmonary embolism in patients with deep venous thrombosis. JAMA 1994;271:223-5. [Erratum, JAMA 1994;271:1908.]
21.
Galle C, Papazyan JP, Miron MJ, Slosman D, Bounameaux H, Perrier A. Prediction of pulmonary embolism extent by clinical findings, D-dimer level and deep vein thrombosis shown by ultrasound. Thromb Haemost 2002;86:1156-60.
22.
Hirsh J, Hoak J. Management of deep vein thrombosis and pulmonary embolism: a statement for healthcare professionals. Circulation 1996;93:2212-45.
23.
Kearon C, Julian JA, Newman TE, Ginsberg JS. Noninvasive diagnosis of deep venous thrombosis. Ann Intern Med 1998;128:663-77. [Erratum, Ann Intern Med 1998;129:425.]
24.
Brandjes DPM, Heijboer H, Buller HR, de Rijk M, Jagt H, ten Cate JW. Acenocoumarol and heparin compared with acenocoumarol alone in the initial treatment of proximal-vein thrombosis. N Engl J Med 1992;327:1485-9.
25.
Abrams J, Frishman WH, Bates SM, Weitz JI, Opie LH. Pharmacologic options for treatment of ischemic disease. In: Antman EM, ed. Cardiovascular therapeutics: a companion to Braunwald's Heart Disease. 2nd ed. Philadelphia: W.B. Saunders, 2002:97-153.

26.
Hirsh J, Warkentin TE, Shaughnessy SG, et al. Heparin and low-molecular-weight heparin: mechanisms of action, pharmacokinetics, dosing, monitoring, efficacy, and safety. Chest 2001;119: Suppl:64S-94S.

27.
Pettila V, Leinonen P, Markkola A, Hiilesmaa V, Kaaja R. Postpartum bone mineral density in women treated for thromboprophylaxis with unfractionated heparin or LMW heparin. Thromb Haemost 2002;87:182-6.

28.
Monreal M, Lafoz E, Olive A, del Rio L, Vedia C. Comparison of subcutaneous unfractionated heparin with a low molecular weight heparin (Fragmin) in patients with venous thromboembolism and contraindications to coumarin. Thromb Haemost 1994;71:7-11.

29.
Warkentin TE, Levine MN, Hirsh J, et al. Heparin-induced thrombocytopenia in patients treated with low-molecular-weight heparin or unfractionated heparin. N Engl J Med 1995;332:1330-5.

30.
Gould MK, Dembitzer AD, Doyle RL, Hastie TJ, Garber AM. Low-molecular-weight heparins compared with unfractionated heparin for treatment of acute venous thrombosis: a meta-analysis of randomized, controlled trials. Ann Intern Med 1999;130:800-9.

31.
Levine MN, Hirsh J, Gent M, et al. A randomized trial comparing activated thromboplastin time with heparin assay in patients with acute venous thromboembolism requiring large daily doses of heparin. Arch Intern Med 1994;154:49-56.

32.
Levine M, Gent M, Hirsh J, et al. A comparison of low-molecular-weight heparin administered primarily at home with unfractionated heparin administered in the hospital for proximal deep-vein thrombosis. N Engl J Med 1996;334:677-81.

33.
Koopman MMW, Prandoni P, Piovella F, et al. Treatment of venous thrombosis with intravenous unfractionated heparin administered in the hospital as compared with subcutaneous low-molecular-weight heparin administered at home. N Engl J Med 1996; 334:682-7. [Erratum, N Engl J Med 1997;337:1251.]

34.
Rodger M, Bredeson C, Wells PS, Beck J, Kearns B, Huebsch LB. Cost-effectiveness of low-molecular-weight heparin and unfractionated heparin in treatment of deep vein thrombosis. CMAJ 1998;159:931-8.

35.
Wells PS, Forster AJ. Thrombolysis in deep vein thrombosis: is there still an indication? Thromb Haemost 2001;86:499-508.

36.
Hyers TM, Agnelli G, Hull RD, et al. Antithrombotic therapy for venous thromboembolic disease. Chest 2001;119:Suppl:176S-193S.

37.
Prins MN, Hutten BA, Koopman MMW, Buller HR. Long-term treatment of venous thromboembolic disease. Thromb Haemost 1999;82:892-8.

38.
Schulman S. Care of patients receiving long-term anticoagulant therapy. N Engl J Med 2003;349:675-83.

39.
Lee AYY, Levine MN, Baker RI, et al. Low-molecular-weight heparin versus a coumarin for the prevention of recurrent venous thromboembolism in patients with cancer. N Engl J Med 2003;349:146-53.

40.
van der Heijden JF, Hutten BA, Buller HR, Prins MH. Vitamin K antagonists or low-molecular-weight heparin for the long term treatment of symptomatic venous thromboembolism. Cochrane Database Syst Rev 2000;4:CD002001.

41.
Decousus H, Leizorovicz A, Parent F, et al. A clinical trial of vena caval filters in the prevention of pulmonary embolism in patients with proximal deep vein thrombosis. N Engl J Med 1998;338: 409-15.

42.
Linkins L, Choi PT, Douketis JD. Clinical impact of bleeding in patients taking oral anticoagulant therapy for venous thromboembolism: a meta-analysis. Ann Intern Med 2003;139: 893-900.

43.
Douketis JD, Kearon C, Bates S, Duku EK, Ginsberg JS. Risk of fatal pulmonary embolism in patients with treated venous thromboembolism. JAMA 1998;279:458-62.

44.
Kearon C. Duration of anticoagulation for venous thromboembolism. J Thromb Thrombolysis 2001;12:59-65.

45.
Ridker PM, Goldhaber SZ, Danielson E, et al. Long-term, low-intensity warfarin therapy for the prevention of recurrent venous thromboembolism. N Engl J Med 2003;348:1425-34.

46.
Kearon C, Ginsberg JS, Kovacs M, et al. Comparison of low-intensity warfarin therapy with conventional-intensity warfarin therapy for long-term prevention of recurrent venous thromboembolism. N Engl J Med 2003;349:631-9.

47.
The MATISSE Investigators. The MATISSE-DVT trial, a randomized, double-blind study comparing once-daily fondaparinux (Arixtra) with low-molecular-weight heparin (LMWH) enoxaparin, twice daily, in the initial treatment of symptomatic deep vein thrombosis (DVT). In: Program and abstracts of the XIX Congress of the International Society on Thrombosis and Haemostasis, Birmingham, England, July 12–18, 2003. Malden, Mass.: Blackwell Publishing, 2003. abstract (computer disk).

48.
Francis CW, Ginsberg JS, Berkowitz SD, et al. Efficacy and safety of the oral direct thrombin inhibitor ximelagatran compared with current standard therapy for acute symptomatic deep vein thrombosis, with or without pulmonary embolism: the THRIVE Treatment Study. Blood 2003;102:6a. abstract.

49.
Schulman S, Wahlander K, Lundstrom T, Clason SB, Eriksson H. Secondary prevention of venous thromboembolism with the oral direct thrombin inhibitor ximelagatran. N Engl J Med 2003;349:1713-21.

50.
Christiansen S, Koster T, Vandenbroucke JP, Rosendaal FR. Risk factors for recurrent venous thrombosis: a prospective follow-up of the Leiden thrombophilia study (LETS). In: Program and abstracts of the XIX Congress of the International Society on Thrombosis and Haemostasis, Birmingham, England, July 12–18, 2003. Malden, Mass.: Blackwell Publishing, 2003. abstract (computer disk).

51.
Baglin T, Luddington R, Brown K, Baglin C. Incidence of recurrent venous thromboembolism in relation to clinical and thrombophilic risk factors. In: Program and abstracts of the XIX Congress of the International Society on Thrombosis and Haemostasis, Birmingham, England, July 12–18, 2003. Malden, Mass.: Blackwell Publishing, 2003. abstract (computer disk).

52.
Margaglinone M, D'Andrea G, Colaizzo D, et al. Coexistence of factor V Leiden and factor II A20210 mutations and recurrent venous thromboembolism. Thromb Haemost 1999;82:1583-7.

53.
Kyrle P, Minar E, Bialonczyk C, Hirschl M, Weltermann A, Eichinger S. The risk of recurrent venous thromboembolism in men and women. N Engl J Med 2004;350:2558-63.

Addendum

Since publication of this article in July 2004, fondaparinux has been approved by the Food and Drug Administration for the initial treatment of venous thromboembolism. However, citing concerns about hepatic toxicity, both the Food and Drug Administration and the French Regulatory Authority (acting as the Reference Member State for the European Mutual Recognition Procedure) have declined to approve ximelagatran for the treatment of venous thrombosis.

A randomized trial evaluating the efficacy of early application of below-knee elastic stockings after the diagnosis of venous thrombosis was published shortly after our paper.[1] The authors concluded that compression stockings reduce the risk of post-thrombotic syndrome by 50 percent. However, given the unblinded design of the study and the lack of specificity and subjective nature of the scale used to diagnose post-thrombotic syndrome, the role of routine stocking therapy remains controversial.

1. Prandoni P, Lensing AW, Prins MH, et al. Below-knee elastic compression stockings to prevent the post-thrombotic syndrome: a randomized, controlled trial. Ann Intern Med 2004;141:249-56.

Bell's Palsy

DONALD H. GILDEN, M.D.

A healthy 50-year-old man notices that his face is drooping on the right side. On examination, facial asymmetry is evident, and some saliva has accumulated on the right side of the patient's mouth. When the patient attempts to close his eyes, his right eye does not close, although it rolls upward, and he is unable to show his teeth or inflate his cheek on the right. How should the patient be evaluated? Does he need immediate treatment?

THE CLINICAL PROBLEM

The most common causes of the abrupt onset of unilateral facial weakness are stroke and Bell's palsy. The patient's history and neurologic examination will determine whether facial weakness is central or peripheral. If weakness is central, brain magnetic resonance imaging (MRI) is required to evaluate the patient for ischemia and for infectious and inflammatory diseases. Other tests — such as examination of the cerebrospinal fluid, sedimentation rate, and glucose level; a blood count; and serologic studies to identify syphilis, the human immunodeficiency virus (HIV), and vasculitis — may be necessary.

If facial weakness is peripheral, no apparent cause will be found in most instances (in the case of Bell's palsy), and no tests are immediately indicated. The incidence of Bell's palsy is 20 to 30 cases per 100,000 people per year[1]; it accounts for 60 to 75 percent of all cases of unilateral facial paralysis.[2] The sexes are affected equally. The median age at onset is 40 years, but the disease may occur at any age.[3] The incidence is lowest in children under 10 years old, increases from the ages of 10 to 29, remains stable at the ages of 30 to 69, and is highest in people over the age of 70. The left and right sides of the face are involved with equal frequency. Most patients recover completely, although some have permanent disfiguring facial weakness.[4] Poor prognostic factors include older age,[1] hypertension,[5] impairment of taste,[6] pain other than in the ear, and complete facial weakness.[7] In the first three days, electrical studies reveal no changes in involved facial muscles, whereas a steady decline in electrical activity is often noted on days 4 to 10. When excitability is retained, 90 percent of patients recover completely; in the absence of excitability, only 20 percent of patients recover completely.[8,9]

Other causes of acquired peripheral facial weakness are much less common. Associated conditions include diabetes mellitus, hypertension, HIV infection, Lyme disease, the Ramsay Hunt syndrome (facial palsy with zoster oticus caused by varicella–zoster virus), sarcoidosis, Sjögren's syndrome, parotid-nerve tumors, eclampsia, and amyloidosis. Peripheral-facial-nerve palsy has also been reported among recipients of inactivated intranasal influenza vaccine.[10]

Bell's palsy rarely recurs. Recurrent or bilateral facial palsy should prompt consideration of myasthenia gravis or lesions at the base of the brain, where the facial nerve exits the pons; such types of palsy occur in lymphoma, sarcoidosis, and Lyme disease.[11] In rare cases, patients with inflammatory demyelinating polyneuropathy (the Guillain–Barré syndrome) present with bilateral facial palsy but relatively little weakness of the extremities. In immunocompetent people, the Ramsay Hunt syndrome is neither recurrent nor bilateral.

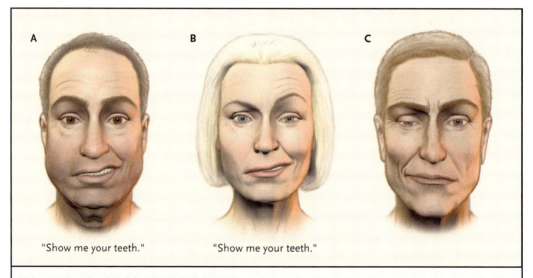

"Show me your teeth."   "Show me your teeth."

Figure 1. Central and Peripheral Facial Weakness.

In response to the request "Show me your teeth," subjects in both Panel A and Panel B demonstrate right lower facial weakness. The man in Panel A has central facial weakness, as demonstrated by the furrows on both sides of the forehead, indicating intact upper facial muscles bilaterally, and he can close both eyes. The woman in Panel B has no furrows on the right side of the forehead, and her right eye is open wider than her left, indicating weak right upper facial muscles. She has peripheral facial weakness caused by a lesion of the facial nerve or in the pons. The man in Panel C has right hemifacial spasm, which can develop not only after peripheral facial paralysis but also with any space-occupying lesion (e.g., a tumor or an ectatic artery) that irritates the facial nerve. Hemifacial spasm produces contraction of his orbicularis oculi muscles, with eye closure and retraction of the muscles of the right lower face. Casual inspection may give the false impression of facial weakness on the opposite (left) side.

Diagnosis

The first step in diagnosis is to determine whether facial weakness is due to a problem in the central nervous system or one in the peripheral nervous system. This is done rapidly with observation and a few questions (Figure 1, Figure 2, Figure 3, and Table 1). Central weakness of the unilateral lower facial area (Figure 1A), which is always due to a lesion above the level of the facial nucleus in the pons of the contralateral hemisphere, is explained by the fact that cells of the facial nucleus that innervate the lower face receive corticobulbar fibers primarily from the contralateral cerebral hemisphere. In contrast, cells of the facial nucleus that innervate the upper face receive corticobulbar fibers originating from both cerebral hemispheres. Thus, a unilateral lesion in the cortex or underlying corticobulbar

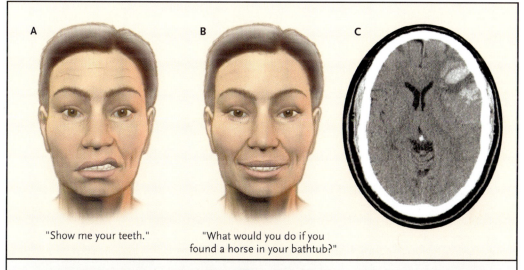

"Show me your teeth."

"What would you do if you found a horse in your bathtub?"

Figure 2. Voluntary Central Facial Weakness That Is Greater Than Mimetic (Involuntary) Central Facial Weakness.

Central facial weakness can be voluntary, mimetic (involuntary), or both. If it is both, it is due to an extensive contralateral hemispheric lesion. When facial weakness is either mostly voluntary or mostly mimetic, the brain site involved can be determined on the basis of the patient's response to a simple request such as "Show me your teeth" (which requires a voluntary response) or a question such as "What would you do if you found a horse in your bathtub?" (which usually elicits a spontaneous smile — i.e., a mimetic response). The examiner should not ask the patient to smile, since that usually elicits a voluntary response. Weakness that is greater during a voluntary contraction than after an involuntary response (i.e., spontaneous laughter) indicates either cortical involvement of the contralateral lower third of the precentral gyrus or subcortical involvement of motor fibers that project from the cortex to the facial nucleus. In response to the request "Show me your teeth," the subject in Panel A shows right lower (central) facial weakness. With a spontaneous smile elicited by the question "What would you do if you found a horse in your bathtub?" (Panel B), no facial weakness is evident; even in the presence of a voluntary central facial palsy, muscles of the lower face contract symmetrically after an involuntary emotional response. In such a case, axial computed tomography of the brain revealed a left hemispheric infarct involving cortical and subcortical structures (Panel C). Because voluntary central facial weakness is greater than mimetic central facial weakness, the cerebral cortex is functionally more damaged than are subcortical structures.

fibers usually produces contralateral voluntary central-type facial paralysis and a contralateral hemiplegia but does not affect salivary and lacrimal secretions or the sense of taste (Table 2).

Peripheral facial palsy, or a weakness or paralysis of all muscles of facial expression (Figure 1B), is usually due to a lesion of the ipsilateral facial nerve but can also be produced by a lesion of the ipsilateral facial nucleus or facial nerve in the pons. Although it appears paradoxical that a "central" lesion in the pons produces peripheral facial weakness, the nomenclature is not likely to change. Facial weakness is best demonstrated by the patient's response to the requests "Close your eyes" (for testing the upper facial area) and "Show me your teeth" (for testing the lower facial area). Denervation of the orbicularis oculi muscles will result in the inability of the patient to close the eyelids effectively, and denervation of the risorius muscle will result in limited retraction of the angle of the mouth (Figure 1B).

Hyperacusis results from paralysis of the stapedius muscle, which dampens vibrations of the ear ossicles and causes sounds to be abnormally loud on the affected side; there is no hearing loss. Also, because the nervus intermedius carries parasympathetic fibers that stimulate salivation and lacrimation, patients with lesions proximal to the geniculate

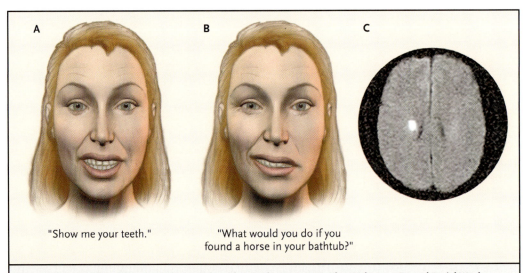

"Show me your teeth."   "What would you do if you found a horse in your bathtub?"

Figure 3. Mimetic (Involuntary) Central Facial Weakness That Is Greater Than Voluntary Central Facial Weakness.

In response to the request "Show me your teeth," the subject in Panel A retracts the muscles of the lower face on both sides. The retraction is slightly greater on the right, a feature suggestive of mild left central facial weakness. With a spontaneous smile elicited by the question "What would you do if you found a horse in your bathtub?" (Panel B), the left central facial weakness is increased, indicative of a deep-seated contralateral hemispheric lesion. In such a case, brain MRI revealed a deep-seated right hemispheric infarct (Panel C). It is not known which pathways mediate mimetic innervation of facial muscles.

Table 1. Diagnosis of Peripheral or Central Facial Weakness and Site of Injury.			
Characteristic	Peripheral*	Central†	
		Voluntary	Mimetic
Weakness in the upper facial area	Yes	No	No
Weakness in the lower facial area	Yes	Yes‡	Yes§
Site of injury¶	Peripheral nerve, pons	Contralateral hemisphere	

* The lesion is ipsilateral to the facial weakness.
† The lesion is contralateral to the weakness in the lower facial area.
‡ The weakness in the lower facial area is greater when the patient responds to the request "Show me your teeth" than when the patient smiles spontaneously.
§ The weakness in the lower facial area is greater when the patient smiles spontaneously than when the patient responds to the request "Show me your teeth."
¶ A facial twitch or spasm preceding the onset of paralysis suggests a tumor, usually outside the pons, that has irritated the facial nerve.

ganglion often have a permanent loss of taste and are unable to produce tears (Figure 4 and Table 2). Rapid recognition of the latter symptom is important, since these patients require artificial tears to lubricate the cornea and may need to have the eye taped shut to prevent drying and infection. Peripheral facial weakness may be confused with hemifacial spasm, in which the corner of the mouth is drawn up and the eye is partially or completely closed because of involuntary contraction of the risorius and orbicularis oculi muscles (Figure 1C). After acute facial paralysis, preganglionic parasympathetic fibers that previously projected to the submandibular ganglion may regrow and enter the major superficial petrosal nerve. Such aberrant regeneration may lead to lacrimation after a salivary stimulus (the syndrome of crocodile tears).

Brain MRI

Brain MRI is not routinely indicated, but if it is performed, the most common abnormality seen is contrast enhancement of the distal intracanalicular and labyrinthine segments of the facial nerve; the geniculate ganglion, as well as the proximal and distal tympanic and mastoid portions of the facial nerve, may also be involved (Figure 5A).[12] A central pontine lesion (e.g., an infarct, as shown in Figure 5B) may also produce facial weakness and is often associated with additional neurologic symptoms and signs.

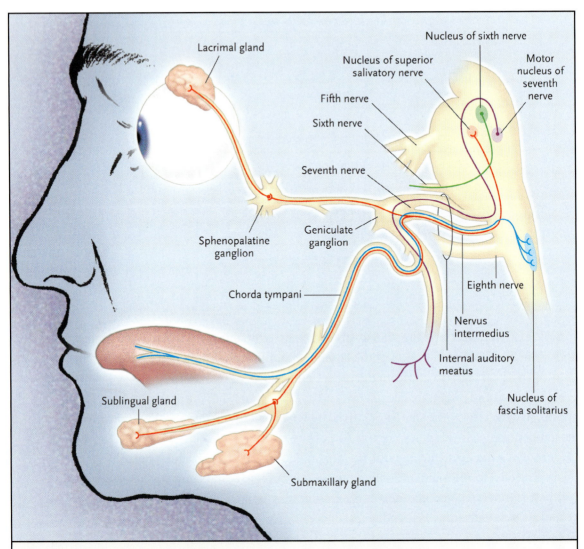

Figure 4. Functional Anatomy of the Facial Nerve and Diagnosis of Peripheral Facial Weakness.

Although the facial nerve has a long, circuitous path, the site of involvement can be deduced from the patient's clinical deficit. The facial, or seventh cranial, nerve is predominantly motor in function. Its nucleus is in the caudal pons. The facial nerve courses dorso-medially and encircles the nucleus of the abducens (sixth) cranial nerve. After bending around the abducens nucleus, the facial nerve lies close to the sixth nerve. The facial nerve exits the pons in the cerebellopontine angle close to the fifth, sixth, and eighth cranial nerves. The eighth nerve, the motor root of the seventh nerve, and the nervus intermedius (the sensory and parasympathetic root of the facial nerve) enter the internal auditory meatus. Sensory cells located in the geniculate ganglion continue distally as the chorda tympani nerve, which carries taste fibers. Peripheral fibers of the nervus intermedius portion of the facial nerve initiate salivary, lacrimal, and mucous secretion.

Electrodiagnostic Studies

Incomplete return of facial motor function and synkinesis (involuntary movement of facial muscles accompanying voluntary facial movement) are long-term sequelae in some patients. These sequelae are predicted by a lack of early clinical improvement in complete facial paralysis and by results of electroneurography; such testing may be clinically useful in patients with complete paralysis. Electroneurography uses a maximal electrically evoked stimulus and recording technique to measure the amplitude of the compound action potential of the facial muscle[13]; the extent of nerve degeneration can be determined by comparing the paralyzed side of the face with the normal side. After facial-nerve compression or complete transection by trauma, axonal degeneration is not evident for a few days. Thus, electrical testing should not be performed until three days after the onset of complete paralysis.

Among patients who do not have 90 percent degeneration within the first three weeks, 80 to 100 percent regain excellent function, with a grade of either 1 (normal strength) or 2 (minimal facial weakness) on the House–Brackmann scale. Among patients who have 90 percent or more degeneration within the first three weeks, only 50 percent have a good recovery of facial function.[14] The rate of degeneration also predicts prognosis; for example, patients with 90 percent degeneration on day 5 have a worse prognosis than

Table 2. Clinical and Anatomical Features of Facial-Nerve Damage.

Site of Damage	Facial-Nerve Signs	Common Associated Features	Common Causes
Cortex, subcortical region	Contralateral central facial weakness; lacrimation, salivation, and taste intact	Contralateral hemiparesis and spasticity	Cortical or subcortical infarct
Pons	Ipsilateral peripheral facial weakness; lacrimation, salivation, and taste intact	Contralateral hemiparesis, sensory loss, ataxia, nystagmus, ipsilateral abducens palsy, ophthalmoparesis	Pontine infarction, glioma, multiple sclerosis
Cerebellopontine angle	Ipsilateral peripheral facial weakness; lacrimation, salivation, and taste usually intact	Tinnitus, facial numbness, ataxia, nystagmus	Acoustic or facial neuroma, meningioma, cholesteatoma, lymphoma, aneurysm, sarcoidosis
Facial nerve in internal auditory canal proximal to or involving geniculate ganglion	Ipsilateral peripheral facial weakness; lacrimation, salivation, and taste likely to be involved	Tinnitus, nystagmus, hearing loss	Bell's palsy, the Ramsay Hunt syndrome, acoustic or facial neuroma
Facial nerve distal to internal auditory canal and geniculate ganglion	Ipsilateral peripheral facial weakness; lacrimation intact but salivation and taste impaired	Tinnitus, nystagmus, hearing loss	Bell's palsy, temporal-bone fracture, cholesteatoma or glomus tumor, middle-ear infection
Facial nerve in stylomastoid foramen	Ipsilateral peripheral facial weakness; lacrimation, salivation, and taste intact	Head injury, parotid mass	Head injury, parotid tumor

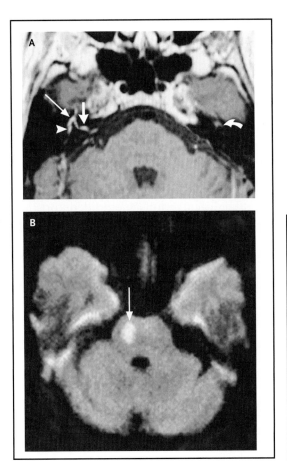

Figure 5. Brain MRIs Contrasting Bell's Palsy with a Central Pontine Infarct.

A T_1-weighted gadolinium-enhanced axial image (Panel A) shows the temporal bones at the level of the facial nerve in a patient with Bell's palsy on the right side. There is enhancement in the geniculate ganglion (long arrow) as well as in the intracanalicular segment (short arrow) and the tympanic segment (arrowhead) of the facial nerve on the right. There is minimal physiologic enhancement of the left geniculate ganglion (curved arrow). Panel B shows a central pontine infarct (arrow) that produced not only ipsilateral peripheral facial weakness and ataxia, but also ophthalmoparesis and contralateral hemisensory loss. (Image showing Bell's palsy courtesy of Dr. Enrique Palacios, Department of Radiology, Louisiana State University Health Science Center, New Orleans.)

those with 90 percent degeneration on day 14. Electroneurography is most useful when performed within two weeks after a complete loss of voluntary facial function.

Medical Treatment

Any evaluation must consider that 71 percent of untreated patients recover completely and 84 percent achieve near-normal function.[5] Thus, the 20 to 30 percent who do not recover fully remain the focus of treatment. Various findings provide a rationale for early and aggressive treatment. First, for more than half a century, surgeons who perform decompression operations on patients with Bell's palsy have described facial-nerve swelling,[15] a finding confirmed by MRI. Second, the detection of herpes simplex virus (HSV) in endoneurial fluid in patients with Bell's palsy[16] has implicated the virus in the pathogenesis of the disease.

Numerous studies of patients with Bell's palsy have compared treatment with glucocorticoids with treatment with acyclovir or placebo; studies comparing antiviral treatment with no treatment have not been performed. One large observational study compared 194 patients treated with prednisone for 12 days (40 mg for 4 days tapered to 8 mg daily by day 12) with 110 untreated patients in a historical control group; complete facial paralysis was observed at follow-up in no patient in the treated group as compared with 10 percent of patients in the untreated group.[17] A later randomized, double-blind, placebo-controlled trial demonstrated a higher rate of recovery of facial function (as assessed by the House–Brackmann grading system) among 35 patients treated with prednisone (30 mg twice daily for five days tapered to 5 mg daily by day 10), as compared with 41 patients given placebo; all the patients in the study were treated within five days after the onset of paralysis.[18] In diabetic patients with complete Bell's palsy who were treated with prednisolone (200 mg for two days tapered to 70 mg by day 7), the rate of cure (i.e., a return to normal facial function) was 97 percent, as compared with 58 percent in untreated patients (P<0.01).[19]

Meta-analyses have also been performed comparing glucocorticoids with placebo. One such analysis, which combined findings from four published studies (one of which was neither blinded nor placebo-controlled), showed significant improvement of facial weakness with glucocorticoid therapy.[20] A second meta-analysis (including only randomized, controlled trials) showed that treatment with glucocorticoids that was started within seven days after the onset of complete facial paralysis increased the likelihood of complete facial recovery by 17 percent (P=0.005), as compared with placebo.[21]

However, not all studies have shown a benefit to glucocorticoid therapy. In one controlled, double-blind trial, rates of recovery were not significantly different between the prednisone and placebo groups after six months[22]; this finding was considered to be potentially attributable to a small sample as well as to a high percentage of patients with initially severe weakness. Another study of 239 patients with Bell's palsy who were randomly assigned to receive either prednisone or placebo showed complete recovery of facial strength in 88 percent of glucocorticoid-treated patients and in 80 percent of the patients in the control group, a difference that was not statistically significant,[23] which is perhaps explained by the fact that patients were followed until complete recovery or for one year.

One randomized trial with no placebo group included 101 patients and compared oral prednisone (1 mg per kilogram of body weight for 10 days tapered to 0 by day 16) with acyclovir (800 mg three times daily for 10 days); the administration of both study drugs was initiated within 4 days after the onset of facial weakness. This study indicated that at three months or later, facial-muscle strength was better after treatment with prednisone than it was after treatment with acyclovir.[24] In another randomized, double-blind trial that included 99 patients, a combination of prednisone and acyclovir (the latter at a dose of 400 mg five times daily) was superior to a combination of prednisone and placebo in restoring the function of voluntary facial muscles (P=0.02) and in preventing partial nerve degeneration (P=0.05).[25] Overall, the data suggest that glucocorticoids decrease the incidence of permanent facial paralysis, although more studies are required to determine whether antiviral therapy confers additional benefit.

Surgical Decompression

Some patients with Bell's palsy may be candidates for surgery. The facial nerve may be compressed (and its conduction blocked) at its narrowest point, the entrance to the meatal foramen, occupied by the labyrinthine segment and geniculate ganglion. Among 12 patients with facial-nerve paralysis who underwent decompression surgery, bulbous swelling of the facial nerve was seen proximal to the geniculate ganglion in 11, and intraoperative evoked-potential electromyography performed in 3 documented conduction block proximal to the geniculate ganglion.[26]

The role of surgical decompression in management remains controversial. In a prospective observational study of 31 patients with complete paralysis and 90 percent or more nerve degeneration as determined by electroneurography, 91 percent of those who underwent decompression had a good outcome (i.e., a grade 1 or 2 on the House–Brackmann scale) by the seventh month, as compared with 42 percent of those who were treated with glucocorticoids.[27] Other observational studies comparing outcomes at 6 to 36 months after prednisone treatment with outcomes after decompression[28-31] have not confirmed a benefit of surgery, however. Data from randomized trials are lacking to compare surgery with medical therapy, and available data are limited by small samples, possible bias in the selection of patients for surgery, the use of varying surgical approaches and systems to assess facial function, and a lack of blinding in studies assessing functional outcomes.

After decompression surgery, permanent unilateral deafness may occur, with estimates ranging from less than 1 percent[27] to 15 percent[29] of patients. Because severe degeneration of the facial nerve is probably irreversible after 2 to 3 weeks,[32] decompression should not be performed 14 days or more after the onset of paralysis.

Cause of Bell's Palsy

Some cases of Bell's palsy have been attributed to ischemia from diabetes and arteriosclerosis, which helps to explain the increased incidence of Bell's palsy in elderly patients; the disorder is analogous to ischemic mononeuropathy of other cranial nerves in patients with diabetes.[33,34] However, HSV type 1 (HSV-1) is probably the cause of most cases of Bell's palsy. Virologic analysis of endoneurial fluid obtained during decompression surgery[16] revealed HSV-1 DNA in 11 of 14 patients with Bell's palsy. HSV-1 DNA appeared to be specific to Bell's palsy, since it was not found in anyone with the Ramsay Hunt syndrome or other neurologic diseases. The rising incidence of Bell's palsy with increasing age parallels seroconversion to HSV-1.[35] Because seropositivity to HSV is well established by adult life, when Bell's palsy is most common, the disease probably reflects virus reactivation from latency in the geniculate ganglion,[36] rather than primary infection. How the virus damages the facial nerve is uncertain.

Treatment

Large randomized, double-blind trials are needed to better assess the effectiveness of glucocorticoids, antiviral agents, or both as compared with placebo, as well as to assess the benefit of surgical decompression among patients considered to be at high risk for permanent paralysis.[37] In particular, studies are needed to determine the time after which medical treatment or surgery is of no value. Furthermore, additional data are needed to determine whether a combination of antiviral and corticosteroid therapy is better than treatment with corticosteroids alone. Of note is the recent observation that long-term recovery of peripheral vestibular function in patients with vestibular neuritis, a condition also attributed to HSV infection, is significantly improved by treatment with corticosteroids but not with valacyclovir.[38]

The Quality Standards Subcommittee of the American Academy of Neurology states that early treatment with oral corticosteroids is probably effective in improving facial-function outcomes in Bell's palsy, that the addition of acyclovir to prednisone is possibly effective, and that insufficient evidence exists to recommend facial-nerve decompression.[37]

SUMMARY AND RECOMMENDATIONS

The first step in evaluating patients with acute facial paralysis is to determine whether the paralysis is central or peripheral. If it is peripheral without any apparent cause (and is thus Bell's palsy), and is diagnosed within one week after the onset of symptoms, as in the patient described in the vignette, no tests are indicated unless other cranial-nerve deficits develop (indicating more widespread disease), there is no recovery three to six weeks after the onset of symptoms, or a facial twitch or spasm preceded Bell's palsy (indicating continuous facial-nerve irritation suggestive of a tumor). The collective findings of facial-nerve swelling, MRI changes consistent with inflammation, and available data regarding clinical outcomes support the use of a short course of prednisone within 2 to 14 days after the onset of symptoms. Because Bell's palsy is associated with HSV infection, antiviral treatment may help, although data are lacking to show that such treatment speeds recovery or leads to a better long-term outcome. In the case described in the vignette, I would treat the patient with oral valacyclovir (1 g twice daily for seven days) or famciclovir (750 mg three times daily) and oral prednisone (1 mg per kilogram per day for seven days). Prednisone should be used cautiously in patients with diabetes, peptic ulcer disease, renal or hepatic dysfunction, or severe hypertension. Either valacyclovir or famciclovir is preferable to acyclovir because adherence to treatment is better than with acyclovir, which requires five daily doses of 800 mg. In children, the dose of prednisone and antiviral agents must be adjusted for weight. The same treatment can be given during pregnancy, although the safety of antiviral agents in pregnancy has not been established. There is no need to taper the dose of prednisone after only one week of treatment.

If complete facial paralysis is still present after one week of medical treatment, electroneurography should be performed. If electroneurography documents 90 percent nerve degeneration, decompression may be considered, although there are no data from clinical trials to support its use.[27] If decompression is performed, timing is critical. The destiny of the facial nerve in Bell's palsy is probably decided within the first two to three weeks after the onset of symptoms.[32] Finally, for patients with permanent facial paralysis, various surgical procedures exist for dynamic reconstruction of the facial nerve.[39]

Supported in part by grants from the National Institutes of Health (NS32623 and AG06127).

I am indebted to Helen MacFarlane for assistance with the figures; to Drs. Nadine Girard, Bodo Kress, Toshibumi Kinoshita, and Enrique Palacios for reviewing the section on brain MRI; to Dr. Steven Deitch for help with computer diagrams; to Drs. Steven Deitch, Deborah Hall, Adam Gilden Tsai, and Kenneth Tyler for a careful critique; to Marina Hoffman for editorial review; and to Cathy Allen for assistance in the preparation of the manuscript.

This article first appeared in the September 23, 2004, issue of the New England Journal of Medicine.

REFERENCES

1.
Hauser WA, Karnes WE, Annis J, Kurland LT. Incidence and prognosis of Bell's palsy in the population of Rochester, Minnesota. Mayo Clin Proc 1971;46: 258-64.

2.
Adour KK, Byl FM, Hilsinger RL Jr, Kahn ZM, Sheldon MI. The true nature of Bell's palsy: analysis of 1,000 consecutive patients. Laryngoscope 1978;88: 787-801.

3.
Katusic SK, Beard CM, Wiederholt WC, Bergstralh EJ, Kurland LT. Incidence, clinical features, and prognosis in Bell's palsy, Rochester, Minnesota 1968-1982. Ann Neurol 1986;20:622-7.

4.
Peitersen E. The natural history of Bell's palsy. Am J Otol 1982;4:107-11.

5.
Adour KK, Wingerd J. Idiopathic facial paralysis (Bell's palsy): factors affecting severity and outcome in 446 patients. Neurology 1974;24:1112-6.

6.
Diamant H, Ekstrand T, Wiberg A. Prognosis of idiopathic Bell's palsy. Arch Otolaryngol 1972;95:431-3.

7.
Cawthorne T, Wilson T. Indications for intratemporal facial nerve surgery. Arch Otolaryngol 1963;78: 429-34.

8.
Campbell EDR, Hickey RP, Nixon KH, Richardson AT. Value of nerve-excitability measurements in prognosis of facial palsy. Br Med J 1962;2:7-10.

9.
Richardson AT. Electrodiagnosis of facial palsies. Ann Otol Rhinol Laryngol 1963;72:569-80.

10.
Mutsch M, Zhou W, Rhodes P, et al. Use of the inactivated intranasal influenza vaccine and the risk of Bell's palsy in Switzerland. N Engl J Med 2004;350: 896-903.

11.
Keane JR. Bilateral seventh nerve palsy: analysis of 43 cases and review of the literature. Neurology 1994;44:1198-202.

12.
Sartoretti-Schefer S, Wichmann W, Valavanis A. Idiopathic, herpetic, and HIV-associated facial nerve palsies: abnormal MR enhancement patterns. AJNR Am J Neuroradiol 1994;15:479-85.

13.
Gantz BJ, Gmuer AA, Holliday M, Fisch U. Electroneurographic evaluation of the facial nerve: method and technical problems. Ann Otol Rhinol Laryngol 1984;93:394-8.

14.
Fisch U. Total facial nerve decompression and electroneuronography. In: Silverstein H, Norrel H, eds. Neurological surgery of the ear. Birmingham, Ala.: Aesculapius, 1977:31-3.

15.
Cawthorne T. The pathology and surgical treatment of Bell's palsy. Proc R Soc Med 1950;4:565-72.

16.
Murakami S, Mizobuchi M, Nakashiro Y, Doi T, Hato N, Yanagihara N. Bell palsy and herpes simplex virus: identification of viral DNA in endoneurial fluid and muscle. Ann Intern Med 1996;124:27-30.

17.
Adour KK, Wingerd J, Bell DN, Manning JJ, Hurley JP. Prednisone treatment for idiopathic facial paralysis (Bell's palsy). N Engl J Med 1972;287: 1268-72.

18.
Austin JR, Peskind SP, Austin SG, Rice DH. Idiopathic facial nerve paralysis: a randomized double blind controlled study of placebo versus prednisone. Laryngoscope 1993;103:1326-33.

19.
Saito O, Aoyagi M, Tojima H, Koike Y. Diagnosis and treatment for Bell's palsy associated with diabetes mellitus. Acta Otolaryngol Suppl 1994;551:153-5.

20.
Williamson IG, Whelan TR. The clinical problem of Bell's palsy: is treatment with steroids effective? Br J Gen Pract 1996;46:743-7.

21.
Ramsey MJ, DerSimonian R, Holtel MR, Burgess LPA. Corticosteroid treatment for idiopathic facial nerve paralysis: a meta-analysis. Laryngoscope 2000;110: 335-41.

22.
May M, Wette R, Hardin WB Jr, Sullivan J. The use of steroids in Bell's palsy: a prospective controlled study. Laryngoscope 1976;86:1111-22.

23.
Wolf SM, Wagner JH, Davidson S, Forsythe A. Treatment of Bell palsy with prednisone: a prospective, randomized study. Neurology 1978;28:158-61.

24.
De Diego JI, Prim MP, De Sarria MJ, Madero R, Gavilan J. Idiopathic facial paralysis: a randomized, prospective, and controlled study using single-dose prednisone versus acyclovir three times daily. Laryngoscope 1998;108:573-5.

25.
Adour KK, Ruboyianes JM, Von Doersten PG, et al. Bell's palsy treatment with acyclovir and prednisone compared with prednisone alone: a double-blind, randomized, controlled trial. Ann Otol Rhinol Laryngol 1996;105:371-8.

26.
Fisch U, Esslen E. Total intratemporal exposure of the facial nerve: pathologic findings in Bell's palsy. Arch Otolaryngol 1972;95:335-41.

27.
Gantz BJ, Rubinstein JT, Gidley P, Woodworth GG. Surgical management of Bell's palsy. Laryngoscope 1999;109:1177-88.

28.
Fisch U. Surgery for Bell's palsy. Arch Otolaryngol 1981;107:1-11.

29.
Brown JS. Bell's palsy: a 5 year review of 174 consecutive cases: an attempted double blind study. Laryngoscope 1982;92:1369-73.

30.
May M, Taylor FH. Bell's palsy: surgery based upon prognostic indicators and results. Laryngoscope 1981;91:2092-103.

31.
May M, Klein SR, Taylor FH. Idiopathic (Bell's) facial palsy: natural history defies steroid or surgical treatment. Laryngoscope 1985;95:406-9.

32.
Fisch U. Prognostic value of electrical tests in acute facial paralysis. Am J Otol 1984;5:494-8.

33.
Merwarth HR. The occurrence of peripheral facial paralysis in hypertensive vascular disease. Ann Intern Med 1942;17:298-307.

34.
Raff MC, Asbury AK. Ischemic mononeuropathy and mononeuropathy multiplex in diabetes mellitus. N Engl J Med 1968;279: 17-22.

35.
Wentworth BB, Alexander ER. Seroepidemiology of infections due to members of the herpesvirus group. Am J Epidemiol 1971;94:496-507.

36.
Furuta Y, Takasu T, Sato KC, Fukuda S, Inuyama Y, Nagashima K. Latent herpes simplex virus type 1 in human geniculate ganglia. Acta Neuropathol (Berl) 1992;84:39-44.

37.
Grogan PM, Gronseth GS. Practice parameter: steroids, acyclovir, and surgery for Bell's palsy (an evidence-based review): report of the Quality Standards Subcommittee of the American Academy of Neurology. Neurology 2001;56:830-6.

38.
Strupp M, Zingler V, Arbusow V, et al. Methylprednisolone, valacyclovir, or the combination for vestibular neuritis. N Engl J Med 2004;351:354-61.

39.
Snyder MC, Johnson PJ. Facial nerve paralysis, dynamic reconstruction. (Accessed January 31, 2006, at http://www.emedicine.com/plastic/topic218.htm.)

The Thyroid Nodule

LASZLO HEGEDÜS, M.D.

A 42-year-old woman presents with a palpable mass on the left side of her neck. She has no neck pain and no symptoms of thyroid dysfunction. Physical examination reveals a solitary, mobile thyroid nodule, 2 cm by 3 cm, without lymphadenopathy. The patient has no family history of thyroid disease and no history of external irradiation. Which investigations should be performed? Assuming that the nodule is benign, which, if any, treatment should be recommended?

THE CLINICAL PROBLEM

In the United States, 4 to 7 percent of the adult population have a palpable thyroid nodule.[1] However, only 1 of 20 clinically identified nodules is malignant. This corresponds to approximately 2 to 4 per 100,000 people per year, constituting only 1 percent of all cancers and 0.5 percent of all cancer deaths.[2] Nodules are more common in women and increase in frequency with age and with decreasing iodine intake. The prevalence is much greater with the inclusion of nodules that are detected by ultrasonography or at autopsy. By the latter assessment, approximately 50 percent of 60-year-old persons have thyroid nodules.[3]

The clinical spectrum ranges from the incidental, asymptomatic, small, solitary nodule, in which the exclusion of cancer is the major concern, to the large, partly intrathoracic nodule that causes pressure symptoms, for which treatment is warranted regardless of cause.[3] The most common diagnoses and their approximate distributions are colloid nodules, cysts, and thyroiditis (in 80 percent of cases); benign follicular neoplasms (in 10 to 15 percent); and thyroid carcinoma (in 5 percent).

The management of a solitary thyroid nodule remains controversial.[3-5] This review will focus on the management of a solitary thyroid nodule that is detected on physical examination, regardless of the finding of additional nodules by radionuclide scanning or ultrasonography, since such a finding does not alter the risk of cancer.[3]

Table 1. Clinical Findings Suggesting the Diagnosis of Thyroid Carcinoma in a Euthyroid Patient with a Solitary Nodule, According to the Degree of Suspicion.

High suspicion

Family history of medullary thyroid carcinoma or multiple endocrine neoplasia

Rapid tumor growth, especially during levothyroxine therapy

A nodule that is very firm or hard

Fixation of the nodule to adjacent structures

Paralysis of vocal cords

Regional lymphadenopathy

Distant metastases

Moderate suspicion

Age of either <20 years or >70 years

Male sex

History of head and neck irradiation

A nodule >4 cm in diameter or partially cystic

Symptoms of compression, including dysphagia, dysphonia, hoarseness, dyspnea, and cough

STRATEGIES AND EVIDENCE

History and Physical Examination

The history and physical examination remain the diagnostic cornerstones in evaluating the patient with a thyroid nodule and may be suggestive of thyroid carcinoma (Table 1). However, a minority of patients with malignant nodules have suggestive findings, which often also occur in patients with benign thyroid disorders. There is also substantial variation among practitioners in evaluating nodules,[2,6] a finding that may explain why an increasing number of thyroid specialists use imaging as part of the evaluation.[4,5]

The risk of thyroid cancer seems nearly as high in incidental nodules (<10 mm), the majority of which escape detection by palpation, as in larger nodules.[7] However, the vast majority of these microcarcinomas do not grow during long-term follow-up and do not cause clinically significant thyroid cancer.[8] The fact that ultrasonography detects nodules (a third of which are more than 20 mm in diameter) in up to 50 percent of patients with a normal neck examination underscores the low specificity and sensitivity of clinical examination.[9] When two or more risk factors that indicate a high clinical suspicion are present, the likelihood of cancer approaches 100 percent.[10] In such cases, biopsy is still useful to guide the type of surgery[1,2] (Figure 1).

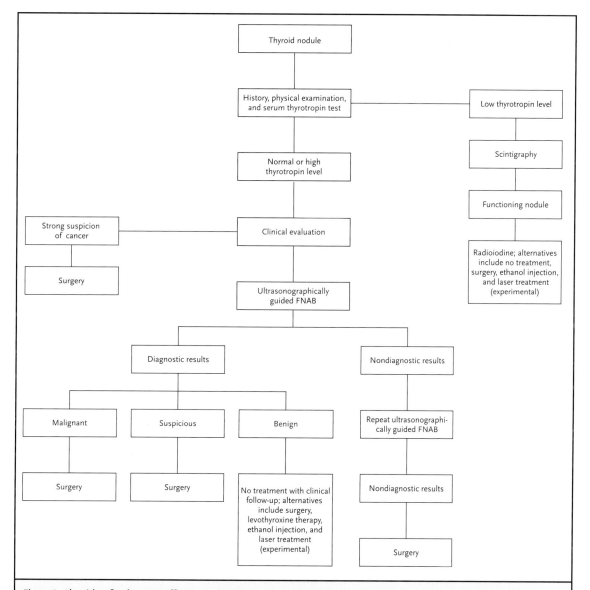

Figure 1. Algorithm for the Cost-Effective Evaluation and Treatment of a Clinically Detectable Solitary Thyroid Nodule.

In the case of a strong clinical suspicion of cancer, surgery is recommended, regardless of the results of fine-needle aspiration biopsy (FNAB). In the case of a suppressed level of serum thyrotropin, thyroid scintigraphy should be performed, since a functioning nodule almost invariably rules out cancer. In the case of a nondiagnostic FNAB, a repeated biopsy yields a satisfactory aspirate in 50 percent of cases. If ultrasonography reveals additional nodules that are more than 10 mm in diameter, FNAB could be performed on one other nodule, in addition to the one that is clinically detectable. The therapeutic options shown cover both solid and cystic nodules. In the case of a recurrent cyst, the possibilities of treatment are repeated FNAB, surgery, and ethanol injection. I do not recommend levothyroxine therapy for the thyroid nodule.

Laboratory Investigations

Because clinical examination is not sensitive for identifying thyroid dysfunction,[6] laboratory evaluation of thyroid function is routinely warranted. The only biochemical test routinely needed is measurement of the serum thyrotropin level. If this level is subnormal, levels of free thyroxine or free triiodothyronine should be measured to document the presence and degree of hyperthyroidism. Approximately 10 percent of patients with a solitary nodule have a suppressed level of serum thyrotropin, which suggests a benign hyperfunctioning nodule.[2] If the serum thyrotropin concentration is elevated, a serum antithyroperoxidase antibody level should be obtained to confirm Hashimoto's thyroiditis. However, the finding of an elevated level does not obviate the need for a fine-needle aspiration biopsy, since the practitioner must rule out a coexisting cancer, including lymphoma, which accounts for only 5 percent of thyroid cancers but is associated with Hashimoto's thyroiditis.[11] Nearly all patients with thyroid cancer are euthyroid.[1]

If a patient has a family history of medullary thyroid cancer or multiple endocrine neoplasia type 2, a basal serum calcitonin level should be obtained; an elevated level suggests medullary thyroid cancer. Before surgery is performed, investigation for primary hyperparathyroidism and pheochromocytoma should be carried out. Serum calcitonin is not routinely measured in patients who have no suggestive family history, since medullary carcinoma is present in only about 1 of 250 patients with a thyroid nodule.[12]

Imaging of the Thyroid Nodule

Radionuclide Scanning   Radionuclide scanning, which is performed much more commonly in Europe than in the United States,[3-5] may be used to identify whether a nodule is functioning (Figure 2). A functioning nodule, with or without suppression of extranodular uptake, is nearly always benign, whereas a nonfunctioning nodule, constituting approximately 90 percent of nodules, has a 5 percent risk of being malignant. Thus, in the patient with a suppressed level of serum thyrotropin, radionuclide confirmation of a functioning nodule may obviate the need for biopsy. A scan can also indicate whether a clinically solitary nodule is a dominant nodule in an otherwise multinodular gland and can reveal substernal extension of the thyroid. A scan can be performed with iodine-123, iodine-131, or technetium-99m–labeled pertechnetate. Iodine isotopes, which are both trapped and bound organically in the thyroid, are preferred, since 3 to 8 percent of nodules that appear functioning on pertechnetate scanning may appear nonfunctioning on radioiodine scanning, and a few of those nodules may be thyroid cancers.[13] A scan cannot be used to measure the size of a nodule accurately.

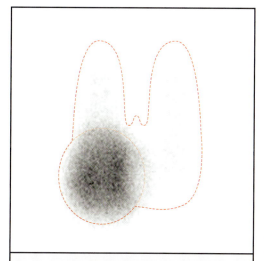

Figure 2. Scintigram of a Solitary Functioning Nodule in the Right Thyroid Lobe.

Scintigraphy that was performed with the use of technetium-99m–labeled pertechnetate shows suppression of extranodular uptake in thyroid tissue.

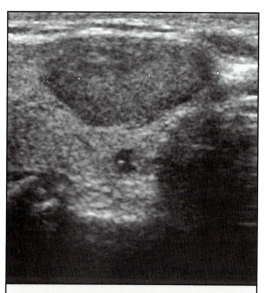

Figure 3. Cross-Sectional Ultrasonogram Showing a Solid, Hypoechoic Nodule (Dark Gray) in the Right Thyroid Lobe.

Ultrasonography Ultrasonography can accurately detect nonpalpable nodules, estimate the size of the nodule and the volume of the goiter, and differentiate simple cysts, which have a low risk of being malignant, from solid nodules or from mixed cystic and solid nodules, which have a 5 percent risk of being malignant (Figure 3). Ultrasonography also provides guidance for diagnostic procedures (e.g., fine-needle aspiration biopsy) as well as therapeutic procedures (e.g., cyst aspiration, ethanol injection, or laser therapy) and facilitates the monitoring of the effects of treatment.[9] In one study, among patients who had been referred for evaluation of a palpable thyroid abnormality, ultrasonography altered the clinical management in two thirds of cases,[14] mainly by identifying nodules that were smaller than 1 cm (which were not considered to require further evaluation) in 20 percent of the patients and by discovering additional nodules (which required biopsy) in 24 percent of the patients. Characteristics revealed by ultrasonography — such as hypoechogenicity, microcalcifications, irregular margins, increased nodular flow visualized by Doppler, and, especially, the evidence of invasion or regional lymphadenopathy — are associated with an increased risk of cancer; however, sonographic findings cannot reliably distinguish between benign and cancerous lesions.[9]

Other Methods   Computed tomography (CT) and magnetic resonance imaging also cannot reliably differentiate between malignant and benign nodules. These tests are rarely indicated in the evaluation of a nodule. An exception is in the diagnosis and evaluation of substernal goiters, since these imaging techniques can assess the extent of the goiter more precisely than can other techniques and can evaluate tracheal compression.[3,15] Evaluation of glucose metabolism by positron-emission tomography using fludeoxyglucose (fluorodeoxyglucose) F 18 may help in distinguishing benign from malignant nodules, but its use is limited by cost and accessibility[16] and it cannot replace biopsy.

Fine-Needle Aspiration Biopsy

Independent of morphology, fine-needle aspiration provides the most direct and specific information about a thyroid nodule. It is performed on an outpatient basis,[1,4,5] is relatively inexpensive, and is easy to learn. Complications are rare and primarily involve local discomfort. The use of anticoagulants or salicylates does not preclude biopsy. In centers with experience in fine-needle aspiration, the use of this technique has been estimated to reduce the number of thyroidectomies by approximately 50 percent, to roughly double the surgical confirmation of carcinoma, and to reduce the overall cost of medical care by 25 percent,[17] as compared with surgery performed on the basis of clinical findings alone.

Fine-needle aspiration has diagnostically useful results in about 80 percent of cases,[18] typically with two to four passes of the needle. The number of cases in which sufficient samples are obtained increases if aspiration is guided by ultrasonography, especially in nodules that are partly cystic, and repeated biopsy reduces by half the rate of insufficient samples (to about 10 percent).[19,20] The diagnostic accuracy of fine-needle aspiration depends on the way in which suspicious lesions are handled. Viewing them as "positive" increases sensitivity (rate of false negative results, 1 percent), but decreases specificity.[21] If fine-needle aspiration reveals a follicular neoplasm (which occurs in approximately 15 percent of nodules, of which only 20 percent turn out to be malignant), radionuclide scanning should be performed.[1-3] If such scanning shows a functioning nodule with or without complete suppression of the rest of the thyroid, surgery can be avoided, since the risk of cancer is negligible.[17] In a cystic lesion or one that is a mixture of cystic and solid components, fine-needle aspiration of a possible solid component should be performed, since the risk of cancer is the same as that for a solid nonfunctioning nodule.[2,20,21] With the exception of calcitonin immunostaining for medullary carcinoma, there are no reliable immunohistologic or molecular tests for distinguishing between benign and malignant nodules.[3]

Table 2. Treatment of the Single Nonmalignant Thyroid Nodule.

Treatment Type	Advantages	Disadvantages
Surgery	Nodule ablation, complete relief of symptoms, definite histologic diagnosis	Need for hospitalization, high cost, risks associated with surgery, vocal-cord paralysis (approximately 1% of patients), hypoparathyroidism (<1%), hypothyroidism (approximately 1%*)
Levothyroxine	No need for hospitalization, low cost, may slow nodule growth, may prevent new nodule formation	Low efficacy, need for lifelong treatment, regrowth of nodule after cessation of treatment, cardiac tachyarrhythmias, reduced bone density, not feasible when thyrotropin level is suppressed
Radioiodine†	No need for hospitalization, low cost, few subjective side effects, nodule reduced by 40% in 1 yr	Use of contraceptives needed in fertile women, only gradual reduction of the nodule, hypothyroidism within 5 yr (10% of patients), risk of radiation thyroiditis and thyrotoxicosis
Ethanol injection	No need for hospitalization, relatively low cost, no hypothyroidism, nodule reduced by 45% in 6 mo	Limited experience with treatment, decreasing efficacy with increasing nodule size, success dependent on operator's skill, painful (reducing compliance), risk of thyrotoxicosis and vocal-cord paralysis (approximately 1–2%), seepage of ethanol,‡ interpretation of cytologic and histologic findings impeded in treated nodules
Laser therapy§		

* This risk applies only to the case of hemithyroidectomy.
† This treatment is used only for the functioning thyroid nodule.
‡ Side effects due to the seepage of ethanol outside the nodule, which are rare (occurring in about 1 percent of patients), comprise nerve damage, perinodular or periglandular fibrosis jeopardizing subsequent surgery, thrombosis of the jugular vein, and neck hematomas.
§ Laser therapy is still experimental, and experience with it is limited. The advantages are the same as those of ethanol injection, but side effects are probably more limited because the higher degree of control with laser therapy limits the risk of extranodular damage.

Treatment of the Solitary Thyroid Nodule

The natural history of solitary thyroid nodules is poorly understood, mainly because nodules that are suspicious for cancer, cause pressure, or prompt reports of cosmetic problems are rarely left untreated. With this reservation, it seems that the majority of benign nonfunctioning nodules grow, particularly those that are solid.[22-24] In one study, 89 percent of nodules that were followed for five years increased by 15 percent or more in volume.[24] The annual rate of evolution of a solitary functioning nodule into a hyperfunctioning nodule is as high as 6 percent; the risk is positively related to the size of the nodule and negatively related to the serum thyrotropin level.[25,26] There is controversy as to whether a solitary nodule should be treated and, if so, how.[4,5] Table 2 summarizes the advantages and disadvantages of potential treatment options. Figure 1 shows a management algorithm.

Levothyroxine Treatment with levothyroxine at a dose sufficient to keep the serum thyrotropin at a level below 0.3 mU per liter has been suggested as a way to prevent growth of an apparently benign nodule. However, this approach has clear limitations. A recent meta-analysis showed no significant difference in the size of nodules after 6 to 12 months of suppressive therapy with levothyroxine, as compared with no treatment, although the size of the nodules decreased by more than 50 percent in a larger proportion of levothyroxine-treated patients than in patients who had no treatment.[27] The likelihood of such shrinkage is greater when serum thyrotropin is suppressed to a level below 0.1 mU per liter than it is when the level is below 0.3 mU.[27-29] In a five-year, randomized trial, suppression to below 0.1 mU per liter significantly reduced the frequency with which new nodules developed (i.e., 8 percent of patients who were treated with levothyroxine as compared with 29 percent of untreated patients).[29] However, therapy with levothyroxine to reduce thyrotropin levels below 0.1 mU per liter is associated with an increased risk of atrial fibrillation, other cardiac abnormalities,[30,31] and reduced bone density.[32] Regrowth of nodules occurs after cessation of therapy. Levothyroxine has no effect on the recurrence of thyroid cysts after aspiration.[33]

Surgery   The main indications for surgery are clinical or cytologic features suggestive of cancer or symptoms due to the nodule (Table 1).[4,5] If preoperative cytology suggests a benign lesion, hemithyroidectomy is generally preferred.[4,5,18] Postoperative administration of levothyroxine is indicated only in cases of hypothyroidism.[34] When surgery is performed by a specialist, the incidence of complications is low (i.e., postoperative hypoparathyroidism in 1 percent of cases and injuries to the recurrent laryngeal nerve in about 1 percent), but the complication rate is higher for less experienced surgeons and those without special training.[35]

Radioiodine   Radioiodine is an option for treatment of a functioning nodule, with or without biochemical hyperthyroidism. It is contraindicated in pregnant and breast-feeding women. Normalization of the results of thyroid radionuclide scanning and the serum thyrotropin level (often referred to as a "cure") is achieved in 75 percent of patients, and thyroid volume is reduced an average of 40 percent, after a single dose of iodine-131 aiming at a level of 100 Gy, independent of pretreatment thyroid function.[36,37] The main side effect is hypothyroidism, which occurs in approximately 10 percent of patients within five years after treatment and increases in frequency over time. This risk is unrelated to dose but is greater in patients with thyroid peroxidase antibodies and with iodine uptake in extranodular thyroid tissue.[36,37] Most nodules do not disappear after radioiodine therapy but may become harder on palpation and may reveal unusual cytologic features as a result of irradiation. Thyroid function should be checked regularly during the first year and yearly thereafter in order to detect hypothyroidism. Nodules are unlikely to grow after radioiodine therapy, but if growth occurs, a biopsy may be warranted.

Percutaneous Ethanol Injection   A number of studies have suggested a benefit of ultraso-nographically guided ethanol injection in the treatment of benign functioning and non-functioning solid thyroid nodules as well as cystic nodules.[38-40] The mechanism of effect involves coagulative necrosis and small-vessel thrombosis. The procedure requires prior documentation of benign cytology, skill, and experience[3,9]; drawbacks include local pain and a potential risk of serious side effects (Table 2). There are few data from controlled trials to support this approach.

Available data suggest that multiple injections of ethanol (a median of four) can achieve a complete cure (i.e., a normalization of results of radionuclide scanning and serum thyro-tropin measures) in two thirds of patients with hyperfunctioning nodules and three quar-ters of patients with functioning nodules without hyperthyroidism.[38,39] In solid nonfunc-tioning nodules that are solitary and cytologically benign, a single ethanol injection has been shown to reduce the volume of nodules by approximately 50 percent.[3,23] Additional ethanol injections have only a limited effect.[41,42] Recently, data from a preliminary study suggested that the use of laser photocoagulation may be as effective as ethanol injection, with fewer adverse effects.[43] However, controlled trials are needed.

In thyroid cysts, the recurrence rate after aspiration is high. Tetracycline, a sclerosing agent, had no effect in a randomized study.[44] Uncontrolled studies have suggested that ethanol injection may prevent the recurrence of cysts.[39,40] A recent randomized, double-blind study[45] involving a six-month follow-up period reported that 21 of 33 patients (64 percent) who were treated with ethanol were cured after one session, as compared with 6 of 33 patients (18 percent) who were treated with saline.

AREAS OF UNCERTAINTY

There are no data from studies comparing the outcome and cost-effectiveness of various strategies of evaluating a nodule (e.g., using radionuclide imaging and ultrasonographic guidance for fine-needle aspiration). There are also insufficient data comparing the outcome (including quality of life) of various management approaches in the absence of cancer.

GUIDELINES FROM PROFESSIONAL SOCIETIES

Clinical-practice guidelines were published in 1996 by the American Thyroid Association[1] (http://www.thyroid.org/professionals/publications/guidelines.html) and the Ameri-can Association of Clinical Endocrinologists[46] (http://www.aace.com/clin/guidelines/thyroid_nodules.pdf). The recommendations of both organizations correspond with those provided here. Radionuclide scanning is not routinely recommended, but it is advocated in the case of a suppressed level of serum thyrotropin or the finding of follicular neo-plasia with the use of fine-needle aspiration. Thyroid ultrasonography is recommended to guide fine-needle aspiration, especially in nodules that are small and incidental or are partly cystic or from which primary fine-needle aspiration has yielded insufficient material. Fine-needle biopsy of all possibly malignant nodules (which are not defined in the guidelines) is advocated. If the cytology is benign, repeated biopsy is seldom indicated.

In the case of a benign nodule, periodic lifelong follow-up every 6 to 24 months (including measurement of serum thyrotropin levels, neck palpation, and fine-needle aspiration in case of growth or other suspicious signs) is recommended. For a functioning benign nodule, iodine-131 is considered the treatment of choice, with surgery as an alternative, especially if the nodule is very large or partly cystic or if the patient is young; treatment is more strongly recommended if the serum thyrotropin level is decreased or overt hyperthyroidism is present, because of adverse effects on bone and the cardiovascular system. For a nonfunctional benign nodule, there is no clear recommendation on the use of levothyroxine, although this therapy is considered contraindicated when the serum thyrotropin level is suppressed, in patients more than 60 years old, and in postmenopausal women. If levothyroxine therapy is used, regular reassessment (the interval is not defined in the guidelines) is recommended, with monitoring of serum thyrotropin levels, which should be subnormal but measurable. The guidelines do not address ethanol injection and laser therapy.

CONCLUSIONS AND RECOMMENDATIONS

For the patient who presents with a nodule, as in the case described in the vignette, the main concern is to exclude the possibility of thyroid cancer, even though the vast majority of nodules are benign (Figure 1). The initial evaluation should include measurement of the serum thyrotropin level and a fine-needle aspiration, preferably guided by ultrasonography. If the patient has a family history of medullary thyroid carcinoma or multiple endocrine neoplasia type 2, the serum calcitonin level should also be checked. If the thyrotropin level is suppressed, radionuclide scanning should be performed. In patients less than 20 years old, and in the case of a high clinical suspicion for cancer (e.g., follicular neoplasia as diagnosed by fine-needle aspiration and a nonfunctioning nodule revealed on scanning), the patient should be offered hemithyroidectomy regardless of the results of fine-needle aspiration.

In the case of a functioning benign nodule, iodine-131 is generally the therapy of choice, independent of concomitant hyperthyroidism. For nonfunctioning cystic nodules, aspiration and ethanol injection therapy may be considered, and ethanol injection or laser therapy if the nodules are solid, but data to support the use of these therapies are limited. My usual approach after documenting benign cytology is to follow the patient yearly with neck palpation and measurement of the serum thyrotropin level, with repeated ultrasonography and fine-needle aspiration if there is evidence of growth of the nodule. I do not recommend levothyroxine therapy to shrink or prevent growth of benign nodules because of the drug's low efficacy and potential side effects.

Dr. Hegedüs reports having received grants from the Agnes and Knut Mørk Foundation, the Novo Nordisk Foundation, and the A.P. Møller Relief Foundation.

I am indebted to Dr. Steen J. Bonnema and Dr. Finn N. Bennedbæk for their helpful comments.

This article first appeared in the October 21, 2004, issue of the New England Journal of Medicine.

REFERENCES

1.
Singer PA, Cooper DS, Daniels GH, et al. Treatment guidelines for patients with thyroid nodules and well-differentiated thyroid cancer. Arch Intern Med 1996;156:2165-72.
2.
Wong CKM, Wheeler MH. Thyroid nodules: rational management. World J Surg 2000;24:934-41.
3.
Hegedüs L, Bonnema SJ, Bennedbæk FN. Management of simple nodular goiter: current status and future perspectives. Endocr Rev 2003;24:102-32.
4.
Bennedbæk FN, Perrild H, Hegedüs L. Diagnosis and treatment of the solitary thyroid nodule: results of a European survey. Clin Endocrinol (Oxf) 1999;50:357-63.
5.
Bennedbæk FN, Hegedüs L. Management of the solitary thyroid nodule: results of a North American survey. J Clin Endocrinol Metab 2000;85:2493-8.
6.
Jarløv AE, Nygaard B, Hegedüs L, Hartling SG, Hansen JM. Observer variation in the clinical and laboratory evaluation of patients with thyroid dysfunction and goiter. Thyroid 1998;8:393-8.

7.
Papini E, Guglielmi R, Bianchini A, et al. Risk of malignancy in nonpalpable thyroid nodules: predictive value of ultrasound and color-Doppler features. J Clin Endocrinol Metab 2002;87:1941-6.
8.
Ito Y, Uruno T, Nakano K, et al. An observation trial without surgical treatment in patients with papillary microcarcinoma of the thyroid. Thyroid 2003;13:381-7.
9.
Hegedüs L. Thyroid ultrasound. Endocrinol Metab Clin North Am 2001;30:339-60.
10.
Hamming JF, Goslings BM, van Steenis FJ, van Ravenswaay Claasen H, Hermans J, van de Velde CJ. The value of fine-needle aspiration biopsy in patients with nodular thyroid disease divided into groups of suspicion of malignant neoplasms on clinical grounds. Arch Intern Med 1990;150:113-6. [Erratum, Arch Intern Med 1990;150:1088.]
11.
Pasieka JL. Hashimoto's disease and thyroid lymphoma: role of the surgeon. World J Surg 2000;24:966-70.

12.
Elisei R, Bottici V, Luchetti F, et al. Impact of routine measurement of serum calcitonin on the diagnosis and the outcome of medullary thyroid cancer: experience in 10,864 patients with nodular thyroid disorders. J Clin Endocrinol Metab 2004;89:163-8.
13.
Shambaugh GE III, Quinn JL, Oyasu R, Freinkel N. Disparate thyroid imaging: combined studies with sodium pertechnetate Tc 99m and radioactive iodine. JAMA 1974;228:866-9.
14.
Marqusee E, Benson CB, Frates MC, et al. Usefulness of ultrasonography in the management of nodular thyroid disease. Ann Intern Med 2000;133:696-700.
15.
Jennings A. Evaluation of substernal goiters using computed tomography and MR imaging. Endocrinol Metab Clin North Am 2001;30:401-14.
16.
Kang KW, Kim S-K, Kang H-S, et al. Prevalence and risk of cancer of focal thyroid incidentaloma identified by 18F-fluorodeoxyglucose positron emission tomography for metastasis evaluation and cancer screening in healthy subjects. J Clin Endocrinol Metab 2003;88:4100-4.
17.
Mazzaferri EL. Management of a solitary thyroid nodule. N Engl J Med 1993;328:553-9.
18.
Burch HB. Evaluation and management of the solid thyroid nodule. Endocrinol Metab Clin North Am 1995;24:663-710.

19.
Danese D, Sciacchitano S, Farsetti A, Andreoli M, Pontecorvi A. Diagnostic accuracy of conventional vs. sonography-guided fine-needle aspiration biopsy of thyroid nodules. Thyroid 1998;8:15-21.
20.
Gharib H, Goellner JR. Fine-needle aspiration biopsy of the thyroid: an appraisal. Ann Intern Med 1993;118:282-9.
21.
Hamburger JI. Diagnosis of thyroid nodules by fine needle biopsy: use and abuse. J Clin Endocrinol Metab 1994;79:335-9.
22.
Kuma K, Matsuzuka F, Kobayashi A, et al. Outcome of long standing solitary thyroid nodules. World J Surg 1992;16:583-7.
23.
Bennedbæk FN, Nielsen LK, Hegedüs L. Effect of percutaneous ethanol injection therapy vs. suppressive doses of L-thyroxine on benign solitary solid cold thyroid nodules: a randomised trial. J Clin Endocrinol Metab 1998;83:30-5.
24.
Alexander EK, Hurwitz S, Heering JP, et al. Natural history of benign solid and cystic thyroid nodules. Ann Intern Med 2003;138:315-8.
25.
Hamburger JI. Evolution of toxicity in solitary nontoxic autonomously functioning thyroid nodules. J Clin Endocrinol Metab 1980;50:1089-93.
26.
Sandrock D, Olbricht T, Emrich D, Benker G, Reinwein D. Long-term follow-up in patients with autonomous thyroid adenoma. Acta Endocrinol (Copenh) 1993;128:51-5.

27.
Castro MR, Caraballo PJ, Morris JC. Effectiveness of thyroid hormone suppressive therapy in benign solitary thyroid nodules: a meta-analysis. J Clin Endocrinol Metab 2002;87:4154-9.

28.
Zelmanovitz F, Genro S, Gross JL. Suppressive therapy with levothyroxine for solitary thyroid nodules: a double-blind controlled clinical study and cumulative meta-analyses. J Clin Endocrinol Metab 1998;83:3881-5.

29.
Papini E, Petrucci L, Guglielmi R, et al. Long-term changes in nodular goiter: a 5-year prospective randomised trial of levothyroxine suppressive therapy for benign cold thyroid nodules. J Clin Endocrinol Metab 1998;83:780-3.

30.
Sawin CT, Geller A, Wolf PA, et al. Low serum thyrotropin concentrations as a risk factor for atrial fibrillation in older persons. N Engl J Med 1994;331:1249-52.

31.
Surks MI, Ortiz E, Daniels GH, et al. Subclinical thyroid disease: scientific review and guidelines for diagnosis and management. JAMA 2004;291:228-38.

32.
Uzzan B, Campos J, Cucherat M, Nony P, Boissel JP, Perret GY. Effects on bone mass of long term treatment with thyroid hormones: a meta-analysis. J Clin Endocrinol Metab 1996;81:4278-89.

33.
McCowen KD, Reed JW, Fariss BL. The role of thyroid therapy in patients with thyroid cysts. Am J Med 1980;68:853-5.

34.
Hegedüs L, Nygaard B, Hansen JM. Is routine thyroxine treatment to hinder postoperative recurrence of nontoxic goiter justified? J Clin Endocrinol Metab 1999;84:756-60.

35.
Songun I, Kievit J, Wobbes T, Peerdeman A, van de Velde CJ. Extent of thyroidectomy in nodular thyroid disease. Eur J Surg 1999;165:839-42.

36.
Ferrari C, Reschini E, Paracchi A. Treatment of the autonomous thyroid nodule: a review. Eur J Endocrinol 1996;135:383-90.

37.
Nygaard B, Hegedüs L, Nielsen KG, Ulriksen P, Hansen JM. Long-term effect of radioactive iodine on thyroid function and size in patients with solitary autonomously functioning toxic thyroid nodules. Clin Endocrinol (Oxf) 1999;50:197-202.

38.
Lippi F, Ferrari C, Manetti L, et al. Treatment of solitary autonomous thyroid nodules by percutaneous ethanol injection: results of an Italian multicenter study. J Clin Endocrinol Metab 1996;81:3261-4.

39.
Bennedbæk FN, Karstrup S, Hegedüs L. Percutaneous ethanol injection therapy in the treatment of thyroid and parathyroid diseases. Eur J Endocrinol 1997;136:240-50.

40.
Verde G, Papini E, Pacella CM, et al. Ultrasound guided percutaneous ethanol injection in the treatment of cystic thyroid nodules. Clin Endocrinol (Oxf) 1994;41:719-24.

41.
Bennedbæk FN, Hegedüs L. Percutaneous ethanol injection therapy in benign solitary solid cold thyroid nodules: a randomised trial comparing one injection with three injections. Thyroid 1999;9:225-33.

42.
Zingrillo M, Collura D, Ghiggi MR, Nirchio V, Trischitta V. Treatment of large cold benign thyroid nodules not eligible for surgery with percutaneous ethanol injection. J Clin Endocrinol Metab 1998;83:3905-7.

43.
Døssing H, Bennedbæk FN, Karstrup S, Hegedüs L. Benign solitary solid cold thyroid nodules: US-guided interstitial laser photocoagulation — initial experience. Radiology 2002;225:53-7.

44.
Hegedüs L, Hansen JM, Karstrup S, Torp-Pedersen S, Juul N. Tetracycline for sclerosis of thyroid cysts: a randomized study. Arch Intern Med 1988;148:1116-8.

45.
Bennedbæk FN, Hegedüs L. Treatment of recurrent thyroid cysts with ethanol: a randomized double-blind controlled trial. J Clin Endocrinol Metab 2003;88:5773-7.

46.
Feld S, Garcia M, Baskin HJ, et al. AACE clinical practice guidelines for the diagnosis and management of thyroid nodules. Endocr Pract 1996;2:78-84.

Hypersensitivity to Hymenoptera Stings

THEODORE M. FREEMAN, M.D.

A 29-year-old man reported that he was stung by a flying hymenopteran — he does not know what type — outside his door, where he had previously noted a nest. Skin itching, diffuse hives, swelling of his arms and legs, tightness in his throat, dizziness, and difficulty talking developed immediately, and he was taken to a local clinic where he received epinephrine and antihistamines. He was observed for two hours, and all symptoms resolved. How should his case be managed subsequently?

THE CLINICAL PROBLEM

Insects of the order Hymenoptera, which includes ants, bees, hornets, wasps, and yellow jackets, have a stinging apparatus at the tail end of their abdominal segment and are capable of delivering between 100 ng (fire ants)[1] and 50 μg (bees)[2] of venom (Table 1 and Figure 1). Although the venoms have various peptide and protein components, some of which are capable of inducing toxic or vasoactive responses, it has been estimated that about 1500 stings would be required to deliver a lethal dose of hymenoptera venom for a nonallergic adult who weighs 70 kg.[5] Despite this estimate, about 40 deaths a year are attributed to hymenoptera stings[6]; these deaths are ascribed to anaphylaxis occurring in persons with a history of prior stings in whom specific IgE antibodies developed to various venom components. Due to the vasoactive components of the venoms, most people experience a local reaction to hymenoptera stings consisting of redness, swelling, tenderness, and pain at the site of the sting. This reaction is self-limited and will resolve within hours. If the sting occurs near or within the oral cavity, there is a potential for respiratory compromise.

Fire-ant venom is composed primarily of a transpiperidine alkaloid that causes tissue necrosis. Most fire-ant stings produce a blister within 24 hours, which often fills with necrotic material, giving the appearance of a pustule (Figure 2). Despite their appearance, these blisters are not infected and should be left intact.

Occasionally, persons will have swelling from a hymenoptera sting that may involve a large area and persist for up to a week. These large local reactions are not life threatening

Table 1. Characteristics of Hymenoptera.

Common Name	Taxonomic Classification	Size	Nesting Habits	Feeding Habits	Aggressiveness	Venom Protein per Sting*	Avoidance Techniques
Honeybee	Family Apidae *Apis mellifera*	15–20 mm	Man-made hives	Nectar and pollen	Nonaggressive	50 µg	Avoid flower-print clothing Avoid flowery scents Wear shoes and socks outdoors
Africanized honey-bee†	Family Apidae *Apis mellifera scutellata*	15–20 mm	Natural hives	Nectar and pollen	Aggressive	Approximately 50 µg	Avoid flower-print clothing Avoid flowery scents Wear shoes and socks outdoors Remove nests near homes
Fire ant	Family Formicidae *Solenopsis invicta*	4–6 mm	Mounds in disturbed soil	Omnivorous	Aggressive in defense of mounds	10–100 ng	Wear shoes and socks outdoors Wear gloves and pants when gardening Remove mounds near homes
Paper wasp	Family Vespidae Subfamily Polistinae Polistes species	20–25 mm	Single layer hanging from eaves, porches	Nectar and arthropods	Aggressive in defense of nests	NA	Avoid flower-print clothing Avoid flowery scents Remove nests near homes
Yellow jacket	Family Vespidae Subfamily Vespinae Vespula species	15–20 mm	Multilayered, usually underground	Scavengers	Very aggressive	2–20 µg	Avoid open food sources, picnic areas, garbage Remove nests near homes
White-faced or bald-faced hornet	Family Vespidae Subfamily Vespinae Dolichovespula species	25–35 mm	Multilayered, usually in open areas	Nectar and arthropods	Aggressive in defense of nests	NA	Avoid flower-print clothing Avoid flowery scents Remove nests near homes
European hornet	Family Vespidae Subfamily Vespinae Vespa species	25–35 mm	Multilayered, usually in open areas	Nectar and arthropods	Aggressive in defense of nests	NA	Avoid flower-print clothing Avoid flowery scents Remove nests near homes

* NA denotes that data are not available.
† The subspecies of honeybee called "Africanized" is more aggressive than the parent species and has caused some clinical problems in South and Central America and in south Texas. The venom is similar to honeybee venom, which may therefore be used in testing and treating patients who have had anaphylaxis after being stung by this subspecies.[3,4]

unless they involve the airway. They may result in considerable morbidity because of a temporary loss of function, such as occurs when the sting involves a foot or hand or is near an eye. Secondary infections can frequently complicate fire-ant stings when the pseudopustule is opened, and they can sometimes complicate other hymenoptera stings. Although it may be difficult in some cases to distinguish a secondary infection from a large local reaction, in the latter event the swelling usually peaks within 48 hours, whereas progression of swelling for more than two days, accompanied by fever or lymphadenitis, suggests secondary infection.

The reactions that lead to anaphylaxis, however, are of more concern than secondary infections. Some anaphylactic events are restricted to cutaneous findings (pruritus, urticaria, and angioedema). Others have a broader effect, with systemic symptoms that may involve the gastrointestinal tract (metallic taste, nausea, vomiting, diarrhea, and abdominal cramping), genitourinary tract (uterine cramps), or nervous system (sense of impend-

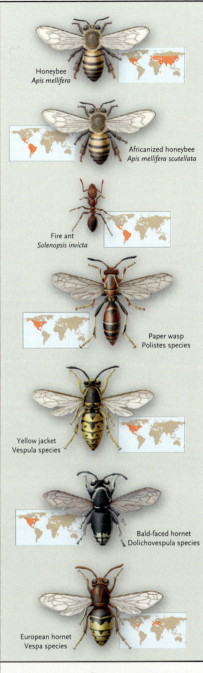

Figure 1. Species of Hymenoptera and Their Geographical Distribution.

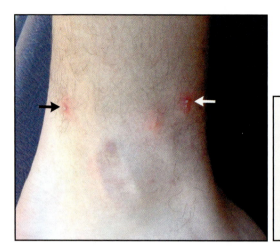

Figure 2. Stings from a Fire Ant on an Ankle, Showing the Pseudopustule.

The clustering of the stings (white arrow) contrasts with the single sting (black arrow) in the photograph, which was taken 24 hours after the event. This pattern is typical of fire-ant stings, as one ant will often inflict multiple stings in a semicircular arc if given time to do so. Also, the pseudopustule is typical of fire-ant stings; it is not a pustule. The stings occurred just above the level of the ankle sock the patient was wearing on the day of the event.

ing doom, light-headedness, and dizziness). Reactions that involve the cardiopulmonary system (breathing difficulties, bronchospasm, hypotension, and arrhythmia) pose the greatest risk. Initial subjective symptoms may progress rapidly (in seconds to minutes) to life-threatening cardiopulmonary collapse. The risk of anaphylaxis with any event is dependent on the nature of the most severe previous reaction experienced by a patient (Table 2). Neuropathic and vasculitic responses and reactions that resemble serum sickness have in rare cases been reported after insect stings.[15,16]

STRATEGIES AND EVIDENCE

Immediate Therapy

The optimal choice of immediate therapy for insect stings depends on the type of reaction. Strategies are based on anecdotal evidence. Local reactions are best treated symptomatically with nonsteroidal antiinflammatory agents, antihistamines, and cold compresses. Topical antihistamines and corticosteroids may also be used. When large local reactions occur, oral steroids are often added to the therapeutic mix.

The definitive therapy for anaphylaxis is epinephrine by injection (0.01 mg per kilogram of body weight; maximum, 0.3 and 0.5 mg per dose, for children and adults, respectively), and this should be administered to any patient who has more than a cutaneous reaction. Antihistamines are often added to treat cutaneous signs and symptoms. Supplemental oxygen, beta-agonists for bronchospasm, and intravenous fluids for hypotension are sometimes indicated. Occasionally, for a reaction that does not respond to the initial dose of epinephrine, steroids (oral or intravenous) are added, although definitive support for their addition is lacking.

Table 2. Risk of Anaphylactic Reactions to Hymenoptera Stings after an Initial Event.

Patient History*	Approximate Risk of Anaphylaxis (%)†	Immunotherapy If Skin Test or in Vitro Test Is Positive for Antibodies
Unknown history	3	No
Large local reactions	10	No
Cutaneous anaphylaxis in child	10	No
Systemic anaphylaxis in child	50–60	Yes
Anaphylaxis in adult	50–60	Yes
Receiving immunotherapy	2	Not applicable

* The risk in the general population refers to the risk in adults; the risk may be lower in children. Large local reactions are defined as persistent swelling of up to a week's duration; cutaneous anaphylaxis in a child is characterized by pruritus, urticaria, or angioedema. The risk of anaphylaxis for adults with cutaneous reactions only may be as low as it is for children, but this is yet to be determined.

† The data in this table are from Golden,[7] Settipane and Boyd,[8] Chaffee,[9] Golden et al.,[10] Graft et al.,[11] Schuberth et al.,[12] Hunt et al.,[13] and Golden et al.[14]

There is a distressing tendency by both patients and physicians to treat anaphylaxis without using epinephrine,[17,18] perhaps because of concern about adverse effects of epinephrine on the heart. However, anaphylaxis itself has been associated with coronary vasospasm.[19-22] The fact that available data suggest that a failure or delay in administering epinephrine increases the chance of a fatal outcome in anaphylaxis[23] underscores the prevailing opinion that epinephrine must be considered the definitive therapy for anaphylaxis.

Epinephrine auto-injectors should be prescribed for any patient who has had an anaphylactic reaction to a hymenoptera sting. The instructions for use are printed on the side of each injector, but these should be reviewed with the patient when prescribing the medication. Patients should be educated to use epinephrine if signs or symptoms beyond a cutaneous reaction develop after a hymenoptera sting, and always to seek additional medical care after using an injector.

Long-Term Therapy

Avoidance   The long-term goal is to prevent future systemic anaphylactic events. The optimal approach to prevent IgE-mediated disease is avoidance of the antigen, but this may not be feasible in practice. Current recommendations for avoidance are summarized in Table 1. The proximity of the habitats of wasps and fire ants to those of humans makes these insects the most likely members of the order to cause anaphylaxis.[24]

Immunotherapy   If avoidance of hymenoptera cannot be ensured, the next step is to minimize the potential for anaphylaxis if a sting should occur. Immunotherapy with hymenoptera venom has been shown to reduce the potential risk of anaphylaxis with subsequent stings significantly[13,14] (Table 2). Although the administration of whole-body extracts is no more effective than placebo therapy for treating the stings of flying hymenoptera,[13] whole-body extracts of fire ants appear to be as useful in preventing future reactions as is venom immunotherapy for flying hymenoptera,[25] perhaps because whole-body extracts of fire ants (in contrast to those of flying hymenoptera) contain adequate amounts of venom.[26] Whole-body extract therapy for fire ants has not been compared directly with fire-ant venom immunotherapy.

Evaluation   The evaluation of patients for whom immunotherapy is considered begins with a review of the history of stings and reactions. The circumstances of the sting may suggest a particular agent (Table 1). The presence of a stinger or a venom sac at the site of a sting suggests, but is not definitive of, a honeybee sting, as occasionally other hymenoptera may leave a stinger in place. Fire ants are usually easy to identify since they do not fly away and will grasp victims with their mandibles and inflict multiple stings if allowed (Figure 2).

The clinical course is also reviewed to verify the diagnosis of anaphylaxis. It is sometimes difficult to separate anxiety symptoms from true anaphylaxis in the setting of a sting. This is especially true if there are no documented objective findings, such as urticaria, hypotension, or air-flow reduction. However, when patients are concerned enough to seek an evaluation even with an unclear or remote history, it is appropriate to test them for specific IgE antibodies. If the results of these tests are negative, patients can be reassured; if they are positive, immunotherapy should be offered. Age is also important. Studies have shown that in children under the age of 16 years who have cutaneous anaphylaxis (urticaria, angioedema, or both), the risk of systemic (in addition to cutaneous) anaphylaxis in response to future stings is only slightly greater than the risk in the general population[6] (Table 2). It is uncertain whether the same is true in adults.

Subsequent evaluation involves testing for the presence of specific IgE antibodies.[27,28] Initial testing is usually delayed for four to six weeks after the sting event to eliminate the possibility of a false negative result caused by a depletion of mediators in the setting of anaphylaxis. If the particular agent is known, then testing includes only that insect. It is often unclear which insect was the perpetrator, in which case testing of sensitivity to each of the flying hymenoptera is warranted.

Typically, testing involves in vivo skin testing for specific IgE antibodies; this is more sensitive than in vitro methods, which are an alternative. The prick method (a needle pricks the skin through a drop of the antigen) is used as the first step (a dilution of 1:1000 weight/volume [wt/vol] for fire-ant venom; 1 μg per milliliter for venom from other hymenoptera). If the result of this test is negative, testing proceeds with an intradermal method (antigen is injected into the dermis), usually using about 0.001 μg per milliliter (1:1,000,000 wt/vol for fire-ant venom) and increases sequentially by 10 times the previous amount to 1.0 μg per milliliter (1:1000 wt/vol for fire-ant venom); above these concentrations, false positive test results may occur. Testing is stopped when the skin test is positive (the reaction is equivalent to or greater than a histamine control). If the maximal intradermal dose is reached without a positive response, the test result is considered negative. If a false negative result is suspected (on the basis of a history suggestive of anaphylaxis), or for patients who cannot be skin-tested (those who have severe dermatitis or who are receiving medications that suppress the histamine response), in vitro methods are reasonable alternatives. Immunotherapy is then offered to anyone who has both a history consistent with anaphylaxis after a sting and specific IgE antibodies to the potential agent, as demonstrated by positive results on skin testing or in vitro testing.

Whereas there may be extensive cross-reactivity between some venom components, such as antigen 5 (one of the more potent vespid antigens), there are enough highly specific components of the venoms (including differences between molecules common to all the venoms, such as phospholipases)[29] to support the recommendation that all venoms for which skin testing yields positive results should be used in treatment. Treatment with more than one venom can be administered concurrently, but this generally requires multiple injections per visit; an exception is the commercial preparation that is a mixture of venoms from the yellow jacket, white-faced hornet, and yellow hornet (maximal dose, 100 μg of each species' venom).

Therapy Immunotherapy starts at 0.1 μg per milliliter for most hymenoptera venoms (1:100,000 wt/vol for fire-ant venom). Each subsequent dose increases the amount of venom delivered to the patient, generally until a dose of 100 μg per milliliter for the venom of flying hymenoptera (0.5 ml of 1:100 wt/vol for fire-ant venom) is reached; 100 μg is twice the dose to which a patient would be exposed in a routine sting, and it is the dose used in initial studies showing the effectiveness of venom immunotherapy. Usually the doses are delivered once a week. This means there is a three-to-six-month period required to reach the maintenance dose. So-called rush protocols have been published,[30-32] in which a shorter dosing interval is used to reach maintenance doses in weeks or even days, and they appear to provide good protection from sting challenges. These are particularly useful when the risk of exposure is high and ongoing, as may occur with patients who must work or play outdoors.[33] These protocols have not been compared directly with standard immunotherapy protocols in randomized controlled trials, but they have been found to give reasonably equivalent protection against direct sting challenges.

When a maintenance level is reached, the interval between injections is often expanded to one month. Some observational data suggest that the interval may be expanded to 8 or even 12 weeks without losing protection.[34,35] The maintenance dose and interval may be adjusted on the basis of clinical criteria. For instance, if a patient receives a sting that results in symptoms while receiving maintenance immunotherapy, the dose interval may be shortened or the dose increased to more than 100 μg.[36]

Protection after a course of immunotherapy appears to last a long time. In a recent report involving a follow-up evaluation of children 10 to 20 years after they had received immunotherapy, only 5 percent of the children with a history of a moderate-to-severe sting reactions who reported a subsequent sting had had a recurrent systemic reaction, as compared with 32 percent of untreated children with a similar history.[37]

The risks associated with hymenoptera immunotherapy are the same as for other allergen immunotherapy. The risk of anaphylaxis after an immunotherapy injection is low (fewer than 1.6 reactions per 100 injections).[13] The majority (88 percent) of patients complete an immunotherapy course without reactions, and most reactions that occur are mild.[38] Rarely, more severe reactions occur, including death (about 1 in 5 million injections for all types of immunotherapy).[39] Therefore, immunotherapy should be administered only in a medical setting by trained personnel capable of recognizing and treating anaphylaxis.

AREAS OF UNCERTAINTY

An important unanswered question relates to the optimal duration of maintenance immunotherapy. The package insert that comes with the venom immunotherapy recommends indefinite use, whereas current clinical guidelines recommend discontinuing immunotherapy after three to five years of the maintenance-level dose,[40,41] especially if the patient no longer has specific IgE antibodies (as evaluated by repeated skin testing).[42,43] However, data from patients who have not received immunotherapy indicate that the loss of these antibodies is no guarantee that anaphylaxis will not occur. In one report, 98 patients (including patients with and patients without a history of anaphylaxis) who had positive tests for specific IgE antibodies at baseline slowly lost their positive responses over time. However, the risk of anaphylaxis was not eliminated; at a mean of four years after initial evaluation, approximately 17 percent of patients (11 of 65) who had subsequent stings had anaphylactic reactions, despite the presumed loss of specific IgE antibodies.[44] Other reports have documented reactions to hymenoptera stings after discontinuing immunotherapy.[37,45] Given these data, some allergists extend venom immunotherapy longer than the suggested three to five years. Consideration of an extended course may be warranted particularly for patients who have had a severe reaction (for such patients, some allergists might continue immunotherapy indefinitely).

Another area that requires additional research is the treatment of patients who have a history of a reaction suggestive of anaphylaxis but in whom testing for specific IgE antibodies yields negative results. One potential explanation is that the earlier reaction was not to hymenoptera; the stings or bites of other insects (mosquitoes, biting flies, and reduvids) and arthropods (spiders, scorpions, and ticks) may also result in anaphylaxis. In rare cases, people with mastocytosis may have an anaphylactoid response to hymenoptera stings without actually having specific IgE antibodies.[46] A more common explanation is the imperfect sensitivity of tests for specific IgE antibodies.[10,47,48] Twenty percent of patients with negative in vitro tests will have positive results on skin testing, and 10 percent of patients whose skin test is negative will have positive results on in vitro testing.[49] In cases in which the suspicion of hymenoptera hypersensitivity is high, and initial tests are negative, it has been recommended that repeated testing be undertaken with both in vivo and in vitro methods.[50,51]

GUIDELINES

Under the joint auspices of the American Academy of Allergy, Asthma and Immunology and the American College of Allergy, Asthma and Immunology, the *Journal of Allergy and Clinical Immunology* published the newest set of guidelines for insect hypersensitivity in 2004.[52] In general, the recommendations presented here are consistent with these guidelines.

SUMMARY AND CONCLUSIONS

For patients with a clear history of anaphylaxis, such as the one described in the vignette, information should be provided on avoidance and on the use of emergency treatment with epinephrine auto-injectors. Patients should be advised to carry an auto-injector and to wear a medical alert bracelet. Referral to an allergist is warranted, and skin testing should be performed for sensitivity to honeybees, wasps, white-faced hornets, yellow hornets, and yellow jackets. Venom immunotherapy should be administered for all venoms for which testing results are positive. The protective benefit is expected from the immunotherapy by the time maintenance dose is reached, usually by three to six months with standard protocols. A rush protocol would be recommended if the patient's risk of being stung again before standard immunotherapy could work were considered high. Although immunotherapy is often administered by allergists, it may be delivered by any practitioner who is willing to observe the patient and to treat anaphylaxis if it should occur.

This article first appeared in the November 4, 2004, issue of the New England Journal of Medicine.

REFERENCES

1.
Hoffman DR, Dove DE, Jacobson RS. Allergens in Hymenoptera venom. XX. Isolation of four allergens from imported fire ant (Solenopsis invicta) venom. J Allergy Clin Immunol 1988;82:818-27.

2.
Hoffman DR, Jacobson RS. Allergens in Hymenoptera venom. XII. How much protein in a sting? Ann Allergy 1984;52:276-8.

3.
Guralnick MW, Benton AW. Entomological aspects of insect sting allergy. In: Levin MI, Lockey RF, eds. Monograph on insect allergy. 4th ed. Milwaukee: American Academy of Allergy, Asthma and Immunology, 2003:11-26.

4.
McKenna WR. Africanized honeybees. In: Levin MI, Lockey RF, eds. Monograph on insect allergy. 4th ed. Milwaukee: American Academy of Allergy, Asthma and Immunology, 2003:27-36.

5.
Goddard J. Physician's guide to arthropods of medical importance. 4th ed. Boca Raton, Fla.: CRC Press, 2003:4.

6.
Barnard JH. Studies of 400 Hymenoptera sting deaths in the United States. J Allergy Clin Immunol 1973;52:259-64.

7.
Golden DBK. Epidemiology of allergy to insect venoms and stings. Allergy Proc 1989;10:103-7.

8.
Settipane GA, Boyd GK. Prevalence of bee sting allergy in 4,992 Boy Scouts. Acta Allergol 1970;25:286-91.

9.
Chaffee F. The prevalence of bee sting allergy in an allergic population. Acta Allergol 1970;25:292-3.

10.
Golden DBK, Marsh DG, Kagey-Sobotka A, et al. Epidemiology of insect venom sensitivity. JAMA 1989;262:240-4.

11.
Graft DF, Schuberth KC, Kagey-Sobotka A, et al. A prospective study of the natural history of large local reactions after Hymenoptera stings in children. J Pediatr 1984;104:664-8.

12.
Schuberth KC, Lichtenstein LM, Kagey-Sobotka A, Szklo M, Kwiterovich KA, Valentine MD. Epidemiologic study of insect allergy in children. II. Effect of accidental stings in allergic children. J Pediatr 1983;102:361-5.

13.
Hunt KJ, Valentine MD, Sobotka AK, Benton AW, Amodio FJ, Lichtenstein LM. A controlled trial of immunotherapy in insect hypersensitivity. N Engl J Med 1978;299:157-61.

14.
Golden DBK, Valentine MD, Kagey-Sobotka A, Lichtenstein LM. Regimens of Hymenoptera venom immunotherapy. Ann Intern Med 1980;92:620-4.

15.
Light WC, Reisman RE, Shimizu M, Arbesman CE. Unusual reactions following insect stings: clinical features and immunologic analysis. J Allergy Clin Immunol 1977;59:391-7.

16.
Reisman RE, Livingston A. Late-onset allergic reactions, including serum sickness, after insect stings. J Allergy Clin Immunol 1989;84:331-7.

17.
Clark S, Bock SA, Gaeta TJ, Brenner BE, Cydulka RK, Camargo CA. Multicenter study of emergency department visits for food allergies. J Allergy Clin Immunol 2004;113:347-52.

18.
Simons FE. First-aid treatment of anaphylaxis to food: focus on epinephrine. J Allergy Clin Immunol 2004;113:837-44. [Erratum, J Allergy Clin Immunol 2004;113:1039.]

19.
Fujita Y, Chikamitsu M, Kimura M, Toriumi T, Endoh S, Sari A. An anaphylactic reaction possibly associated with an intraoperative coronary artery spasm during general anesthesia. J Clin Anesth 2001;13:221-6.

20.
Matucci RO, Cecchi L, Vultaggio A, et al. Coronary vasospasm during an acute allergic reaction. Allergy 2002;57:867-8.

21.
Conraads VM, Jorens PG, Ebo DG, Claeys MJ, Bosmans JM, Vrints CJ. Coronary artery spasm complicating anaphylaxis secondary to skin disinfectant. Chest 1998;113:1417-9.

22.
Machiels JP, Jacques JM, de Meester A. Coronary artery spasm during anaphylaxis. Ann Emerg Med 1996;27:674-5.

23.
Bock SA, Muñoz-Furlong A, Sampson HA. Fatalities due to anaphylactic reactions to foods. J Allergy Clin Immunol 2001;107:191-3.

24.
Freeman TM. Hymenoptera hypersensitivity in an imported fire ant endemic area. Ann Allergy Asthma Immunol 1997;78:369-72.

25.
Freeman TM, Hylander RD, Ortiz AA, Martin MF. Imported fire ant immunotherapy: effectiveness of whole body extracts. J Allergy Clin Immunol 1992;90:210-5.

26.
Hoffman DR, Jacobson RS, Schmidt M, Smith AM. Allergens in Hymenoptera venoms. XXIII. The venom content of imported fire ant whole body extracts. Ann Allergy 1991;66:29-31.

27.
Hunt KJ, Valentine MD, Sobotka AK, Lichtenstein LM. Diagnosis of allergy to stinging insects by skin testing with Hymenoptera venoms. Ann Intern Med 1976;85:56-9.

28.
Georgitis J, Reisman RE. Venom skin tests in insect-allergic and insect-nonallergic populations. J Allergy Clin Immunol 1985;76:803-7.

29.
Hoffman DR. Hymenoptera venoms: composition, standardization, stability. In: Levin MI, Lockey RF, eds. Monograph on insect allergy. 4th ed. Milwaukee: American Academy of Allergy, Asthma and Immunology, 2003:37-54.

30. Yunginger JW, Paull BR, Jones RT, Santrach PJ. Rush venom immunotherapy program for honeybee sting sensitivity. J Allergy Clin Immunol 1979;63:340-7.

31. Bernstein JA, Kagen SL, Bernstein DI, Bernstein IL. Rapid venom immunotherapy is safe for routine use in the treatment of patients with Hymenoptera anaphylaxis. Ann Allergy 1994;73:423-8.

32. Tankersley MS, Walker RL, Butler WK, Hagan LL, Napoli DC, Freeman TM. Safety and efficacy of an imported fire ant rush immunotherapy protocol with and without prophylactic treatment. J Allergy Clin Immunol 2002;109:556-62.

33. Duplantier JE, Freeman TM, Bahna SL, Good RA, Sher MR. Successful rush immunotherapy for anaphylaxis to imported fire ants. J Allergy Clin Immunol 1998;101:855-6.

34. Golden DB, Kagey-Sobotka A, Valentine MD, Lichtenstein LM. Prolonged maintenance interval in Hymenoptera venom immunotherapy. J Allergy Clin Immunol 1981;67:482-4.

35. Goldberg A, Confino-Cohen R. Maintenance venom immunotherapy administered at 3-month intervals is both safe and efficacious. J Allergy Clin Immunol 2001;107:902-6.

36. Rueff F, Wenderoth A, Przybilla B. Patients still reacting to a sting challenge while receiving conventional Hymenoptera venom immunotherapy are protected by increased venom doses. J Allergy Clin Immunol 2001;108:1027-32.

37. Golden DBK, Kagey-Sobotka A, Norman PS, Hamilton RG, Lichtenstein LM. Outcomes of allergy to insect stings in children, with and without venom immunotherapy. N Engl J Med 2004;351:668-74.

38. Lockey RF, Turkeltaub PC, Olive ES, Hubbard JM, Baird-Warren IA, Bukantz SC. The Hymenoptera venom study. III. Safety of venom immunotherapy. J Allergy Clin Immunol 1990;86:775-80.

39. Lockey RF, Benedict LM, Turkeltaub PC, Bukantz SC. Fatalities from immunotherapy (IT) and skin testing (ST). J Allergy Clin Immunol 1987;79:660-77.

40. Golden D, Kwiterovich K, Kagey-Sobotka A, Valentine MD, Lichtenstein LM. Discontinuing venom immunotherapy: outcome after five years. J Allergy Clin Immunol 1996;97:579-87.

41. Haugaard L, Norregaard O, Dahl R. In-hospital sting challenge in insect venom-allergic patients after stopping venom immunotherapy. J Allergy Clin Immunol 1991;87:699-702.

42. Reisman RE. Duration of venom immunotherapy: relationship to the severity of symptoms of initial insect sting anaphylaxis. J Allergy Clin Immunol 1993;92:831-6.

43. Lerch E, Müller UR. Long-term protection after stopping venom immunotherapy: results of re-stings in 200 patients. J Allergy Clin Immunol 1998;101:606-12.

44. Golden DB, Marsh DG, Freidhoff LR, et al. Natural history of Hymenoptera venom sensitivity in adults. J Allergy Clin Immunol 1997;100:760-6.

45. Golden DBK, Kwiterovich KA, Kagey-Sobotka A, Lichtenstein LM. Discontinuing venom immunotherapy: extended observations. J Allergy Clin Immunol 1998;101:298-305.

46. Kontou-Fili K. Patients with negative skin tests. Curr Opin Allergy Clin Immunol 2002;2:353-7.

47. Parker JL, Santrach PJ, Dahlberg MJE, Yunginger JW. Evaluation of Hymenoptera-sting sensitivity with deliberate sting challenges: inadequacy of present diagnostic methods. J Allergy Clin Immunol 1982;69:200-7.

48. Sobotka AK, Adkinson NF Jr, Valentine MD, Lichtenstein LM. Allergy to insect stings. IV. Diagnosis by radioallergosorbent tests (RAST). J Immunol 1978;121:2477-84.

49. Golden DBK. Diagnostic methods in insect allergy. In Levin MI, Lockey RF, eds. Monograph on insect allergy. 4th ed. Milwaukee: American Academy of Allergy, Asthma and Immunology, 2003:63-74.

50. Reisman RE. Insect sting allergy: the dilemma of the negative skin test reactor. J Allergy Clin Immunol 2001;107:781-2.

51. Golden DB, Tracy JM, Freeman TM, Hoffman DR. Negative venom skin test results in patients with histories of systemic reaction to a sting. J Allergy Clin Immunol 2003;112:495-8.

52. Moffitt JE, Golden DBK, Reisman RE, et al. Stinging insect hypersensitivity: a practice parameter update. J Allergy Clin Immunol 2004;114:869-86.

Newly Diagnosed Atrial Fibrillation

RICHARD L. PAGE, M.D.

A 77-year-old woman with a history of hypertension treated with metoprolol presents for her annual examination. She reports no new symptoms. The examination is remarkable only for the finding of an irregular heart rate. Electrocardiographic testing reveals atrial fibrillation at an average rate of 75 beats per minute. She has no history of arrhythmia, coronary disease, valvular disease, diabetes, alcohol abuse, transient ischemic attack, or stroke. For the past several months, she has exercised on a treadmill without difficulty, although she notes that the machine does not always measure her heart rate. What should her physician advise?

THE CLINICAL PROBLEM

Atrial fibrillation is the most common arrhythmia that requires treatment, with an estimated prevalence in the United States of 2.3 million patients in 2001.[1] The prevalence increases with age — atrial fibrillation occurs in 3.8 percent of people 60 years of age and older and in 9.0 percent of those 80 years of age and older.[1]

Risk of Stroke and Death

The most devastating consequence of atrial fibrillation is stroke as a result of thromboembolism typically emanating from the left atrial appendage.[2] The rate of stroke varies but may range from 5.0 percent to 9.6 percent per year among patients at high risk who are taking aspirin (but not warfarin).[3,4]

Patients with paroxysmal (i.e., self-terminating) and persistent atrial fibrillation (i.e., that lasts more than seven days or requires cardioversion) appear to have a risk of stroke that is similar to that of patients with permanent atrial fibrillation.[5] In the Stroke Prevention in Atrial Fibrillation studies of patients with atrial fibrillation, the risk of stroke among those with sinus rhythm that had been documented within the 12 months before enrollment (3.2 percent per year) was similar to that among those with permanent atrial fibrillation (3.3 percent per year).[5] The duration of episodes of atrial fibrillation and the overall time spent in atrial fibrillation (i.e., burden) have not been established as determining the risk of stroke. Atrial fibrillation is associated with an increase in the relative risk of death ranging from 1.3 to twice that value, independent of other risk factors.[6,7] This risk may be greater for women than for men.[7]

Associated Diseases and Predisposing Conditions

In most cases, atrial fibrillation is associated with cardiovascular disease, in particular hypertension, coronary artery disease, cardiomyopathy, and valvular disease (primarily mitral); it also occurs after cardiac surgery and in the presence of myocarditis or pericarditis. When atrial fibrillation complicates severe mitral regurgitation, valve repair or replacement is indicated.[8] In some cases, atrial fibrillation results from another supraventricular tachycardia. When it is associated with the Wolff–Parkinson–White syndrome, rapid conduction down the accessory pathway may result in hemodynamic collapse.[9]

Other predisposing conditions include excessive alcohol intake, hyperthyroidism, and pulmonary disorders, including pulmonary embolism. Obstructive sleep apnea may also be related, in which case the provision of continuous positive airway pressure reduces the risk of the recurrence of atrial fibrillation.[10] Both vagal and sympathetic mechanisms of paroxysmal atrial fibrillation have been described (neurogenic atrial fibrillation),[11] as have familial forms of the condition.[12] "Lone" atrial fibrillation (i.e., that occurring in the absence of a cardiac or other explanation) is common, particularly in patients with paroxysmal atrial fibrillation — up to 45 percent of such patients have no underlying cardiac disease.[13]

Evaluation

The patient's history and the physical examination should focus on these potential causes of atrial fibrillation. The "minimum evaluation" recommended at diagnosis should include 12-lead electrocardiography, chest radiography, transthoracic echocardiography, and serologic tests of thyroid function.[11] Echocardiographic testing is used to assess valve function, chamber size, and the peak right ventricular pressure and to detect hypertrophy and pericardial disease. Additional tests may be warranted, including exercise testing to determine whether the patient has symptoms and to assess the heart rate with exercise, 24-hour ambulatory monitoring to evaluate heart-rate control, transesophageal echocardiography to screen for a left atrial thrombus and to guide cardioversion, and, rarely, an electrophysiological study to detect predisposing arrhythmias.[11]

Symptoms and Hemodynamic Consequences

Patients with atrial fibrillation may have palpitations, dyspnea, fatigue, light-headedness, and syncope. These symptoms are usually related to the elevated heart rate and, in most patients, can be mitigated with the use of drugs to control the heart rate. Exceptions are due, presumably, to an irregular ventricular response or a reduction of cardiac output.

The hemodynamic consequences of atrial fibrillation are related to the loss of atrial mechanical function, irregularity of ventricular response, and high heart rate. These consequences are magnified in the presence of impaired diastolic ventricular filling, hypertension, mitral stenosis, left ventricular hypertrophy, and restrictive cardiomyopathy.[11] Irregularity of the cardiac cycle, especially when accompanied by short coupling intervals, and rapid heart rates in atrial fibrillation lead to a reduction in diastolic filling, stroke volume, and cardiac output. In a study of patients who were evaluated while in atrial fibrillation and again during ventricular pacing at the same overall heart rate, the irregular rhythm was associated with a lower cardiac output (4.4 vs. 5.2 liters per minute) and higher pulmonary-capillary wedge pressure (17 vs. 14 mm Hg).[14]

A chronically elevated heart rate of 130 beats per minute or more may result in secondary cardiomyopathy,[15] a type of left ventricular dysfunction that may largely be reversed when control of the ventricular rate is achieved.[15,16] A report by Hsu et al.[17] indicates that, in patients with atrial fibrillation, heart-rate control and rhythm control with the use of radiofrequency catheter ablation improve left ventricular function in both those with and those without congestive heart failure.

Asymptomatic Atrial Fibrillation

Asymptomatic, or "silent," atrial fibrillation occurs frequently.[18] Among patients in the Canadian Registry of Atrial Fibrillation, 21 percent in whom the condition was newly diagnosed were asymptomatic.[19] The first presentation of asymptomatic atrial fibrillation may be catastrophic; in the Framingham Study, among patients with stroke that was associated with atrial fibrillation, the arrhythmia was newly diagnosed in 24 percent.[20] Even among patients with documented symptomatic atrial fibrillation, asymptomatic recurrences are common. In one study of patients with symptomatic paroxysmal atrial fibrillation, asymptomatic episodes were 12 times more common than symptomatic episodes.[21] In a recent trial,[22] among untreated patients, 17 percent had asymptomatic episodes before they noted symptoms, and the percentage was probably an underestimation, because the monitoring of these patients was intermittent. Some antiarrhythmic agents, by reducing conduction in the atrioventricular node, may increase the likelihood of the occurrence of asymptomatic atrial fibrillation. Both propafenone and propranolol have been associated with frequent asymptomatic atrial fibrillation,[23] and the risk may be similar with other agents that block atrioventricular nodal conduction.[24] Among patients with a pacemaker and a history of atrial fibrillation, one in six had silent recurrences lasting 48 hours or longer.[25]

Anticoagulant Therapy

The need for anticoagulation to reduce the risk of stroke among patients with atrial fibrillation due to mitral stenosis is well recognized.[11] Several randomized, prospective trials involving patients with nonvalvular atrial fibrillation[26-32] have confirmed a significant reduction in the risk of stroke with warfarin. These studies defined the patients at greatest risk as the elderly, variably defined as those older than 60, 65, and 75 years of age, and those with a history of thromboembolism, diabetes mellitus, coronary artery disease, hypertension, heart failure, and thyrotoxicosis.[11,33] These trials have provided a basis for two important guidelines for the use of warfarin in such patients[11,33,34] (Table 1). Recently, an index based on the assignment of points for five risk factors (i.e., congestive heart failure, hypertension, age, diabetes, and transient ischemic attack or stroke) was reported to be accurate in predicting stroke when it was used to evaluate the risk among patients in the Medicare database[4]; it is the basis for yet another guideline for antithrombotic therapy in atrial fibrillation[35] (Table 1). In addition, complex aortic plaques detected by transesophageal echocardiography that are associated with an increased risk of stroke in patients with atrial fibrillation also warrant the institution of anticoagulant therapy.[36]

An international normalized ratio (INR) value in the range of 2.0 to 3.0 is recommended. The risk of stroke doubles when the INR falls to 1.7, although values up to 3.5 do not convey an increased risk of bleeding complications.[37] INR values of 2.0 or greater are associated with a reduced severity of stroke and, if stroke occurs, a lower likelihood that it will result in death.[38]

Certain patients are at relatively low risk for a thromboembolic event and do not require intensive anticoagulant therapy[11,33,35] (Table 1). Aspirin is often recommended for these patients, although their risk is so low that even aspirin may not be necessary. Alternative antiplatelet agents, such as clopidogrel, have not been tested adequately in this clinical situation.

The duration of atrial fibrillation becomes important when cardioversion (with the use of electric or pharmacologic means) is being considered. It is generally accepted that patients who have had an episode of atrial fibrillation lasting less than 48 hours may safely undergo cardioversion without anticoagulant therapy, although the data supporting this practice are scant.[11] For episodes lasting longer than 48 hours, adequate anticoagulant therapy is warranted, both before cardioversion and for four weeks afterward. A recent report concluded that a strategy of initiating anticoagulant therapy and ruling out left atrial thrombus with the use of transesophageal echocardiography was a possible alternative to the usual strategy of anticoagulant therapy for three weeks before cardioversion.[39]

Table 1. Guidelines for Antithrombotic Therapy in Atrial Fibrillation.

Characteristic	Therapy Recommended by the ACC–AHA and ESC	Differences in ACCP Guidelines
Age		
<60 yr, no heart disease	Aspirin at a dose of 325 mg per day, or no therapy	Aspirin at a dose of 325 mg for patients <65 yr of age with no risk factor†
<60 yr, with heart disease but no risk factors*	Aspirin at a dose of 325 mg per day	No divergence
≥60–75 yr, no risk factors*	Aspirin at a dose of 325 mg per day	Option of aspirin at a dose of 325 mg per day or warfarin (INR, 2.0–3.0) for patients 65–75 yr of age
≥60 yr, with diabetes mellitus or coronary artery disease	Warfarin (INR, 2.0–3.0), aspirin optional in addition (at a dose of 81–162 mg per day)	Option of aspirin at a dose of 325 mg per day or warfarin (INR, 2.0–3.0) for patients with diabetes alone or coronary artery disease alone who are <65 yr of age
>75 yr, especially among women	Warfarin (INR, approximately 2.0; target INR, 1.6–2.5)	Warfarin (INR, 2.0–3.0), but no recommendation for INR value <2.0
Heart failure, left ventricular ejection fraction ≤0.35, thyrotoxicosis, and hypertension	Warfarin (INR, 2.0–3.0)	No divergence
Rheumatic heart disease (mitral stenosis)	Warfarin (INR, 2.5–3.5 or higher) may be appropriate	Other than for patients with mechanical valves, no INR recommended above target, 2.5 (range, 2.0–3.0)
Previous thromboembolism	Warfarin (INR, 2.5–3.5 or higher) may be appropriate	Other than for patients with mechanical valves, no INR recommended above target, 2.5 (range, 2.0–3.0)
Persistent atrial thrombus on transesophageal echocardiography	Warfarin (INR, 2.5–3.5 or higher) may be appropriate	Other than for patients with mechanical valves, no INR recommended above target, 2.5 (range, 2.0–3.0)
Prosthetic heart valves	Warfarin (INR, 2.5–3.5 or higher) may be appropriate	Depending on the type of prosthetic valve, warfarin (INR, 2.5 [range, 2.0–3.0] or INR, 3.0 [range, 2.5 to 3.5]) with or without additional aspirin, at a dose of 80 to 100 mg[34]
Warfarin recommended but contraindicated or refused	Aspirin at a dose of 325 mg per day	No divergence

* According to the guidelines of the American College of Cardiology and American Heart Association (ACC–AHA) Task Force on Practice and the European Society of Cardiology (ESC) Committee for Practice, the risk factors for thromboembolism include heart failure, a left ventricular ejection fraction of less than 35 percent, and a history of hypertension.[11] INR denotes international normalized ratio.

† According to the American College of Chest Physicians (ACCP), moderate risk factors include an age of 65 to 75 years, diabetes mellitus, and coronary artery disease with preserved left ventricular function; high risk factors include previous stroke, transient ischemic attack, or systemic embolus; a history of hypertension; poor left ventricular systolic function; an age of 75 years or older; rheumatic mitral-valve disease; and the presence of a prosthetic heart valve.[33]

Table 2. Pharmacologic Agents to Control Heart Rate and Rhythm.*

Drug (Class)†	Purpose	Usual Maintenance Dose	Adverse Effects	Cautions and Contraindications
Metoprolol (II)	Rate control (rhythm in some cases)	50–200 mg daily, divided doses or sustained-release formulation	Hypotension, heart block, bradycardia, asthma, congestive heart failure	—
Propranolol (II)	Rate control (rhythm in some cases)	80–240 mg daily, divided doses or sustained-release formulation	Hypotension, heart block, bradycardia, asthma, congestive heart failure	—
Diltiazem (IV)	Rate control	120–360 mg daily, divided doses or sustained-release formulation	Hypotension, heart block, congestive heart failure	—
Verapamil (IV)	Rate control	120–360 mg daily, divided doses or sustained-release formulation	Hypotension, heart block, congestive heart failure, interaction with digoxin	—
Digoxin	Rate control	0.125–0.375 mg daily	Toxic effects of digitalis, heart block, bradycardia	—
Amiodarone (III)	Rhythm control (rate in some cases)	100–400 mg daily	Pulmonary toxic effects, skin discoloration, hypothyroidism, gastrointestinal upset, hepatic toxic effects, corneal deposits, optic neuropathy, interaction with warfarin, torsades de pointes (rare)	—
Quinidine (IA)	Rhythm control	600–1500 mg daily, divided doses	Torsades de pointes, gastrointestinal upset, enhanced atrioventricular nodal conduction	Prolongs QT interval; avoid with left ventricular wall thickness ≥1.4 cm
Procainamide (IA)	Rhythm control	1000–4000 mg daily, divided doses	Torsades de pointes, lupus-like syndrome, gastrointestinal symptoms	Prolongs QT interval; avoid with left ventricular wall thickness ≥1.4 cm
Disopyramide (IA)	Rhythm control	400–750 mg daily, divided doses	Torsades de pointes, congestive heart failure, glaucoma, urinary retention, dry mouth	Prolongs QT interval; avoid with left ventricular wall thickness ≥1.4 cm
Flecainide (IC)	Rhythm control	200–300 mg daily, divided doses	Ventricular tachycardia, congestive heart failure, enhanced atrioventricular nodal conduction (conversion to atrial flutter)	Contraindicated in patients with ischemic and structural heart disease
Propafenone (IC)	Rhythm control	450–900 mg daily, divided doses	Ventricular tachycardia, congestive heart failure, enhanced atrioventricular nodal conduction (conversion to atrial flutter)	Contraindicated in patients with ischemic and structural heart disease
Sotalol (III)	Rhythm control	240–320 mg daily, divided doses	Torsades de pointes, congestive heart failure, bradycardia, exacerbation of chronic obstructive or bronchospastic lung disease	Prolongs QT interval; avoid with left ventricular wall thickness ≥1.4 cm
Dofetilide (III)	Rhythm control	500–1000 µg daily, divided doses	Torsades de pointes	Prolongs QT interval; avoid with left ventricular wall thickness ≥1.4 cm

* The information in the table is adapted from Fuster et al.[11]
† The Vaughn Williams class of antiarrhythmic drugs is given for those classified. Digoxin is not classified in this system.

Table 3. Choice of Antiarrhythmic Agent According to the Underlying Cardiac Disorder.*

Underlying Disorder	Rate Control†	Rhythm Control		
		First Choice	Second Choice	Third Choice
Minimal or no heart disease	β-adrenergic blocker or calcium-channel blocker	Flecainide, propafenone, sotalol	Amiodarone, dofetilide	Disopyramide, procainamide, quinidine (or nonpharmacologic options)
Adrenergic atrial fibrillation with minimal or no heart disease	β-adrenergic blocker	β-adrenergic blocker or sotalol	Amiodarone, dofetilide	—
Heart failure	β-adrenergic blocker, if tolerated; digoxin	Amiodarone, dofetilide	—	—
Coronary artery disease	β-adrenergic blocker	Sotalol	Amiodarone, dofetilide	Disopyramide, procainamide, quinidine
Hypertension with LVH but wall thickness <1.4 cm	β-adrenergic blocker or calcium-channel blocker	Flecainide, propafenone	Amiodarone, dofetilide, sotalol	Disopyramide, procainamide, quinidine
Hypertension with LVH and wall thickness ≥1.4 cm	β-adrenergic blocker or calcium-channel blocker	Amiodarone	—	—

* LVH denotes left ventricular hypertrophy. The information in this table is adapted from Fuster et al.[11]
† β-adrenergic blockers include metoprolol and propranolol; calcium-channel blockers includes diltiazem and verapamil.

Rate Control

Current guidelines recommend a ventricular rate during atrial fibrillation of 60 to 80 beats per minute at rest and 90 to 115 beats per minute during exercise.[11] A number of pharmacologic agents are available to control the heart rate and rhythm (Tables 2 and 3). Digoxin has been replaced as first-line therapy for rate control by β-adrenergic blockers and calcium-channel blockers, largely owing to improved rate control during exertion with the use of these alternative agents.[11] In one study, during peak exercise, the mean heart rate was 175 beats per minute in patients receiving digoxin, as compared with 130 in those receiving a β-adrenergic blocker and 151 in those receiving a calcium-channel blocker.[40] Digoxin is useful in combination with other agents[40] or when β-adrenergic–blocking agents and calcium-channel blockers are not tolerated. In some patients, particularly the elderly, the ventricular rate during atrial fibrillation may be intrinsically controlled, so that no atrioventricular nodal–blocking agent is required. Among patients with a pause that causes symptoms after the spontaneous conversion of atrial fibrillation, or those whose symptoms are due to low heart rates in spite of their having high heart rates at other times, a pacemaker may be necessary to permit therapy with atrioventricular nodal–blocking agents (as in the "tachy-brady" or the sick sinus syndrome).

Rhythm Control

A number of agents may maintain sinus rhythm (Tables 2 and 3). The use of β-adrenergic agents may be effective in adrenergically mediated and paroxysmal atrial fibrillation[41] (although the effects may be related to the conversion of symptomatic atrial fibrillation into asymptomatic atrial fibrillation).[24] With the exception of the β-adrenergic–blocking agents, most antiarrhythmic drugs carry a risk of serious adverse effects. Antiarrhythmic therapy should be chosen on the basis of the patient's underlying cardiac condition (Table 3).[11] Antiarrhythmic agents classified according to the Vaughn Williams system as class IC are reserved to treat patients without a structural cardiac abnormality, and as described elsewhere,[42] may be prescribed for outpatients with acute conversion of paroxysmal atrial fibrillation (i.e., the so-called pill-in-the-pocket approach). Agents in classes IA and III should be avoided by patients with prolongation of the QT interval or left ventricular hypertrophy because of the potential for torsades de pointes. On the one hand, amiodarone, which has a low risk of proarrhythmia (less than 1 percent per year),[43] causes substantial noncardiac toxic effects and is therefore generally reserved for second-line therapy except in the treatment of patients with severe cardiomyopathy. On the other hand, it is the most effective antifibrillatory agent; in one trial, 65 percent of patients treated with amiodarone were free from recurrence after 16 months of therapy (as compared with 37 percent of those who were treated with propafenone or sotalol).[44]

Rate Control versus Rhythm Control

In recent randomized studies, rate control was compared with rhythm control in patients with persistent atrial fibrillation.[45-47] The Pharmacological Intervention in Atrial Fibrillation trial found no difference between the treatment groups in the primary end point of the quality of life, although a secondary analysis showed improvement in the distance walked in six minutes among patients in the rhythm-control group.[45] The Rate Control versus Electrical Cardioversion for Persistent Atrial Fibrillation (RACE) trial found that rate control was not inferior to rhythm control in the effects on a composite end point (consisting of death from cardiovascular causes, heart failure, thromboembolic complications, bleeding, implantation of a pacemaker, and serious adverse effects of drugs) over a period of 2.3 years (rate control, 17.2 percent, vs. rhythm control, 22.6 percent).[46] The largest of these trials, the Atrial Fibrillation Follow-up Investigation of Rhythm Management trial, which was designed to assess mortality, found no significant difference in this end point between the groups at five years (rhythm control, 23.8 percent, vs. rate control, 21.3 percent).[47] Thus, the evidence suggests that the strategy used to treat atrial fibrillation — rate control versus rhythm control — does not have a substantial effect on the quality of life or on cardiovascular end points, including death.

Nonetheless, some questions remain. All three of these trials compared strategies with the use of an intention-to-treat analysis. The success rate for maintaining sinus rhythm was as low as 39 percent after 2.3 years of treatment[46] and as high as 73 percent at 3 years.[47] A secondary analysis of the data from the RACE trial showed that for patients with symptoms related to atrial fibrillation and those who were in sinus mechanism at the end of the follow-up period, regardless of the treatment randomly assigned, the quality of life had improved.[48] All three studies enrolled only patients for whom rhythm control was considered to be an option by both the patient and the physician; in highly symptomatic patients, rhythm control may still be preferable. For patients who have minimal symptoms or when sinus rhythm cannot be maintained, however, a strategy of rate control is safe and appropriate. Anticoagulant therapy should be continued, irrespective of the strategy used.

Ablation

In the past decade, ablation for atrial fibrillation has become a therapeutic option. The initial efforts involved the creation of radiofrequency lines of conduction block, rather than surgical incisions.[49] The subsequent discovery that paroxysmal atrial fibrillation primarily emanates from the pulmonary veins[50] led to the use of focal-vein ablation and then to techniques to isolate the firing foci with the use of circumferential or segmental ablation near the ostia of the pulmonary veins.[51]

Recently, the use of anatomical ablation with lesions placed circumferentially around the right and left veins, with or without additional left atrial linear lesions, has been successful in patients with paroxysmal atrial fibrillation and those with persistent atrial fibrillation. In an observational study of 1171 patients, those who underwent ablation had significantly lower rates of recurrence after one year (16 percent) than those receiving antiarrhythmic drugs (39 percent)[52]; among the patients who underwent ablation, mortality and morbidity also were lower and the quality of life was better.

However, data are needed from a randomized trial to establish whether these differences are attributable to the therapy or to other factors. Early series primarily enrolled patients with normal left ventricular function, but in a recent study of 377 patients, one quarter had an ejection fraction below 40 percent,[53] and 73 percent of this group had no recurrence during a follow-up period of 14 months (as compared with 87 percent of the patients with a left ventricular ejection fraction of 40 percent or greater).[53]

Although new techniques and increased experience are associated with lower complication rates, concern persists about potential stroke and tamponade (events that are estimated to occur in 1 percent of cases among experienced physicians).[54] Furthermore, pulmonary-vein stenosis may occur in 5 to 6 percent of patients,[55,56] even when techniques to minimize the risk are used.[57] When a pulmonary-vein stenosis occurs, conservative management may be appropriate, but dilation with or without stenting may be necessary.[55,56]

AREAS OF UNCERTAINTY

Approaches to prevent the development of atrial fibrillation warrant further attention. Recent randomized trials involving patients with left ventricular dysfunction suggest that angiotensin-converting–enzyme inhibitors reduce the risk of atrial fibrillation.[58,59] These data emphasize the importance of treatment for hypertension and cardiovascular disease in such patients.

The role of ablation, as compared with antiarrhythmic therapy, remains uncertain; its use may increase as tools and techniques are improved. The role of new oral anticoagulant agents that are currently in development, which might obviate the need for dose adjustment and the measurement of INR values, needs to be determined. The direct thrombin inhibitor ximelagatran appears to be as effective as warfarin in the prevention of stroke and systemic embolism in patients with atrial fibrillation.[60] However, clinical use of ximelagatran may be limited by its hepatic toxicity; the elevation of levels of alanine aminotransferase to more than three times the upper limit of normal occurred in 6 percent of the patients taking ximelagatran, as compared with 1 percent of those taking warfarin, and hepatic failure leading to death has been reported with the use of ximelagatran.[61]

GUIDELINES

The American College of Cardiology and American Heart Association (ACC–AHA) Task Force on Practice and the European Society of Cardiology (ESC) Committee for Practice have published guidelines for the management of atrial fibrillation[11] that recommend the "minimum evaluation" of newly discovered atrial fibrillation, mentioned earlier, and advise on the use of antiarrhythmic agents (Tables 2 and 3).[11] These guidelines suggest that there is "no clear advantage"[11] to a strategy of rate control as compared with rhythm control. Their recommendations for antithrombotic therapy are similar to, but not identical with, those published by the American College of Chest Physicians (ACCP)[33,34] (Table 1). A third set of guidelines, proposed by the American Academy of Family Physicians (AAFP) and the American College of Physicians (ACP),[35] recommend less aggressive anticoagulant therapy with warfarin. This set of guidelines defines patients who have no history of stroke or transient ischemic attack and have only a single risk factor for stroke (e.g., an age of 75 years or older, congestive heart failure, hypertension, or diabetes)[35] as at low risk (i.e., not in need of warfarin therapy).

RECOMMENDATIONS

The patient described in the vignette presented with atrial fibrillation that was asymptomatic and may have been present for months (as suggested by the failure of the treadmill monitor to measure her heart rate). The evaluation should include testing with electrocardiography, echocardiography, and chest radiography and measurement of the serum thyrotropin level. On the basis of data from randomized trials, her survival would not be improved by the use of strategies aimed at conversion and the maintenance of sinus rhythm, and no strategy could improve her symptoms since she has none. Thus, I would continue heart-rate–control therapy with the use of her current β-adrenergic–blocking agent. Her age and hypertension place her at elevated risk for thromboembolism, and anticoagulant therapy with warfarin is indicated, with a target INR of 2.0 to 3.0. Because atrial fibrillation represents a marker of risk for atherosclerotic disease and stroke,[62] I would also assess the patient for and aggressively treat other risk factors for cardiovascular disease, including her hypertension.

Dr. Page reports having received honoraria from Berlex and AstraZeneca.

This article first appeared in the December 2, 2004, issue of the New England Journal of Medicine.

REFERENCES

1.
Go AS, Hylek EM, Phillips KA, et al. Prevalence of diagnosed atrial fibrillation in adults: national implications for rhythm management and stroke prevention: the AnTicoagulation and Risk Factors in Atrial Fibrillation (ATRIA) study. JAMA 2001;285: 2370-5.

2.
Halperin JL, Hart RG. Atrial fibrillation and stroke: new ideas, persisting dilemmas. Stroke 1988;19:937-41.

3.
Rockson SG, Albers GW. Comparing the guidelines: anticoagulation therapy to optimize stroke prevention in patients with atrial fibrillation. J Am Coll Cardiol 2004;43:929-35.

4.
Gage BF, Waterman AD, Shannon W, Boechler M, Rich MW, Radford MJ. Validation of clinical classification schemes for predicting stoke: results from the National Registry of Atrial Fibrillation. JAMA 2001;285: 2864-70.

5.
Hart RG, Pearce LA, Rothbart RM, et al. Stroke with intermittent atrial fibrillation: incidence and predictors during aspirin therapy. J Am Coll Cardiol 2000;35: 183-7.

6.
Krahn AD, Manfreda J, Tate RB, Mathewson FA, Cuddy TE. The natural history of atrial fibrillation: incidence, risk factors, and prognosis in the Manitoba Follow-Up Study. Am J Med 1995;98:476-84.

7.
Benjamin EJ, Wolf PA, D'Agostino RB, Silbershatz H, Kannel WB, Levy D. Impact of atrial fibrillation on the risk of death: the Framingham Heart Study. Circulation 1998;98:946-52.

8.
ACC/AHA guidelines for the management of patients with valvular heart disease: a report of the American College of Cardiology/ American Heart Association Task Force on Practice Guidelines (Committee on Management of Patients With Valvular Heart Disease). J Am Coll Cardiol 1998;32:1486-588.

9.
Klein GJ, Bashore TM, Sellers TD, Pritchett EL, Smith WM, Gallagher JJ. Ventricular fibrillation in the Wolff–Parkinson–White syndrome. N Engl J Med 1979;301:1080-5.

10.
Kanagala R, Murali NS, Friedman PA, et al. Obstructive sleep apnea and the recurrence of atrial fibrillation. Circulation 2003;107: 2589-94.

11.
Fuster V, Ryden LE, Asinger RW, et al. ACC/ AHA/ESC guidelines for the management of patients with atrial fibrillation: executive summary: a report of the American College of Cardiology/American Heart Association Task Force on Practice Guidelines and the European Society of Cardiology Committee for Practice Guidelines and Policy Conferences (Committee to Develop Guidelines for the Management of Patients with Atrial Fibrillation): developed in collaboration with the North American Society of Pacing and Electrophysiology. J Am Coll Cardiol 2001;38:1231-66.

12.
Brugada R, Tapscott T, Czernuszewicz GZ, et al. Identification of a genetic locus for familial atrial fibrillation. N Engl J Med 1997;336:905-11.

13.
Levy S, Maarek M, Coumel P, et al. Characterization of different subsets of atrial fibrillation in general practice in France: the ALFA study. Circulation 1999;99: 3028-35.

14.
Clark DM, Plumb VJ, Epstein AE, Kay GN. Hemodynamic effects of an irregular sequence of ventricular cycle lengths during atrial fibrillation. J Am Coll Cardiol 1997;30:1039-45.

15.
Packer DL, Bardy GH, Worley SJ, et al. Tachycardia-induced cardiomyopathy: a reversible form of left ventricular dysfunction. Am J Cardiol 1986;57:563-70.

16.
Lemery R, Brugada P, Cheriex E, Wellens HJ. Reversibility of tachycardia-induced left ventricular dysfunction after closed-chest catheter ablation of the atrioventricular junction for intractable atrial fibrillation. Am J Cardiol 1987;60: 1406-8.

17.
Hsu L-F, Jaïs P, Sanders P, et al. Catheter ablation of atrial fibrillation in congestive heart failure. N Engl J Med 2004;351:2373-83.

18.
Savelieva IA, Camm AJ. Silent atrial fibrillation — another Pandora's box. Pacing Clin Electrophysiol 2000;23:145-8.

19.
Kerr C, Boone J, Connolly S, et al. Follow-up of atrial fibrillation: the initial experience of the Canadian Registry of Atrial Fibrillation. Eur Heart J 1996;17:Suppl C:48-51.

20.
Wolf PA, Kannel WB, McGee DL, Meeks SL, Bharucha NE, McNamara PM. Duration of atrial fibrillation and imminence of stroke: the Framingham Study. Stroke 1983;14:664-7.

21.
Page RL, Wilkinson WE, Clair WK, McCarthy EA, Pritchett ELC. Asymptomatic arrhythmias in patients with symptomatic paroxysmal atrial fibrillation and paroxysmal supraventricular tachycardia. Circulation 1994;89:224-7.

22.
Page RL, Tilsh TW, Connolly SJ, et al. Asymptomatic or "silent" atrial fibrillation: frequency in untreated patients and patients receiving azimilide. Circulation 2003;107: 1141-5.

23.
Wolk R, Kulakowski P, Karczmarewicz S, et al. The incidence of asymptomatic paroxysmal atrial fibrillation in patients treated with propranolol or propafenone. Int J Cardiol 1996;54:207-11.

24.
Page RL. Beta-blockers for atrial fibrillation: must we consider asymptomatic arrhythmias? J Am Coll Cardiol 2000;36:147-50.

25.
Israel CW, Gronefeld G, Ehrlich JR, Li Y-G, Hohnloser SH. Long-term risk of recurrent atrial fibrillation as documented by an implantable monitoring device: implications for optimal patient care. J Am Coll Cardiol 2004;43:47-52.

26.
Petersen P, Boysen G, Godtfredsen J, Andersen ED, Andersen B. Placebo-controlled, randomised trial of warfarin and aspirin for prevention of thromboembolic complications in chronic atrial fibrillation: the Copenhagen AFASAK study. Lancet 1989;1:175-9.

27.
Stroke Prevention in Atrial Fibrillation Study: final results. Circulation 1991;84:527-39.

28.
The Boston Area Anticoagulation Trial for Atrial Fibrillation (BAATAF) Investigators. The effect of low-dose warfarin on the risk of stroke in patients with nonrheumatic atrial fibrillation. N Engl J Med 1990;323:1505-11.

29.
Connolly SJ, Laupacis A, Gent M, Roberts RS, Cairns JA, Joyner C. Canadian Atrial Fibrillation Anticoagulation (CAFA) Study. J Am Coll Cardiol 1991;18:349-55.

30.
Ezekowitz MD, Bridgers SL, James KE, et al. Warfarin in the prevention of stroke associated with nonrheumatic atrial fibrillation. N Engl J Med 1992;327:1406-12. [Erratum, N Engl J Med 1993;328:148.]

31.
Risk factors for stroke and efficacy of antithrombotic therapy in atrial fibrillation: analysis of pooled data from five randomized controlled trials. Arch Intern Med 1994;154:1449-57. [Erratum, Arch Intern Med 1994;154:2254.]

32.
Hart RG, Benavente O, McBride R, Pearce LA. Antithrombotic therapy to prevent stroke in patients with atrial fibrillation: a meta-analysis. Ann Intern Med 1999;131:492-501.

33.
Albers GW, Dalen JE, Laupacis A, Manning WJ, Petersen P, Singer DE. Antithrombotic therapy in atrial fibrillation. Chest 2001;119:Suppl:194S-206S.

34.
Stein PD, Alpert JS, Bussey HI, Dalen JE, Turpie AG. Antithrombotic therapy in patients with mechanical and biological prosthetic heart valves. Chest 2001;119:Suppl 1:220S-75. [Erratum, Chest 2001;120:1044.]

35.
Snow V, Weiss KB, LeFevre M, et al. Management of newly detected atrial fibrillation: a clinical practice guideline from the American Academy of Family Physicians and the American College of Physicians. Ann Intern Med 2003;139:1009-17.

36.
Transesophageal echocardiographic correlates of thromboembolism in high-risk patients with nonvalvular trial fibrillation: the Stroke Prevention in Atrial Fibrillation Investigators Committee on Echocardiography. Ann Intern Med 1998;128:639-47.

37.
Hylek EM, Skates SJ, Sheehan MA, Singer DE. An analysis of the lowest effective intensity of prophylactic anticoagulation for patients with nonrheumatic atrial fibrillation. N Engl J Med 1996;335:540-6.

38.
Hylek EM, Go AS, Chang Y, et al. Effect of intensity of oral anticoagulation on stroke severity and mortality in atrial fibrillation. N Engl J Med 2003;349:1019-26.

39.
Klein AL, Grimm RA, Murray RD, et al. Use of transesophageal echocardiography to guide cardioversion in patients with atrial fibrillation. N Engl J Med 2001;344:1411-20.

40.
Farshi R, Kistner D, Sarma JS, Longmate JA, Singh BN. Ventricular rate control in chronic atrial fibrillation during daily activity and programmed exercise: a crossover open-label study of five drug regimens. J Am Coll Cardiol 1999;33:304-10.

41.
Kuhlkamp V, Schirdewan A, Stangl K, Homberg M, Ploch M, Beck OA. Use of metoprolol CR/XL to maintain sinus rhythm after conversion from persistent atrial fibrillation: a randomized, double-blind, placebo controlled study. J Am Coll Cardiol 2000;36:139-46.

42.
Alboni P, Botto GL, Baldi N, et al. Out-of-hospital treatment of recent-onset atrial fibrillation with the "pill-in-the-pocket" approach. N Engl J Med 2004;351:2384-91.

43.
Hohnloser SH, Singh BN. Proarrhythmia with class III antiarrhythmic drugs: definition, electrophysiologic mechanisms, incidence, predisposing factors, and clinical implications. J Cardiovasc Electrophysiol 1995;6:920-36.

44.
Roy D, Talajic M, Dorian P, et al. Amiodarone to prevent recurrence of atrial fibrillation. N Engl J Med 2000;342:913-20.

45.
Hohnloser SH, Kuck K-H, Lilienthal J. Rhythm or rate control in atrial fibrillation — Pharmacological Intervention in Atrial Fibrillation (PIAF): a randomised trial. Lancet 2000;356:1789-94.

46.
Van Gelder IC, Hagens VE, Bosker HA, et al. A comparison of rate control and rhythm control in patients with recurrent persistent atrial fibrillation. N Engl J Med 2002;347:1834-40.

47.
Wyse DG, Waldo AL, DiMarco JP, et al. A comparison of rate control and rhythm control in patients with atrial fibrillation. N Engl J Med 2002;347:1825-33.

48.
Hagens VE, Ranchor AV, Van Sonderen E, et al. Effect of rate or rhythm control on quality of life in persistent atrial fibrillation: results from the Rate Control versus Electrical Cardioversion (RACE) Study. J Am Coll Cardiol 2004;43:241-7.

49.
Cox JL, Schuessler RB, D'Agostine HJ Jr, et al. The surgical treatment of atrial fibrillation. III. Development of a definitive surgical procedure. J Thorac Cardiovasc Surg 1991;101:569-83.

50.
Haissaguerre M, Jais P, Shah DC, et al. Spontaneous initiation of atrial fibrillation by ectopic beats originating in the pulmonary veins. N Engl J Med 1998;339:659-66.

51.
Oral H, Knight BP, Tada H, et al. Pulmonary vein isolation for paroxysmal and persistent atrial fibrillation. Circulation 2002;105:1077-81.

52.
Pappone C, Rosanio S, Augello G, et al. Mortality, morbidity, and quality of life after circumferential pulmonary vein ablation for atrial fibrillation: outcomes from a controlled nonrandomized long-term study. J Am Coll Cardiol 2003;42:185-97.

53.
Chen MS, Marrouche NF, Khaykin Y, et al. Pulmonary vein isolation for the treatment of atrial fibrillation in patients with impaired systolic function. J Am Coll Cardiol 2004;43:1004-9.

54.
Ellenbogen KA, Wood MA. Ablation of atrial fibrillation: awaiting the new paradigm. J Am Coll Cardiol 2003;42:198-200.

55.
Saad EB, Marrouche NF, Saad CP, et al. Pulmonary vein stenosis after catheter ablation of atrial fibrillation: emergence of a new clinical syndrome. Ann Intern Med 2003;138:634-8.

56.
Purerfellner H, Aichinger J, Martinek M, et al. Incidence, management, and outcome in significant pulmonary vein stenosis complicating ablation for atrial fibrillation. Am J Cardiol 2004;93:1428-31.

57.
Vasamreddy CR, Jayam V, Bluemke DA, Calkins H. Pulmonary vein occlusion: an unanticipated complication of catheter ablation of atrial fibrillation using the anatomic circumferential approach. Heart Rhythm 2004;1:78-81.

58.
Pedersen OD, Bagger H, Køber L, Torp-Pedersen C. Trandolapril reduces the incidence of atrial fibrillation after acute myocardial infarction in patients with left ventricular dysfunction. Circulation 1999;100:376-80.

59.
Vermes E, Tardif J-C, Bourassa MG, et al. Enalapril decreases the incidence of atrial fibrillation in patients with left ventricular dysfunction: insight from the Studies of Left Ventricular Dysfunction (SOLVD) trials. Circulation 2003;107:2926-31.

60.
Olsson SB. Stroke prevention with the oral direct thrombin inhibitor ximelagatran compared with warfarin in patients with non-valvular atrial fibrillation (SPORTIF III): randomised controlled trial. Lancet 2003;362:1691-8.

61.
Desai M. NDA 21-686: ximelagatran (H376/95). Briefing document. (Accessed January 31, 2006, at http://www.fda.gov/ohrms/dockets/ac/04/briefing/2004-4069B1_06_FDA-Backgrounder-C-R-MOR.pdf.)

62.
Wyse DG, Gersh BJ. Atrial fibrillation: a perspective: thinking inside and outside the box. Circulation 2004;109:3089-95.

ADDENDUM

Since publication of this article, atrio-esophageal fistula has been reported as an additional rare complication of percutaneous transcatheter ablation of atrial fibrillation.[1]

1. Pappone C, Oral H, Santinelli V, et al. Atrio-esophageal fistula as a complication of percutaneous transcatheter ablation of atrial fibrillation. Circulation 2004;109:2724-6.

Prophylaxis against Rabies

CHARLES E. RUPPRECHT, V.M.D., M.S., PH.D.,

AND ROBERT V. GIBBONS, M.D., M.P.H.

A six-month-old girl presents for a "well-baby" appointment in New Jersey. The mother is concerned about a dead bat she found in the child's bedroom.

A Virginia businessman relaxing on his patio after work pulls a toy from his puppy's mouth. He notices a dead raccoon within his fenced yard, where his puppy has been playing, and telephones you for advice.

You receive e-mail from a South American colleague, who has been bitten by a stray dog while jogging. She solicits your medical opinion.

How would you manage these situations?

THE CLINICAL PROBLEM

Human rabies is uncommon in developed nations.[1-5] In the United States, scores of deaths from rabies were documented annually in the early 20th century. Now, fewer than three deaths are reported each year, most without a documented exposure (Figure 1 and Table 1). Still, this zoonosis exerts a disproportionate influence on health resources because of the necessity for prophylactic measures, including the administration of biologic agents. Continued apprehension is rooted in ancient superstitions, the dramatic manifestation of hydrophobia, and the extreme case fatality ratio. Cases of the disease in humans are preventable, but enzootic foci are plentiful and are not eliminated easily. The public may not appreciate that their surroundings are a veritable sea of rabies, maintained by common animals (Table 2).

Globally, dogs are the major reservoirs. Bites from rabid dogs cause tens of thousands of deaths per year and prompt prophylactic treatment in millions of persons.[4,5] Recent assessments illustrate that the magnitude of rabies in developing countries is grossly underestimated.[6] Exposures may occur as single events, or one rabid animal may expose multiple people.[7] In the United States, 15,000 to 40,000 people receive prophylaxis annually.[8]

Prophylaxis is effective and safe, but it is expensive and is often used inappropriately.[9,10] As with any pharmaceutical agent, minimal considerations when prophylactic measures

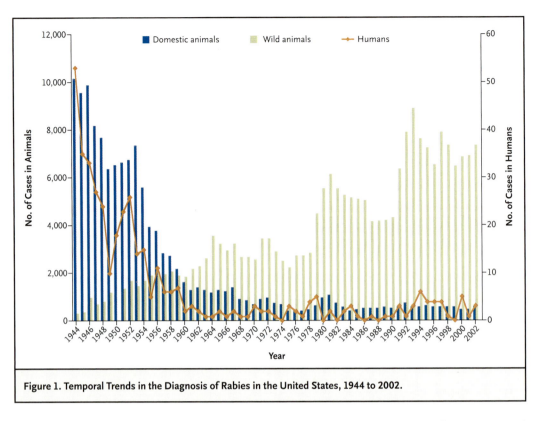

Figure 1. Temporal Trends in the Diagnosis of Rabies in the United States, 1944 to 2002.

are used include proper training, storage, handling, administration, infection-control precautions, and sterile technique.

Nature of the Infection

Rabies is an acute progressive encephalitis caused by RNA viruses in the family Rhabdoviridae, genus Lyssavirus.[11-14] Rabies virus is the only known lyssavirus in the New World. Some locations are considered rabies-free: among them are Hawaii and many islands in the Pacific Ocean and the Caribbean (except Cuba, the Dominican Republic, Haiti, Grenada, and Puerto Rico).[15] However, their continued freedom from rabies depends on effective methods to prevent introduction of the virus and depends on active laboratory-based surveillance.

All mammals are susceptible and can transmit rabies virus, but true reservoirs, which are responsible for ultimate long-term disease maintenance, persist only among Carnivora (mainly carnivorous mammals) and Chiroptera (bats).[15] Specific viruses are adapted to these hosts and typically perpetuate infection within a species before the hosts die. In North America, raccoons, skunks, bats, and foxes are the primary reservoirs responsible

Table 1. Sources of Human Exposure to Rabies in the United States.

Year	Domestic Animal*	Wildlife	Other Sources†	Unknown‡	Total No. of Cases
	number of cases (percent)				
1946–1955	86 (72)	8 (7)	0	26 (22)	120
1956–1965	21 (55)	7 (18)	0	10 (26)	38
1966–1975	6 (38)	7 (44)	1 (6)	2 (12)	16
1976–1985	6 (30)	1 (5)	2 (10)	11 (55)	20
1986–1995	2 (12)	1 (6)	0	14 (82)	17
1996–2003	4 (19)	2 (10)	0	15 (71)	21

* After 1979, there were no cases involving documented exposure to a domestic animal known to be rabid or probably rabid. Thereafter, all cases originated in countries where canine rabies was endemic.
† Other sources of exposure included laboratory aerosol (in 1972 and 1977) and corneal transplantation (in 1978).
‡ If a definitive source of exposure was not identified in the patient's history, the source of exposure was considered to be unknown, regardless of the source suspected on the basis of antigenic or genetic characterization.

for transmission (Table 2). Unvaccinated domestic animals and humans become rabid after exposure to such reservoirs. By definition, all reservoirs are capable of transmitting infection, but not all potential vectors are reservoirs. For example, livestock die of the disease without effective prolonged transmission. Cats (usually infected by dogs or wild animals) are effective vectors but do not sustain the disease.

In developed countries, the incidence of human exposure to rabid domestic animals has decreased as a result of improved canine vaccination.[16] Whereas more than 9000 rabid dogs were reported in the United States in 1944, fewer than 100 were reported in 2002.[15] Because cats are popular but less well supervised and less often vaccinated than dogs, rabid cats now outnumber rabid dogs. Rabies in small mammals (such as mice and squirrels) is rare, and transmission from them to humans remains undocumented.[17] Larger rodents, like woodchucks, are more frequently reported to be rabid (Table 2).

Transmission

In nature, the rabies virus is labile; is inactivated by sunlight, heat, desiccation, and other environmental factors; and is not viable outside the host. Exposure occurs when there is penetration of the skin by teeth or direct transdermal or mucosal contact with infectious material, such as brain tissue or saliva. Almost all cases are caused by bites from infected mammals.

Table 2. Cases of Animal Rabies in the United States.

Animal*	Average No. of Cases, 1998–2002	Geographic Focus†
Raccoon	2962	Eastern United States
Skunk	2257	California, upper and lower Midwest, eastern United States
Bat	1175	Entire United States, except Hawaii
Fox	443	Alaska, Texas, southwestern United States
Cat	276	Entire United States, except Hawaii
Cattle	106	Entire United States, except Hawaii
Dog	105	Entire United States, except Hawaii
Horse or mule	62	Entire United States, except Hawaii
Mongoose	58	Puerto Rico
Woodchuck	50	Eastern United States
Bobcat	30	Entire United States, except Hawaii
Sheep or goat	9	Entire United States, except Hawaii
Other wild animal	24	Entire United States, except Hawaii
Other domestic animal	3	Entire United States, except Hawaii

* All mammals are considered to be susceptible to rabies, and incidental (or spillover) infection from wild-animal reservoirs may occur in any species.
† Rabies may occur in an exposed animal in any location; the geographic foci listed here are based on current epidemiologic trends. No cases of rabies have been reported in Hawaii or in American Samoa, the Commonwealth of the Northern Mariana Islands, Guam, or the U.S. Virgin Islands.

Lyssaviruses are highly neurotropic and travel by retrograde axoplasmic flow from the periphery to the central nervous system.[18] Replication occurs primarily in neurons. There is passive, centrifugal movement from the brain to other organs or glands, such as the salivary glands. The virus is excreted abundantly in saliva. Excretion is concomitant with the development of clinical signs but may begin several days beforehand. The virus may be detected in practically any tissue.

According to experimental data and epidemiologic observations, some domestic species may be observed for signs of rabies. A healthy dog, cat, or ferret that exposes a person may be observed for 10 days.[16] If the animal remains healthy, the patient does not need prophylaxis; only wound care is needed. If the animal sickens with signs compatible with rabies, it should be euthanized and the brain should immediately be examined. If infection is confirmed within 24 to 48 hours after the animal is euthanized, there is adequate

Table 3. Biologic Agents Licensed in the United States for Human Rabies Prevention.*

Product	Dose	Route	Indications
Vaccines†			
RabAvert (Chiron Behring)‡	1 ml	Intramuscular	Preexposure or postexposure§
Rabies vaccine adsorbed (BioPort)¶	1 ml	Intramuscular	Preexposure or postexposure§
Imovax Rabies (Aventis Pasteur)‡‖	1 ml	Intramuscular	Preexposure or postexposure§
Human rabies immune globulins**			
BayRab (Bayer)	20 IU/kg	Local††	Postexposure only
Imogam Rabies-HT (Aventis Pasteur)	20 IU/kg	Local††	Postexposure only

* Adverse reactions include pain, erythema, swelling, or induration (in 15 to 74 percent of recipients); itching or local lymphadenopathy; headache, malaise, myalgia, or dizziness (10 to 25 percent); gastrointestinal symptoms (in less than 10 percent); allergic reactions during primary vaccination (in 0.1 percent [less than 10 percent of whom have anaphylactic reactions]); type III hypersensitivity reactions (in 6 to 10 percent after booster doses of human diploid cell vaccine and in fewer during primary vaccination).[23-26] Precautions should be taken if a serious allergic reaction has been documented after previous administration of a product or component.
† The vaccines are inactivated with beta-propiolactone. Additives (e.g., polygeline) or residual substances used during the manufacturing process (e.g., antibiotics) may be present.
‡ This vaccine is a lyophilized preparation.
§ For postexposure prophylaxis, the vaccine is administered on days 0, 3, 7, 14, and 28 in patients who have not previously been vaccinated and on days 0 and 3 in patients who have been previously vaccinated; for preexposure prophylaxis, the vaccine is administered on days 0, 7, and 21 or 28.
¶ This vaccine is currently not available.
‖ Imovax Rabies I.D., given by the intradermal route, is no longer available in the United States.
** Human rabies immune globulins are purified from the serum of vaccinated donors. Historically, licensed human rabies immune globulins in the United States have been safe. No human infection with adventitious agents has been documented.
†† As much of the product as is anatomically feasible is infiltrated into and around the wound, and any remainder is administered intramuscularly, in the deltoid or quadriceps (at a location other than that used for vaccine inoculation, to minimize potential interference).

time to begin prophylaxis. After exposure to wildlife in which rabies is suspected, prophylaxis is warranted in most circumstances. Vaccination is discontinued if tests of the animal's brain tissue are negative for infection.

STRATEGIES AND EVIDENCE

Prophylaxis

Decisions regarding prophylaxis are complex: they depend on local epidemiology, the nature of the animal involved and its behavior, the degree of contact, and (when possible) the results of diagnostic testing. Procedures include treatment of the patient after exposure as well as vaccination of those at risk for exposure. Efficacy data for prophylaxis are generated by experiments in animals as well as clinical trials.[19]

Postexposure prophylaxis consists of three primary elements: wound care, infiltration of rabies immune globulin, and vaccine administration.[20] Immediate and thorough washing of wounds with a soap solution may considerably reduce the risk of contracting rabies.[21] Other measures, such as the use of tetanus toxoid or antibiotics, are applied as needed.[22] Decisions are urgent, because delays may affect the outcome. Postexposure prophylaxis is highly effective if applied appropriately. In the United States, no failures have been reported since 1979.[1-3]

Vaccines

Three rabies vaccines are licensed in the United States. Table 3 summarizes their uses and potential adverse effects, which are generally minor.[20,27-31] Serious reactions are infrequent[32] and are less common with current cell-culture vaccines than with products derived from nerve tissue.[33] Although associations have been reported between current vaccines and cases of neurologic illness, causality has not been established.[34-39]

When possible, the same product is used for an entire vaccine series. Switching to another product is reasonable if sensitivity to a vaccine or its components develops between doses, although follow-up data are limited.[20,40] Prophylaxis should not be discontinued after the development of local or mild systemic signs.

Modern cell-culture vaccines are potent, but the immunity they afford eventually wanes. After primary vaccination, additional doses are needed after known exposures or as part of routine maintenance of the antibody titer in persons deemed at risk (as discussed below). When booster doses of vaccine are given, complex anamnestic responses occur: they include the stimulation and deployment of existing memory T cells, the differentiation of memory B cells into antibody-secreting cells, elicitation of additional memory B cells, and replenishment of antigen depots at lymphoid germinal centers.

Human Rabies Immune Globulin

Passive administration of virus-neutralizing antibodies, before a patient mounts an active immune response from vaccination, is an important part of postexposure prophylaxis.[20] For patients who have not been vaccinated, human rabies immune globulin is administered only once, concomitantly with vaccine. When there is a visible wound, as much of the dose as is feasible is infiltrated directly into the wound (Table 3). The expense and limited distribution of human rabies immune globulin, however, are problems in the developing world.[4] Equine rabies immune globulin may be an alternative. Multisite intradermal vaccination is another possible strategy to accelerate the immune response.

As compared with unpurified or heterologous serum, modern commercial preparations of human rabies immune globulin are highly safe and are not associated with the acquisition of disease. Human blood products can contain antibodies to other agents and may inhibit immune responses to noninactivated viral vaccines. Interference depends on the amount of specific antibody. Administration of vaccines such as measles and varicella vaccines should be delayed for at least four months after postexposure prophylaxis to allow the degradation of human rabies immune globulin.[41,42] If the interval is shorter, additional vaccination may be necessary, unless serologic testing indicates that the immunologic response has been appropriate.

Preexposure Vaccination

It is recommended that vaccination be provided to persons at risk (laboratory workers, diagnosticians, veterinarians and their staff, animal-control officers, rabies researchers, and some travelers to areas where rabies is prevalent) before exposure.[20] This strategy simplifies the management of a subsequent exposure because fewer doses are needed and because human rabies immune globulin is not required (Table 3). To avoid injury to sciatic nerves and lessen the delivery to adipose depots, it is recommended that the gluteal region not be used for administration.[41] Routine serologic analysis for verification of the presence of virus-neutralizing antibody is unnecessary after primary vaccination, unless major interruptions in the schedule occur or questions arise about immune competence. Thereafter, the need for routine booster vaccination may be monitored by serologic testing performed every six months to two years as long as a person remains at risk. If titers fall below a minimal acceptable level (i.e., complete neutralization at a serum dilution of 1:5), a single vaccine booster is administered. Healthy adults maintain adequate titers for years. No absolute protective level exists, and two booster doses are administered as part of postexposure prophylaxis, regardless of titer. Antibodies are important but are only one means of preventing a productive viral infection. More short-lived immune functions, such as cytokine responses, are reinvigorated in response to vaccination.

AREAS OF UNCERTAINTY

Bats and Rabies

"Cryptic" human cases, in which there is no history of exposure to a rabid animal, are now the norm in the United States (Table 1). Molecular characterization has determined that the majority of these cases are associated with bat rabies viruses.[43] Bat bites are not dramatic and may not be appreciated when they occur or when the patient is examined

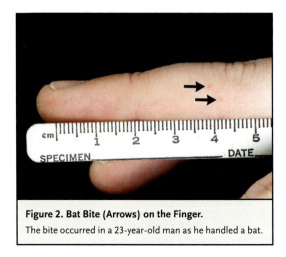

Figure 2. Bat Bite (Arrows) on the Finger.
The bite occurred in a 23-year-old man as he handled a bat.

(Figure 2). In other cases, people may recognize that a bite has occurred but may not comprehend its implications[44] or may believe that the risk of rabies is exceedingly low.[45] Certain persons, such as young children or persons with disabilities, may be unable to provide an accurate history of a bite. When in doubt, attempts should be made to capture animals safely for submission to a laboratory.

Rabies is not commonly reported in free-ranging bats (estimated frequency, less than 1 percent, according to field surveillance) and is diagnosed in approximately 5 to 15 percent of bats submitted for public health evaluation. If test results are negative, postexposure prophylaxis is unnecessary. As with wild-carnivore bites, prophylaxis should begin if the bat is unavailable for examination.[20] Once the risks have been explained, many patients without a definitive exposure (such as healthy adults who are light sleepers or who had body parts covered and would have detected a bat bite) may elect to forgo postexposure prophylaxis.

Exposures Other Than Bites

Since 1960, exposures other than bites have resulted in fewer than 35 well-documented human cases.[46] Most of the reported cases were due to poorly inactivated vaccine (in 18 instances) or transplantation (in 12). Although extremely uncommon, transplantation of tissue from a donor with rabies will have disastrous consequences for the transplant recipient, as has recently been described.[47] No cases in humans after indirect, nonbite exposure, such as touching a pet that may have been exposed to a rabid animal, have been reported. Theoretically, human-to-human transmission is possible, but no cases have been documented among health care workers. Barrier procedures and personal-protection equipment minimize the risk of true exposure.

Many circumstances, though fueled by fear, are not indications for prophylaxis. The medical care of a patient with rabies can cause anxiety on the part of the clinician because of the voluminous production of saliva and the opportunity for unnoticed exposure. Often, postexposure prophylaxis is entertained because the threat of disease is erroneously considered to be greater than unanticipated risks of vaccination. Primum non nocere: if the benefits do not outweigh the risks, postexposure prophylaxis should not be performed.

Schedules and Delays

Clinicians should adhere to prophylaxis schedules. Deviations of a few days are unimportant, but the effect of lapses lasting weeks or months is unknown. Most deviations will not require complete reinitiation of vaccination.[41] For example, if a patient who had begun postexposure prophylaxis missed the dose scheduled for day 14 and attended a clinic visit on day 21, vaccination may be continued with administration of doses at intervals as if the patient had been on schedule. When in doubt, the patient's immune status may be monitored by serologic testing 7 to 14 days after the final dose is given.[20]

Prophylaxis should be instituted whenever exposure is suspected, and it is warranted regardless of the interval between exposure and presentation. Delays in initiating prophylaxis are associated with treatment failure.[48] Typical incubation periods are between one and three months[1-3]; in rare cases, incubation periods are less than two weeks or exceed one year.[49,50] The extent of delay that renders postexposure prophylaxis ineffective is not known.[51]

Travel

Rabies vaccination is not warranted for most routine international travel.[52] Business ventures lasting several days are unlikely to pose a substantive risk. If an exposure does occur, timely access to proper care can be sought on the traveler's return. Concerns related to the rise in ecotourism are minimized by careful planning, tempered with common sense. Minimally, all travelers should receive education about rabies and refrain from contact with animals. Modern biologic agents are not readily available in developing countries. Regardless of the duration of travel, if the location and activity are such that contact with animals is probable but opportunities for intervention are unlikely (especially in the case of travel to a remote region where rabies is endemic), preexposure vaccination should be encouraged.[20] Guidelines related to travel are available from the Centers for Disease Control and Prevention (http://www.cdc.gov/travel/diseases/rabies.htm).

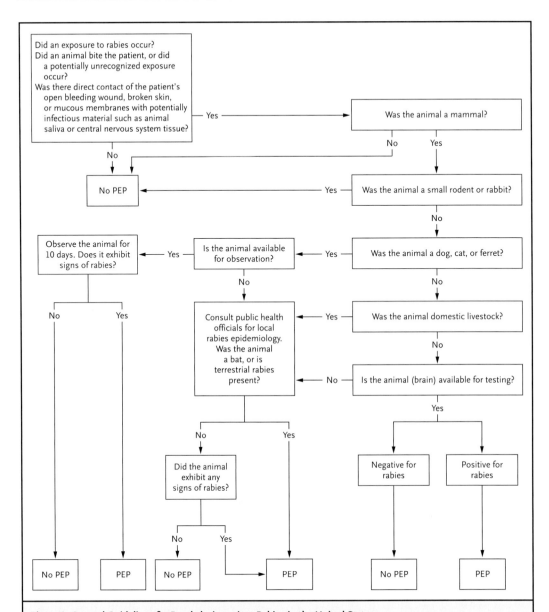

Figure 3. General Guidelines for Prophylaxis against Rabies in the United States.

Bites from bats and high-risk wild carnivores such as raccoons, skunks, foxes, bobcats, coyotes, and mongoose are of great concern and warrant consideration of immediate postexposure prophylaxis (PEP). In the case of direct contact between a human and a bat, the possibility of a bite should be considered unless the exposed person can be reasonably certain that a bite did not occur. PEP should be considered for persons who were in the same room as a bat and who might be unaware, or unable to communicate, that a bite had occurred. Rabies has been reported in large rodents (e.g., woodchucks and beavers) in areas where terrestrial rabies is enzootic. Rabies has rarely been diagnosed in small mammals such as rabbits and small rodents (e.g., squirrels, chipmunks, rats, hamsters, gerbils, guinea pigs, and mice).

(continued on next page)

Pregnancy

Specific testing of reproductive outcomes has not been performed, but pregnancy is not a contraindication to postexposure prophylaxis against rabies. Vaccination has not been associated with adverse outcomes.[53] Prophylaxis is appropriate after exposure to protect the life of the mother and the fetus. Exposure, or the diagnosis of rabies in the mother, is not an indication for termination of the pregnancy.

Treatment

Once symptoms begin, treatment is largely futile. Patients usually die within days to weeks after presentation. Historically, five patients who survived represent unusual occurrences and received some form of prophylaxis before onset. Diagnosis by detection of virus, antigen, antibodies, or nucleic acid in the patient's saliva, tissues, serum, or cerebrospinal fluid warrants attempts to treat,[54] although management is essentially palliative. Experimental trials have included rabies immune globulin, interferon, and ribavirin, without beneficial effect.[45]

GUIDELINES

The Advisory Committee on Immunization Practices (ACIP) publishes routine protocols for prevention of human rabies in the United States (http://www.cdc.gov/nip/publications/acip-list.htm).[20] The information presented in this article is consistent with the ACIP guidelines. The recommendations of the American Academy of Pediatrics are in accord

---

(continued from previous page)

There has never been a documented case of transmission from these small mammals to a human. PEP may be considered for the latter in unusual circumstances (e.g., a bite from a small mammal with a history and clinical signs compatible with rabies), unless the animal is available for testing and is negative. An apparently healthy dog, cat, or ferret that bites a person should be confined and observed daily for 10 days. (The determination of whether a bite was provoked is necessarily subjective. For domestic animals, territorial-defense–related aggression and bites that occur when the animal is surprised, startled, or manipulated are generally viewed as provoked.) The animal should not receive a rabies vaccine during the observation period. A veterinarian should evaluate the animal at the first sign of illness. Management of animals other than dogs, cats, and ferrets depends on the species, the circumstances of the bite, the local rabies epidemiology, and the biting animal's history, current health status, and potential for exposure to rabies. Because prior vaccination of an animal may not be 100 percent effective, current vaccination does not preclude the necessity of a 10-day observation period or, as warranted, euthanasia and testing. State and local authorities should be informed of biting incidents involving cats, dogs, and ferrets. If the animal exhibits signs of rabies during the 10-day observation period, the patient should immediately begin to receive prophylaxis, and the animal should be euthanized and its brain tissue tested for rabies. If the animal is confirmed to have been rabid, PEP should be completed; if test results are negative, PEP can cease. Diagnostic testing of brain tissue should be completed within 24 to 48 hours so that a decision about starting PEP can be made. If the diagnosis cannot be completed within this period, prophylaxis should be started, pending the results of testing. Incubation periods of less than one week have been reported after severe bites on the face, head, and neck. The initiation of PEP should be considered in persons with such exposures before the results of laboratory testing become available.

with those of the ACIP; vaccine doses during postexposure prophylaxis are equivalent in adults and children.[55] The National Association of State Public Health Veterinarians regularly issues a compendium of recommendations for the prevention and control of rabies in animals.[16] As a barrier to human infection, pets and other animals should be vaccinated and receive regular booster doses. Exposed, currently vaccinated animals should receive immediate booster doses, whereas unvaccinated animals should either be euthanized or quarantined. The World Health Organization maintains information on the global distribution of rabies and recommendations for postexposure prophylaxis, including alternative vaccines, schedules, and routes, on its Web site (http://www.who.int/emc-documents/rabies/whocdscsreph200210.html).[5,56] Booster doses of vaccine are suggested when the antibody titer in a patient at risk falls below 0.5 IU per milliliter.

SUMMARY AND RECOMMENDATIONS

Once symptoms develop, rabies is almost invariably fatal. The overarching public health goals are to educate the public about the disease, prevent exposures, offer vaccination to those at increased risk, and administer postexposure prophylaxis appropriately. Figure 3 provides general guidance for the most common circumstances encountered in the United States.

The child described in the first vignette should be examined thoroughly for any evidence of a small lesion compatible with a bite wound. If the bat is available, the carcass should be sent to a diagnostic facility. Postexposure prophylaxis is unnecessary if test results in the bat are negative. However, prophylaxis is needed if the bat is found to have been rabid. If the bat is unavailable, consultation with the local or state health department is appropriate, and prophylaxis should be considered if it is likely that the child was exposed.

In the second vignette, the owner has not been exposed, even if his puppy had contact with the raccoon sometime that morning. Actions should focus on diagnostic testing of the raccoon and pet management, depending on the results and depending on the immune status of the puppy.

In the last vignette, the action to be taken depends on the specific circumstances. If the suspicion of rabies is low (i.e., the dog appeared healthy; the attack was provoked; the woman was bitten on an ankle through her clothing; there were only minor abrasions, which were washed well; and the episode occurred in a major city free of canine rabies in recent years, such as Rio de Janeiro or Montevideo, Uruguay) or if the dog is found alive, prophylaxis is not indicated. If the bite occurred in an area where canine rabies is endemic, immediate postexposure prophylaxis is warranted, either with locally produced biologic agents or those obtained from the closest major urban area or country.

The views expressed in this article are those of the authors and do not necessarily represent the official policies of the Centers for Disease Control and Prevention, the Department of the Army, or the Department of Defense. Use of trade names does not constitute government endorsement.

We are indebted to Jesse Blanton for the photograph used in Figure 2; to the staff in the Viral and Rickettsial Zoonoses Branch, Centers for Disease Control and Prevention, for their valuable insights; and to our many national and international colleagues for their timely devotion to the amelioration of this often ignored disease.

This article first appeared in the December 16, 2004, issue of the New England Journal of Medicine.

REFERENCES

1.
Held JR, Tierkel ES, Steele JH. Rabies in man and animals in the United States, 1946-65. Public Health Rep 1967;82:1009-18.

2.
Anderson LJ, Nicholson KG, Tauxe RV, Winkler WG. Human rabies in the United States, 1960 to 1979: epidemiology, diagnosis, and prevention. Ann Intern Med 1984;100:728-35.

3.
Noah DL, Drenzek CL, Smith JS, et al. Epidemiology of human rabies in the United States, 1980 to 1996. Ann Intern Med 1998;128:922-30.

4.
Warrell MJ, Warrell DA. Rabies and other lyssavirus diseases. Lancet 2004;363:959-69.

5.
World Health Organization. World survey for rabies No. 35 for the year 1999. Geneva: World Health Organization, 2002. (Accessed November 19, 2004, at http://www.who.int/emc-documents/rabies/whocdscsreph200210.html.)

6.
Coleman PG, Fevre EM, Cleaveland S. Estimating the public health impact of rabies. Emerg Infect Dis 2004;10:140-2.

7.
Rotz LD, Hensley JA, Rupprecht CE, Childs JE. Large-scale human exposures to rabid or presumed rabid animals in the United States: 22 cases (1990-1996). J Am Vet Med Assoc 1998;212:1198-200.

8.
Krebs JW, Long-Marin SC, Childs JE. Causes, costs, and estimates of rabies postexposure prophylaxis treatments in the United States. J Public Health Manag Pract 1998;4:56-62.

9.
Moran GJ, Talan DA, Mower W, et al. Appropriateness of rabies postexposure prophylaxis treatment for animal exposures. JAMA 2000;284:1001-7.

10.
Manufacturer's recall of human rabies vaccine. MMWR Morb Mortal Wkly Rep 2004;53(Dispatch, April 2):1-2. (Accessed January 31, 2006, at http://www.cdc.gov/mmwr/preview/mmwrhtml/mm53d402a1.htm.)

11.
King AA, Meredith CD, Thomson GR. The biology of southern African lyssavirus variants. Curr Top Microbiol Immunol 1994;187:267-95.

12.
Hanna JN, Carney IK, Smith GA, et al. Australian bat lyssavirus infection: a second human case, with a long incubation period. Med J Aust 2000;172:597-9.

13.
Fooks AR, Brookes SM, Johnson N, McElhinney LM, Hutson AM. European bat lyssaviruses: an emerging zoonosis. Epidemiol Infect 2003;131:1029-39.

14.
Botvinkin AD, Poleschuk EM, Kuzmin IV, et al. Novel lyssaviruses isolated from bats in Russia. Emerg Infect Dis 2003;9:1623-5.

15.
Krebs JW, Wheeling JT, Childs JE. Rabies surveillance in the United States during 2002. J Am Vet Med Assoc 2003;223:1736-48. [Erratum, J Am Vet Med Assoc 2004;224:705.]

16.
Jenkins SR, Auslander M, Conti L, Leslie MJ, Sorhage FE, Sun B. Compendium of animal rabies prevention and control, 2004. J Am Vet Med Assoc 2004;224:216-22.

17.
Childs JE, Colby L, Krebs JW, et al. Surveillance and spatiotemporal associations of rabies in rodents and lagomorphs in the United States, 1985-1994. J Wildl Dis 1997;33:20-7.

18.
Charlton KM. The pathogenesis of rabies and other lyssaviral infections: recent studies. Curr Top Microbiol Immunol 1994;187:95-119.

19.
Bahmanyar M, Fayaz A, Nour-Salehi S, Mohammadi M, Koprowski H. Successful protection of humans exposed to rabies infection: postexposure treatment with the new human diploid cell rabies vaccine and antirabies serum. JAMA 1976;236:2751-4.

20.
Human rabies prevention — United States, 1999: recommendations of the Immunization Practices Advisory Committee (ACIP). MMWR Recomm Rep 1999;48(RR-1):1-21.

21.
Dean DJ. Pathogenesis and prophylaxis of rabies in man. N Y State J Med 1963;63:3507-13.

22.
Griego RD, Rosen T, Orengo IF, Wolf JE. Dog, cat, and human bites: a review. J Am Acad Dermatol 1995;33:1019-29.

23.
Systemic allergic reactions following immunization with human diploid cell rabies vaccine. MMWR Morb Mortal Wkly Rep 1984;33:185-7.

24.
Dreesen DW, Bernard KW, Parker RA, Deutsch AJ, Brown J. Immune complex-like disease in 23 persons following a booster dose of rabies human diploid cell vaccine. Vaccine 1986;4:45-9.

25.
Swanson MC, Rosanoff E, Gurwith M, Deitch M, Schnurrenberger P, Reed CE. IgE and IgG antibodies to beta-propiolactone and human serum albumin associated with urticarial reactions to rabies vaccine. J Infect Dis 1987;155:909-13.

26.
Fishbein DB, Yenne KM, Dreesen DW, Teplis CF, Mehta N, Briggs DJ. Risk factors for systemic hypersensitivity reactions after booster vaccinations with human diploid cell rabies vaccine: a nationwide prospective study. Vaccine 1993;11:1390-4.

27.
Anderson LJ, Winkler WG, Hafkin B, Keenlyside RA, D'Angelo LJ, Deitch MW. Clinical experience with a human diploid cell rabies vaccine. JAMA 1980;244: 781-4.

28.
Plotkin SA. Rabies vaccine prepared in human cell cultures: progress and perspectives. Rev Infect Dis 1980;2:433-48.

29.
Dreesen DW, Fishbein DB, Kemp DT, Brown J. Two-year comparative trial on the immunogenicity and adverse effects of purified chick embryo cell rabies vaccine for pre-exposure immunization. Vaccine 1989;7: 397-400.

30.
Noah DL, Smith MG, Gotthardt JC, Krebs JW, Green D, Childs JE. Mass human exposure to rabies in New Hampshire: exposures, treatment, and cost. Am J Public Health 1996;86: 1149-51.

31.
Jones RL, Froeschle JE, Atmar RL, et al. Immunogenicity, safety and lot consistency in adults of a chromatographically purified Vero-cell rabies vaccine: a randomized, double-blind trial with human diploid cell rabies vaccine. Vaccine 2001;19:4635-43.

32.
Surveillance for safety after immunization: Vaccine Adverse Event Reporting System (VAERS) — United States, 1991–2001. MMWR Surveill Summ 2003; 52(SS1):1-24.

33.
Parviz S, Luby S, Wilde H. Postexposure treatment of rabies in Pakistan. Clin Infect Dis 1998;27:751-6.

34.
Boe E, Nyland H. Guillain-Barre syndrome after vaccination with human diploid cell rabies vaccine. Scand J Infect Dis 1980;12:231-2.

35.
Bernard KW, Smith PW, Kader FJ, Moran MJ. Neuroparalytic illness and human diploid cell rabies vaccine. JAMA 1982;248:3136-8.

36.
Knittel T, Ramadori G, Mayet WJ, Lohr H, Meyer zum Buschenfelde KH. Guillain-Barre syndrome and human diploid cell rabies vaccine. Lancet 1989;1:1334-5.

37.
Tornatore CS, Richert JR. CNS demyelination associated with diploid cell rabies vaccine. Lancet 1990;335: 1346-7.

38.
Moulignier A, Richer A, Fritzell C, Foulon D, Khoubesserian P, de Recondo J. Meningoradiculitis after injection of an antirabies vaccine: a vaccine from human diploid cell culture. Presse Med 1991;20: 1121-3. (In French.)

39.
Chakravarty A. Neurologic illness following postexposure prophylaxis with purified chick embryo cell antirabies vaccine. J Assoc Physicians India 2001;49: 927-8.

40.
Briggs DJ, Dreesen DW, Nicolay U, et al. Purified Chick Embryo Cell Culture Rabies Vaccine: interchangeability with Human Diploid Cell Culture Rabies Vaccine and comparison of one versus two-dose post-exposure booster regimen for previously immunized persons. Vaccine 2000;19:1055-60.

41.
General recommendations on immunization: recommendations of the Advisory Committee on Immunization Practices (ACIP) and the American Academy of Family Physicians (AAFP). MMWR Recomm Rep 2002;51(RR-2):1-35.

42.
Siber GR, Werner BG, Halsey NA, et al. Interference of immune globulin with measles and rubella immunization. J Pediatr 1993;122:204-11.

43.
Messenger SL, Smith JS, Rupprecht CE. Emerging epidemiology of bat-associated cryptic cases of rabies in humans in the United States. Clin Infect Dis 2002;35:738-47.

44.
Gibbons RV, Holman RC, Mosberg SR, Rupprecht CE. Knowledge of bat rabies and human exposure among United States cavers. Emerg Infect Dis 2002;8:532-4.

45.
Human death associated with bat rabies — California, 2003. MMWR Morb Mortal Wkly Rep 2004;53:33-5.

46.
Gibbons RV. Cryptogenic rabies, bats, and the question of aerosol transmission. Ann Emerg Med 2002;39: 528-36.

47.
Update: investigation of rabies infections in organ donor and transplant recipients — Alabama, Arkansas, Oklahoma, and Texas, 2004. Atlanta: Centers for Disease Control and Prevention, 2004. (Accessed January 31, 2006, at http://www.cdc. gov/mmwr/preview/ mmwrhtml/mm53d709. htm.)

48.
Thraenhart O, Marcus I, Kreuzfelder E. Current and future immunoprophylaxis against human rabies: reduction of treatment failures and errors. Curr Top Microbiol Immunol 1994;187: 173-94.

49.
Smith JS, Fishbein DB, Rupprecht CE, Clark K. Unexplained rabies in three immigrants in the United States: a virologic investigation. N Engl J Med 1991;324: 205-11.

50.
Chhabra M, Ichhpujani RL, Tewari KN, Lal S. Human rabies in Delhi. Indian J Pediatr 2004;71:217-20.

51.
Helmick CG. The epidemiology of human rabies postexposure prophylaxis, 1980-1981. JAMA 1983;250: 1990-6.

52.
LeGuerrier P, Pilon PA, Deshaies D, Allard R. Pre-exposure rabies prophylaxis for the international traveller: a decision analysis. Vaccine 1996;14:167-76.

53.
Chutivongse S, Wilde H, Benjavongkulchai M, Chomchey P, Punthawong S. Postexposure rabies vaccination during pregnancy: effect on 202 women and their infants. Clin Infect Dis 1995;20:818-20.

54.
Jackson AC, Warrell MJ, Rupprecht CE, et al. Management of rabies in humans. Clin Infect Dis 2003;36:60-3.

55.
Rabies. In: Pickering LK, ed. Red Book: 2003 report of the Committee on Infectious Diseases. 26th ed. Elk Grove Village, Ill.: American Academy of Pediatrics, 2003:514-21.

56.
WHO recommendations on rabies post-exposure treatment and the correct technique of intradermal immunization against rabies. Geneva: World Health Organization, 1997. (Accessed November 19, 2004, at http://www.who.int/emc-documents/rabies/whoemczoo966c.htm.)

Addendum

Rabies remains a major global health problem and a consuming medical challenge. Recently, recovery was reported of a patient with rabies after the induction of coma and use of antiviral drugs.[1] Such treatment strategies offer hope but require confirmation in other cases.

1. Willoughby RE Jr, Tieves KS, Hoffman GM, et al. Survival after treatment of rabies with induction of coma. N Engl J Med 2005;352:2508-14.

Attention Deficit–Hyperactivity Disorder

MARSHA D. RAPPLEY, M.D.

A mother brings in her eight-year-old son for evaluation after he is suspended from riding the school bus for jumping out of his seat, teasing other children, and not following directions. He spends two to three hours a night with homework that he never successfully completes. His mother wants to know whether he has attention deficit–hyperactivity disorder. How should he be evaluated and treated?

THE CLINICAL PROBLEM

Attention deficit–hyperactivity disorder (ADHD) is characterized by the inability to marshal and sustain attention, modulate activity level, and moderate impulsive actions. The result is maladaptive behaviors that are inconsistent with age and developmental level. Evidence from neuropsychological, pharmacologic, and brain-imaging studies implicates dopamine and norepinephrine neurotransmitter systems in frontostriatal circuitry in the pathophysiology of the disorder. Genetic factors appear to play an important role.[1-3] Extremely low birth weight (less than 1000 g)[4] and environmental conditions, such as head trauma and exposure to lead, are also associated with symptoms of ADHD.

The diagnosis of ADHD requires the identification of specific behaviors that meet the criteria of the *Diagnostic and Statistical Manual of Mental Disorders*, fourth edition, revised (DSM-IV-R)[5] (Table 1). Three types of ADHD are diagnosed: combined inattentive, hyperactive, and impulsive (about 80 percent of patients); predominantly inattentive (about 10 to 15 percent); and predominantly hyperactive and impulsive (about 5 percent).

The prevalence of ADHD is estimated at 3 to 7 percent of all children. Boys are more often affected than girls (the ratio ranges, according to the population studied, from 9 to 1 to 2.5 to 1), but increasingly, cases involving girls are being identified.[5,6] ADHD is a chronic condition with symptoms experienced over a lifetime.[7] This review focuses on ADHD in children and adolescents.

Table 1. Criteria for the Diagnosis of ADHD.*

The diagnosis requires evidence of inattention or hyperactivity and impulsivity or both

Inattention

Six or more of the following symptoms of inattention have persisted for at least six months to a degree that is maladaptive and inconsistent with developmental level:

Often fails to give close attention to details and makes careless mistakes

Often has difficulty sustaining attention

Often does not seem to listen

Often does not seem to follow through

Often has difficulty organizing tasks

Often avoids tasks that require sustained attention

Often loses things necessary for activities

Often is easily distracted

Often is forgetful

Hyperactivity and impulsivity

Six or more of the following symptoms of hyperactivity and impulsivity have persisted for at least six months to a degree that is maladaptive and inconsistent with developmental level:

Often fidgets

Often leaves seat

Often runs about or climbs excessively

Often has difficulty with quiet leisure activities

Often is "on the go" or "driven by a motor"

Often talks excessively

Often blurts out answers

Often has difficulty awaiting turn

Often interrupts or intrudes

Symptoms that cause impairment:

Are present before 7 years of age

Are present in two or more settings (e.g., home, school, or work)

Do not occur exclusively during the course of a pervasive developmental disorder, schizophrenia, or another psychotic disorder

Are not better accounted for by another mental disorder (e.g., a mood disorder or an anxiety disorder)

* The criteria are adapted from the *Diagnostic and Statistical Manual of Mental Disorders,* fourth edition, revised.[5]

STRATEGIES AND EVIDENCE

Diagnosis

The abilities to focus attention, regulate activity, and control impulses emerge for all children in a developmental process. Thus, the diagnosis of ADHD is based on a comprehensive history that elicits symptoms specific to the diagnosis, the context in which these symptoms occur, and the degree to which these are inconsistent with age and persist to cause impairment.[8]

Evidence of symptoms is obtained directly from the child, the parents, and the teachers. The National Initiative for Children's Healthcare Quality Vanderbilt Assessment Scale

Table 2. Mental Health Conditions That Mimic or Coexist with ADHD.

Disorder	Symptoms Overlapping with ADHD	Features Not Characteristic of ADHD	Diagnostic Problem
Learning disorders	Underachievement in school Disruptive behavior during academic activity Refusal to engage in academic tasks and use academic materials	Underachievement and disruptive behavior in academic work, rather than in multiple settings and activities	It can be difficult to determine which to evaluate first — a learning disorder or ADHD (follow the preponderance of symptoms)
Oppositional defiant disorder	Disruptive behavior, especially regarding rules Failure to follow directions	Defiance, rather than unsuccessful attempts to cooperate	Defiant behavior is often associated with a high level of activity It is difficult to determine the child's effort to comply in instances of a negative parent–child or teacher–child relationship
Conduct disorder	Disruptive behavior Encounters with law-enforcement and legal systems	Lack of remorse Intent to harm or do wrong Aggression and hostility Antisocial behavior	Fighting or running away may be reasonable reactions to adverse social circumstances
Anxiety, obsessive-compulsive disorder, or post-traumatic stress disorder	Poor attention Fidgetiness Difficulty with transitions Physical reactivity to stimuli	Excessive worries Fearfulness Obsessions or compulsions Nightmares Reexperiences of trauma	Anxiety may be a source of high activity and inattention
Depression	Irritability Reactive impulsivity Demoralization	Pervasive and persistent feelings of irritability or sadness	It may be difficult to distinguish depression from a reaction to repeated failure, which is associated with ADHD
Bipolar disorder	Poor attention Hyperactivity Impulsivity Irritability	Expansive mood Grandiosity Manic quality	It is difficult to distinguish severe ADHD from early-onset bipolar disorder
Tic disorder	Poor attention Impulsive verbal or motor actions Disruptive activity	Repetitive vocal or motor movements	Tics may not be apparent to the patient, the family, or a casual observer
Adjustment disorder	Poor attention Hyperactivity Disruptive behavior Impulsivity Poor academic performance	Recent onset Precipitating event	Chronic stressors, such as having a sibling with mental illness, or attachment-and-loss issues may produce symptoms of anxiety and depression

for parents and teachers consists of checklists of behaviors that can help the primary care physician assess the child with ADHD.[9] Parents and teachers rate the child's symptoms on a scale of "never" to "very often" on items derived from the DSM-IV-R criteria for ADHD. They also rate the child's school performance and interpersonal relationships. The scores indicate whether impairment meets the diagnostic criteria for ADHD. Although the checklists reflect subjective impressions, they allow a comparison of the patient with children of the same age and are the best available tool to discern behavior that exceeds normal variation.

Behaviors of ADHD may overlap or coexist with other mental health conditions (Table 2). The most common conditions are learning and language disorders, oppositional defiant disorder, conduct disorder, anxiety, and depression, as well as bipolar, post-traumatic stress, tic, and adjustment disorders.[10]

Table 3. Guidelines for the Diagnosis and Treatment of Patients with ADHD.*

Diagnosis
    Comprehensive developmental, social, and family history
    Standardized checklists to assess behaviors[9,19]
    Consideration of coexisting mental health disorders
    Physical examination, not to diagnose ADHD but to assess genetic and
        other conditions

Treatment
    Management of ADHD as a chronic health condition
    Establishment of treatment goals agreed on by the child, the family, and
        school personnel
    Medication with stimulants to manage symptoms (monotherapy)†
    Behavioral therapy for parent–child discord and persistent oppositional
        behavior

Desired outcomes of treatment
    Improved relationships with family, teachers, and peers
    Decreased frequency of disruptive behavior
    Improved quality of and efficiency in completing academic work, and in-
        creased quantity of work completed
    Increased independence in caring for self and carrying out age-appropriate
        activities
    Improved self-esteem
    Enhanced safety (e.g., care in crossing streets, staying with an adult in
        public places, and reduced risk-taking behavior)

* This information has been compiled from the guidelines of the American
Academy of Pediatrics,[7,13] the American Academy of Child and Adolescent
Psychiatry,[15,16] the European Society for Child and Adolescent Psychiatry,[17]
and the Scottish Intercollegiate Guidelines Network.[18]
† Atomoxetine is recommended by the American Academy of Child and Adoles-
cent Psychiatry as a possible alternative to stimulant medication.[20]

A careful history is warranted of the development of motor, social, and language skills, as well as of temperament, sleep habits, school achievement, moods, worries, and relationships. Furthermore, the primary care physician should be informed about prenatal and birth events, including prematurity and prenatal exposure to substances associated with behavioral and learning problems, such as tobacco and cocaine.[11] The assessment should include circumstances that might influence behavior and school performance, such as frequent moves or bitter custody disputes.[12] It is also important to determine whether there is a family history of ADHD, depression, bipolar disorder, anxiety disorders, or tic disorders. Genetic disorders that may have symptoms similar to those of ADHD (such as the fragile X syndrome) should be considered.

No physical findings are diagnostic of ADHD. Laboratory studies are not routinely obtained. Testing for achievement, intelligence, and specific learning disabilities may aid the differential diagnosis and help with planning for school services; such testing may be obtained through school-based assessment or by referral to a psychologist. Computerized or manual performance tests of attention and impulsivity are not diagnostic of ADHD.[13]

Treatment of the Patient

Treatment of the patient with ADHD focuses on control of the symptoms (which vary with the patient's development), classroom education, interpersonal relationships, and the transition to adult life.[14] Therapy is guided by measurable target outcomes, such as the number of calls in a week from the teacher to report disciplinary action, the amount of time spent on homework assignments, or participation in other activities without disruption (Table 3).[7]

THERAPY

Pharmacologic Interventions

Methylphenidate and Dextroamphetamine   There is strong evidence to support the use of stimulant medication for the management of inattention, impulsivity, and hyperactivity in school-age children.[21] Methylphenidate and dextroamphetamine have consistently shown efficacy and safety when compared with placebo in randomized, controlled trials.[22] Two studies are particularly informative. The Multimodal Treatment Study of ADHD involved 597 children at six centers who were followed for 24 months, including a 14-month treatment phase.[23] The study by Abikoff et al. involved 103 children at two centers who were randomly assigned to 24 months of treatment.[24] The two studies included children seven to nine years of age and involved randomized pharmacologic and psychological interventions. Both studies assessed behavioral outcomes in the settings of the home and the school. Consistent with previous smaller studies, these trials showed that 68 to 80 percent of children treated with stimulants had improvements in behavior such that at the end of the treatment phase the children no longer met the criteria for a diagnosis of ADHD. The benefit of treatment was reduced in the Multimodal Treatment Study of ADHD after the children completed the active-study phase, whereas the benefit was sustained in the study by Abikoff et al. during the 24 months of treatment.

Randomized trials directly comparing methylphenidate and dextroamphetamine have shown similar benefits from the two medications but more frequent mild side effects with dextroamphetamine.[25,26] Evidence supports either medication as a first choice; 70 to 80 percent of children show improved attention with the use of one or the other.[22] Preparations are available as short-, intermediate-, and long-acting, with a duration of 3 to 10

Table 4. Recommended Medications for ADHD.

Medication*	Initial Dose	Usual Dose	Doses per Day	Side Effects	Contraindications
	mg				
Methylphenidate†					
Ritalin, Methylin	5–10	10–20	2–3	Appetite suppression, stomachaches, headaches, irritability, weight loss, deceleration in rate of growth, exacerbation of psychosis, exacerbation of tics, mild increase in blood pressure and pulse	Marked anxiety, tension, agitation, glaucoma, use of monoamine oxidase inhibitors, seizures, tics
Concerta	18–27	27–54	1		
Metadate ER, Metadate CD, Methylin ER	10	10–20	1		
Ritalin LA	20	20–40	1		
Focalin‡	2.5–5	2.5–10	2–3		
MethyPatch§					
Dextroamphetamine (sulfate alone and in combination with amphetamine salts)†					
Dexedrine	5	5–20	2–3	Appetite suppression, weight loss, stomachaches, headaches, irritability, possible growth inhibition, exacerbation of psychosis, exacerbation of tics, mild increase in blood pressure and pulse	Cardiovascular disease, hypertension, hyperthyroidism, glaucoma, drug dependence, use of monoamine oxidase inhibitors
Dexedrine Spansule	5–10	5–15	1–2		
Adderall	5–10	5–30	1–2		
Adderall XR	5–10	10–30	1		
Atomoxetine¶					
Strattera	10–25	18–60	1	Appetite suppression, nausea, vomiting, fatigue, weight loss, deceleration in rate of growth, mild increase in blood pressure and pulse	Jaundice or other clinical or laboratory evidence of liver injury, use of monoamine oxidase inhibitors, narrow-angle glaucoma
Bupropion‖					
Wellbutrin SR	100–150	150	1–2	Weight loss, insomnia, agitation, anxiety, dry mouth, seizures, others	Seizures, bulimia, anorexia nervosa, abrupt discontinuation of alcohol or benzodiazepines, use of monoamine oxidase inhibitors or other bupropion products (e.g., Zyban)
Wellbutrin XL	150	150–300	1		

* For each category the generic drug is given and dosing information for each named marketed drug.
† The manufacturer states that seizures and tic disorder are contraindications; research supports the use of stimulants in children with seizures that have stabilized with the use of anticonvulsants and in children with tic disorder or Tourette's disorder.[27,28] With use of a long-acting methylphenidate or dextroamphetamine product, a short-acting product may be added at 4 p.m. to 6 p.m. for homework or special activities; appetite and sleep onset are then carefully monitored.
‡ Focalin is a dextro isomer of methylphenidate that is given at a lower dose.
§ The MethyPatch is a sustained-action transdermal patch that is not yet available.
¶ Younger children may need two doses a day.
‖ Bupropion has not been approved by the Food and Drug Administration for pediatric use. Only sustained release (twice daily) or extended release (once daily) are recommended for adolescents. There is a higher incidence of side effects with the immediate-release preparation.

hours and similar efficacy (Table 4). The administration of short-acting medications can be timed to correspond to certain of the child's activities. Long-acting medications obviate the need for doses during the school day.

Dosages of methylphenidate and dextroamphetamine are not weight-based. Guidelines consistently recommend starting with lower doses and titrating to an effective dose that does not cause side effects (Table 4).[7,15] Side effects are generally mild and managed by attention to dose and timing. The most common side effects are appetite suppression, stomachache, and headache, leading to discontinuation of the medication in approximately 1 percent to 4 percent of children.[25,29] Delayed onset of sleep, previously thought to be associated with treatment, may be associated with the underlying disorder.[30] In a 24-month follow-up, the Multimodal Treatment Study of ADHD showed a deceleration in growth of approximately 1 cm per year with the use of stimulant medication.[31] However, growth remained within the normal curve for most children, except those at the lowest percentiles of height for age. It is not known whether this effect is cumulative or can be ameliorated by summers off medication, allowing time for growth to catch up.

Follow-up visits in the Multimodal Treatment Study of ADHD[23] and the study by Abikoff et al.[24] were monthly. In general practice, however, once a stable dose of medication has been established, visits every three to four months are reasonable to monitor the effectiveness and potential side effects of the medication. Blood pressure, pulse, height, and weight are followed, given the potential for the medication to affect these measures (Table 4).

Other Medications   Two other medications are effective with core symptoms of ADHD. Atomoxetine, a norepinephrine-reuptake inhibitor, is not classified as a stimulant. Randomized trials including more than 1000 children and adults showed that 58 to 64 percent of children treated during a 6-to-12-week period achieved 25 to 30 percent or greater improvement in symptoms.[32,33] Two recent reports of severe liver injury (which apparently reversed after drug cessation) have led to the addition of a bolded warning to the label indicating that atomoxetine should be discontinued in patients with jaundice or laboratory evidence of liver injury.[34] Side effects such as appetite suppression and weight loss are reported at a frequency similar to that for side effects seen with methylphenidate.[32,35] A study conducted in several countries showed a treatment benefit that was sustained over nine months.[36] Seizures and prolonged QT intervals corrected for heart rate are reported with overdoses of atomoxetine, but not with therapeutic doses.[37] Cases of tics developing during treatment with atomoxetine were recently reported[38] but were not described in randomized trials.

Bupropion, an aminoketone antidepressant, is also effective for inattention and impulsivity, but has not been approved by the Food and Drug Administration for use in children. Two randomized trials comparing bupropion with methylphenidate reported a smaller treatment effect and more side effects with bupropion among a total of 124 children and adolescents (Table 4).[39,40] Atomoxetine and bupropion might be effective for children who require control of symptoms 24 hours a day and for those who do not respond to methylphenidate or dextroamphetamine.[32]

The tricyclic antidepressants imipramine and desipramine, and the alpha-adrenergic agonist clonidine, are not often used in the treatment of ADHD because of concerns about cardiac effects and the availability of safe, effective medications described above. The stimulant pemoline remains available but is no longer recommended owing to reports of fatal hepatotoxicity.

A single medication is generally all that is needed to treat uncomplicated ADHD. Combinations of psychotropic medications have not been well studied and are reserved for very severe ADHD and coexisting mental health disorders.

Nonpharmacologic Interventions

Behavioral Therapy   Behavioral therapy is not routinely recommended as first-line treatment for uncomplicated ADHD in school-age children. Large randomized trials directly compared behavioral therapy with pharmacologic therapy. The trials showed that behavioral therapy alone was less effective than pharmacologic therapy alone, and they showed mixed results for behavioral therapy in combination with medication.

The behavioral-treatment group of the Multimodal Treatment Study of ADHD involved 35 individual and group sessions over 14 months and focused on behavior-management techniques, a summer treatment program, consultation with each child's teacher, and the presence of a behavioral aide in the child's classroom for 12 weeks.[41] This intensive behavioral therapy alone was not as effective as medication alone for improving attention. However, the combination was more effective for oppositional behavior and parent–child discord, among other outcomes, than either of the treatments alone.

The study by Abikoff et al.[24] examined psychosocial treatment, not as the sole treatment, but in addition to medication. The sessions were weekly in the first year and monthly in the second year and included parent training, family therapy, organizational-skills training, individual tutoring, social-skills training, and individual psychotherapy. No benefit was found for adding psychosocial treatment to treatment with medication.

Behavioral treatment that is generally available in communities and schools usually involves 8-to-12-week group sessions with children and parents, provided by psychologists or social workers. Sessions focus on improving the understanding of ADHD, teaching parents skills such as effective use of rewards and disincentives, and modifying the physical and social environment to change the child's behavior, such as structuring daily routines.[7] Behavioral therapy is added to medication for specific indications, such as persistent oppositional behavior and parent–child discord. Psychological treatment is indicated for coexisting mental health conditions, such as depression and anxiety.

Other Interventions   Physicians cannot prescribe an educational assessment, but they can support a parent's request for an assessment when it is indicated by persistent academic problems. In the United States, children with ADHD are entitled to interventions within the school setting if the parents and school officials determine that the child's behavior or condition interferes with his or her ability to participate in the educational process. The interventions might be simple, such as seating the child near the teacher to minimize classroom distractions, or they might involve assigning specific staff members to review daily assignments with the child.[42] Collaboration among the doctor, the parents, and the teacher can be facilitated with very brief lists of target behaviors, rated by the teacher, and taken by parents to appointments; these can be useful in gauging the effectiveness of treatment (Table 3).[7,9]

Other treatment interventions, such as physical exercises, neurofeedback, chelation therapy, systemic antifungal treatment, and vitamins, are often promoted at substantial expense to families. Little evidence supports a role for these interventions in the treatment of ADHD. Diets, including those involving the reduced consumption of sugar, were studied and found to affect behavior in no more than 1 percent of children.[43-45]

Reasons to refer to a specialist such as a developmental or behavioral pediatrician or a child psychiatrist include coexisting mental health conditions, adverse social circumstances that warrant team management, and treatment failure.[7]

Special Populations

Children less than five years of age may demonstrate severely disruptive behaviors; these are probably associated with other chronic physical and mental health conditions.[46,47] Randomized trials show that training parents improves symptoms in preschoolers. In one trial, parents of 87 three-year-olds were randomly assigned to a control group or to 10 to 12 sessions in which they were taught to set consistent limits and positively interact with their preschooler. Children of parents in the intervention group were significantly more likely to achieve at least a 30 percent reduction in negative behaviors than were children of parents in the control group (62 percent vs. 28 percent), and 80 percent of the children in the intervention group showed improvement at one year of follow-up (there was no comparison group at that time).[48] An 8-week randomized trial involving parents of three-year-olds showed that training the parents had a significant benefit on the children, and improvement was sustained 15 weeks after the intervention.[49]

A short-term study (three to four weeks) involving 28 children with ADHD, who were 4 to 5.9 years of age, showed normalization of behavior for 25 children who received stimulant medication as compared with 3 who received a placebo. Irritability and decreased appetite were frequent side effects.[50] Although approximately 1 percent of children two to four years of age may be treated with psychotropic medications, there is little evidence to support or guide this treatment,[51,52] and the overuse of medication is a particular concern in this group.

Children with mental retardation may have symptoms that meet the criteria for a separate diagnosis of ADHD. However, according to DSM-IV-R criteria, symptomatic behaviors should not be diagnosed as ADHD if they can be better explained by another diagnosis.[5] Randomized, controlled trials support the use of stimulant medication to treat children and adults who have symptoms of ADHD and mental retardation.[53,54]

ADHD affects 4 percent of adults; as many as 60 to 80 percent of children continue to have problems in adulthood with inattention and impulsivity, which adversely affect achievement and interpersonal relationships. The diagnosis of ADHD in adults, as in children and adolescents, is established through DSM-IV-R criteria, and coexisting mental health disorders must be considered in the diagnosis and treatment. Short-term studies have indicated improvement in attention and impulsivity with the use of stimulants and atomoxetine, but long-term data are lacking.[55] A detailed discussion of adult ADHD is beyond the scope of this article.

AREAS OF UNCERTAINTY

The subjective nature of judging behavior contributes to concern that ADHD is overdiagnosed and overtreated. Epidemiologic studies consistently show either underdiagnosis or overdiagnosis, with wide geographic and demographic variation.[56,57] Data are not yet available to assess the long-term benefits and risks of medication. Although a concern has been raised regarding a risk of substance abuse in patients treated with stimulant medication, studies indicate that children with ADHD who are treated have a lower risk of substance abuse later in life than children with ADHD who are not treated.[58,59]

GUIDELINES

Guidelines for diagnosing and treating ADHD have been issued by several organizations representing pediatrics and child psychiatry (Table 3). These are consistent, and taken together, establish the standard of care for ADHD.

CONCLUSIONS AND RECOMMENDATIONS

The evaluation of a child for ADHD involves taking a careful history, including the use of a standardized checklist to assess behaviors, and paying attention to the possibility of other mental health conditions or adverse social circumstances causing or exacerbating symptoms (Table 2). If the evaluation reveals behaviors meeting DSM-IV-R criteria for the diagnosis of ADHD (Table 1), a plan for care should take into consideration that ADHD is a chronic health condition and should involve the parents, the child, and the teacher in identifying behaviors to which therapy is targeted (Table 3).

In school-age children such as the one described in the vignette, I begin treatment with methylphenidate, because it is the treatment best supported by research. I prescribe a long-acting preparation, typically a low dose (10 to 18 mg) for a child less than 10 years of age and a midrange dose (20 to 36 mg) for older children or teenagers. A higher starting dose (30 to 54 mg) is reasonable for patients with severe symptoms. If medication is ineffective at the maximal dose or causes intolerable side effects, I try prescribing two to four daily doses of short-acting medication or switching to a long-acting preparation of dextroamphetamine; an alternative is atomoxetine. I see the child and his or her parents every month initially and every three months once a stable dose has been reached, to assess effectiveness and side effects. I recommend behavioral therapy for children and families experiencing conflict with one another and for children with a coexisting mental health condition.

I am indebted to the children, families, and staff of the Collaborative Developmental Clinic and to Sid Shah, Betty Elliott, James Kallman, Nicholas Kuzera, Ellen Perrin, James Perrin, Martin Stein, Esther Wender, and William Weil.

This article first appeared in the January 13, 2005, issue of the New England Journal of Medicine.

REFERENCES

1.
Nigg JT, Quamma JP, Greenberg MT, Kusche CA. A two-year longitudinal study of neuropsychological and cognitive performance in relation to behavioral problems and competencies in elementary school children. J Abnorm Child Psychol 1999;27:51-63.

2.
Durston S. A review of the biological bases of ADHD: what have we learned from imaging studies? Ment Retard Dev Disabil Res Rev 2003;9:184-95.

3.
Castellanos FX, Lee PP, Sharp W, et al. Developmental trajectories of brain volume abnormalities in children and adolescents with attention-deficit/hyperactivity disorder. JAMA 2002;288:1740-8.

4.
Hille ET, den Ouden AL, Saigal S, et al. Behavioural problems in children who weigh 1000 g or less at birth in four countries. Lancet 2001;357:1641-3.

5.
Diagnostic and statistical manual of mental disorders, 4th ed. rev.: DSM-IV-R. Washington, D.C.: American Psychiatric Association, 2000.

6.
Barbaresi WJ, Katusic SK, Colligan RC, et al. How common is attention-deficit/hyperactivity disorder? Incidence in a population-based birth cohort in Rochester, Minn. Arch Pediatr Adolesc Med 2002;156:217-24.

7.
American Academy of Pediatrics, Subcommittee on Attention-Deficit/Hyperactivity Disorder and Committee on Quality Improvement. Clinical practice guideline: treatment of the school-age child with attention-deficit/hyperactivity disorder. Pediatrics 2001;108:1033-44.

8.
Dixon SD, Stein MT. Encounters with children: pediatric behavior and development. 3rd ed. St. Louis: Mosby, 2000.

9.
National Initiative for Children's Healthcare Quality. Caring for children with ADHD: a resource toolkit for clinicians. Elk Grove Village, Ill.: American Academy of Pediatrics, 2002.

10.
Green M, Wong M, Atkins D, et al. Diagnosis of attention deficit/hyperactivity disorder. Technical review. No. 3. Rockville, Md.: Agency for Health Care Policy and Research, August 1999. (AHCPR publication no. 99-0049.)

11.
Linnet KM, Dalsgaard S, Obel C, et al. Maternal lifestyle factors in pregnancy risk of attention deficit hyperactivity disorder and associated behaviors: review of the current evidence. Am J Psychiatry 2003;160:1028-40.

12.
Bussing R, Zima BT, Gary FA, et al. Social networks, caregiver strain, and utilization of mental health services among elementary school students at high risk for ADHD. J Am Acad Child Adolesc Psychiatry 2003;42:842-50.

13.
American Academy of Pediatrics. Clinical practice guideline: diagnosis and evaluation of the child with attention deficit/hyperactivity disorder. Pediatrics 2000;105:1158-70.

14.
Reiff MI, Tippins S. ADHD: a complete and authoritative guide. Elk Grove Village, Ill.: American Academy of Pediatrics, 2004.

15.
Greenhill LL, Pliszka S, Dulcan MK, et al. Practice parameter for the use of stimulant medications in the treatment of children, adolescents, and adults. J Am Acad Child Adolesc Psychiatry 2002;41: Suppl:26S-49S.

16.
Dulcan MK, Benson RS. AACAP official action: summary of the practice parameters for the assessment and treatment of children, adolescents, and adults with ADHD. J Am Acad Child Adolesc Psychiatry 1997;36:1311-7.

17.
Taylor E, Sergeant J, Doepfner M, et al. Clinical guidelines for hyperkinetic disorder. Eur Child Adolesc Psychiatry 1998;7:184-200.

18.
Scottish Intercollegiate Guidelines Network. Attention deficit and hyperkinetic disorders in children and young people: a national clinical guideline. Guideline no. 52. June 2001. (Accessed January 31, 2006, at http://www.sign.ac.uk/pdf/sign52.pdf.)

19.
The revised Conners' Parent Rating Scale. (CPRS-R): factor structure, reliability, and criterion validity. 1998. (Accessed December 17, 2004, at http://www.mhs.com/onlineCat/product.asp?productID=CRS-R.)

20.
American Academy of Child and Adolescent Psychiatry. Guidelines pocketcard managing: attention deficit/hyperactivity disorder, version 1.1. Baltimore: International Guidelines Center, 2003.

21.
2003 InfoPOEM. Key word: attention deficit hyperactivity disorder. (Accessed January 31, 2006, at http://www.infopoems.com.)

22.
Jadad AR, Boyle M, Cunningham C, Kim M, Schachar R. Treatment of attention deficit/hyperactivity disorder. Evidence report/technology assessment. No. 11. Rockville, Md.: Agency for Healthcare Research and Quality, November 1999. (AHRQ publication no. 00-E005.)

23.
MTA Cooperative Group. National Institute of Mental Health Multimodal Treatment Study of ADHD follow-up: 24-month outcomes of treatment strategies for attention-deficit/hyperactivity disorder. Pediatrics 2004;113:754-61.

24.
Abikoff H, Hechtman L, Klein RG, et al. Symptomatic improvement in children with ADHD treated with long-term methylphenidate and multimodal psychosocial treatment. J Am Acad Child Adolesc Psychiatry 2004;43:802-11.

25.
Efron D, Jarman F, Barker M. Side effects of methylphenidate and dexamphetamine in children with attention deficit hyperactivity disorder: a double-blind, crossover trial. Pediatrics 1997;100:662-6.

26.
Efron D, Jarman F, Barker M. Methylphenidate versus dexamphetamine in children with attention deficit hyperactivity disorder: a double-blind, crossover trial. Pediatrics 1997;100:E6.

27.
Tourette's Syndrome Study Group. Treatment of ADHD in children with tics: a randomized controlled trial. Neurology 2002;58:527-36.

28.
Gross-Tsur V, Manor O, van der Meere J, Joseph A, Shalev RS. Epilepsy and attention deficit hyperactivity disorder: is methylphenidate safe and effective? J Pediatr 1997;130:670-4.

29.
Barkley RA, McMurray MB, Edelbrock CS, Robbins K. Side effects of methylphenidate in children with attention deficit hyperactivity disorder: a systemic, placebo-controlled evaluation. Pediatrics 1990;86:184-92.

30.
O'Brien LM, Ivanenko A, Crabtree VM, et al. The effect of stimulants on sleep characteristics in children with attention deficit/hyperactivity disorder. Sleep Med 2003;4:309-16.

31.
National Institute of Mental Health Multimodal Treatment Study of ADHD follow-up: changes in effectiveness and growth after the end of treatment. Pediatrics 2004;113:762-9.

32.
Kelsey DK, Sumner CR, Casat CD, et al. Once-daily atomoxetine treatment for children with attention-deficit/hyperactivity disorder, including an assessment of evening and morning behavior: a double-blind, placebo-controlled trial. Pediatrics 2004;114:e1-e8.

33.
Spencer T, Heiligenstein JH, Biederman J, et al. Results from 2 proof-of-concept, placebo-controlled studies of atomoxetine in children with attention-deficit/hyperactivity disorder. J Clin Psychiatry 2002;63:1140-7.

34.
Abboud L. Lilly warns doctors about Strattera. Wall Street Journal. December 20, 2004:B4.

35.
Kratochvil CJ, Heiligenstein JH, Dittmann R, et al. Atomoxetine and methylphenidate treatment in children with ADHD: a prospective, randomized, open-label trial. J Am Acad Child Adolesc Psychiatry 2002;41:776-84.

36.
Michelson D, Buitelaar JK, Danckaerts M, et al. Relapse prevention in pediatric patients with ADHD treated with atomoxetine: a randomized, double-blind, placebo-controlled study. J Am Acad Child Adolesc Psychiatry 2004;43:896-904.

37.
Sawant S, Daviss SR. Seizures and prolonged QTc with atomoxetine overdose. Am J Psychiatry 2004;161:757.

38.
Lee TS, Lee TD, Lombroso PJ, King RA. Atomoxetine and tics in ADHD. J Am Acad Child Adolesc Psychiatry 2004;43:1068-9.

39.
Barrickman LL, Perry PJ, Allen AJ, et al. Bupropion versus methylphenidate in the treatment of attention-deficit hyperactivity disorder. J Am Acad Child Adolesc Psychiatry 1995;34:649-57.

40.
Conners CK, Casat CD, Gualtieri CT, et al. Bupropion hydrochloride in attention deficit disorder with hyperactivity. J Am Acad Child Adolesc Psychiatry 1996;35:1314-21.

41.
Jensen PS, Hinshaw SP, Swanson JM, et al. Findings from the NIMH Multimodal Treatment Study of ADHD (MTA): implications and applications for primary care providers. J Dev Behav Pediatr 2001;22:60-73.

42.
DuPaul GJ, Stoner G. ADHD in the schools: assessment and intervention strategies. 2nd ed. New York: Guilford Press, 2003.

43.
Wolraich ML, Wilson DB, White JW. The effect of sugar on behavior or cognition in children: a meta-analysis. JAMA 1995;274:1617-21.

44.
Voigt RG, Llorente AM, Jensen CL, Fraley JK, Berretta MC, Heird WC. A randomized, double-blind, placebo-controlled trial of docosahexaenoic acid supplementation in children with attention-deficit/hyperactivity disorder. J Pediatr 2001;139:189-96.

45.
Wolraich ML. Addressing behavior problems among school-aged children: traditional and controversial approaches. Pediatr Rev 1997;18:266-70.

46.
Rappley MD, Mullan PB, Alvarez FJ, Eneli IU, Wang J, Gardiner JC. Diagnosis of attention-deficit/hyperactivity disorder and use of psychotropic medication in very young children. Arch Pediatr Adolesc Med 1999;153:1039-45.

47.
DeBar LL, Lynch F, Powell J, Gale J. Use of psychotropic agents in preschool children: associated symptoms, diagnoses, and health care services in a health maintenance organization. Arch Pediatr Adolesc Med 2003;157:150-7.

48.
Bor W, Sanders MR, Markie-Dadds C. The effects of the Triple P-Positive Parenting Program on preschool children with co-occurring disruptive behavior and attentional/hyperactive difficulties. J Abnorm Child Psychol 2002;30:571-87.

49.
Sonuga-Barke EJ, Daley D, Thompson M, Laver-Bradbury C, Weeks A. Parent-based therapies for preschool attention-deficit/hyperactivity disorder: a randomized, controlled trial with a community sample. J Am Acad Child Adolesc Psychiatry 2001;40:402-8.

50.
Short EJ, Manos MJ, Findling RL, Schubel EA. A prospective study of stimulant response in preschool children: insights from ROC analyses. J Am Acad Child Adolesc Psychiatry 2004;43:251-9.

51.
Rappley MD, Eneli IU, Mullan PB, et al. Patterns of psychotropic medication use in very young children with attention-deficit hyperactivity disorder. J Dev Behav Pediatr 2002;23:23-30.

52.
Zito JM, Safer DJ, dosReis S, Gardner JF, Boles M, Lynch F. Trends in the prescribing of psychotropic medications to preschoolers. JAMA 2000;283:1025-30.

53.
Pearson DA, Santos CW, Roache JD, et al. Treatment effects of methylphenidate on behavioral adjustment in children with mental retardation and ADHD. J Am Acad Child Adolesc Psychiatry 2003;42:209-16.

54.
Aman MG, Buican B, Arnold LE. Methylphenidate treatment in children with borderline IQ and mental retardation: analysis of three aggregated studies. J Child Adolesc Psychopharmacol 2003;13:29-40.

55.
Wilens TE, Faraone SV, Biederman J. Attention-deficit/hyperactivity disorder in adults. JAMA 2004;292:619-23.

56.
Rappley MD, Gardiner JC, Jetton JR, Houang RT. The use of methylphenidate in Michigan. Arch Pediatr Adolesc Med 1995;149:675-9.

57.
LeFever GB, Dawson KV, Morrow AL. The extent of drug therapy for attention deficit-hyperactivity disorder among children in public schools. Am J Public Health 1999;89:1359-64.

58.
Katusic SK, Barbaresi W, Colligan RC, Weaver AL, Mrazek DA, Jacobsen SJ. The impact of psychostimulant treatment on drug/alcohol abuse among children with ADHD. J Dev Behav Pediatr 2003;24:396-7. abstract.

59.
Wilens TE, Faraone SV, Biederman J, Gunawardene S. Does stimulant therapy of attention-deficit/hyperactivity disorder beget later substance abuse? A meta-analytic review of the literature. Pediatrics 2003;111:179-85.

Addendum

On February 9, 2005, Health Canada, the Canadian drug regulatory agency, removed Adderall XR from the Canadian market because of concerns about sudden death, which was reported in 20 patients taking this medication.[1] Other Adderall products had not been previously marketed in Canada. On the same day, the U.S. Food and Drug Administration (FDA) announced that it had reviewed the same postmarketing reports that were reviewed by Health Canada, described 12 pediatric deaths, and concluded that Adderall products should not be removed from the U.S. market.[2] Among these 12 deaths, 5 occurred in children with structural heart defects, and the remaining cases had complicating circumstances of heat exhaustion, dehydration, near drowning, and toxic levels, among others. The FDA also concluded that the number of sudden deaths was not greater than that expected among this population, given the approximately 30 million prescriptions written during the time of these reports (1999 to 2003). The FDA instituted a labeling change for Adderall XR in August 2004 to include a warning that patients with heart disease should not ordinarily be treated with Adderall products. A recent multicenter trial assessing the tolerability and effectiveness of Adderall XR was conducted for 24 months among 273 children 6 to 12 years of age who had been treated for 24 months or longer. The only serious adverse events (defined as events that resulted in death or hospitalization or that were life-threatening or medically significant) reported by this study were two occurrences of seizure.[3]

1. Health Canada suspends the market authorization of Adderall XR®, a drug prescribed for Attention Deficit Hyperactivity Disorder (ADHD) in children. Ottawa, Ont., Canada: Health Canada, 2005. (Accessed January 31, 2006, at www.hc-sc.gc.ca/english/protection/warnings/2005/2005_01.html.)

2. Public health advisory for Adderall and Adderall XR. Rockville, Md.: U.S. Food and Drug Administration, 2005. (Accessed January 31, 2006, at www.fda.gov/cder/drug/advisory/adderall.htm.)

3. McGough JJ, Biederman J, Wigal SB, et al. Long-term tolerability and effectiveness of once-daily mixed amphetamine salts (Adderall XR) in children with ADHD. J Am Acad Child Adolesc Psychiatry 2005;44:530-8.

Hypercalcemia Associated with Cancer

ANDREW F. STEWART, M.D.

A 47-year-old woman with a history of breast cancer presents with confusion and dehydration. The serum calcium level is 18.0 mg per deciliter (4.5 mmol per liter). She has postural hypotension and low central venous pressure on examination of the jugular veins. The serum phosphorus level is 5.0 mg per deciliter (1.6 mmol per liter), the blood urea nitrogen level is 80.0 mg per deciliter (28.6 mmol per liter), the serum creatinine level is 2.0 mg per deciliter (177 mmol per liter), and the albumin level is 3.3 g per deciliter. A bone scintigraphic scan reveals no evidence of skeletal involvement by the tumor. How should she be treated?

THE CLINICAL PROBLEM

Hypercalcemia has been reported to occur in up to 20 to 30 percent of patients with cancer at some time during the course of their disease.[1-4] This incidence may be falling owing to the wide use of bisphosphonates in patients with either multiple myeloma or breast cancer, although data are lacking. Hypercalcemia leads to progressive mental impairment, including coma, as well as renal failure. These complications are particularly common terminal events among patients with cancer. The detection of hypercalcemia in a patient with cancer signifies a very poor prognosis; approximately 50 percent of such patients die within 30 days.[5]

Hypercalcemia associated with cancer can be classified into four types (Table 1).[1-4] In patients with local osteolytic hypercalcemia, the hypercalcemia results from the marked increase in osteoclastic bone resorption in areas surrounding the malignant cells within the marrow space.[3,4,6] The condition known as humoral hypercalcemia of malignancy (HHM) is caused by systemic secretion of parathyroid hormone (PTH)–related protein (PTHrP) by malignant tumors.[1,2,7,8] PTHrP causes increased bone resorption[1,2,7,8] and enhances renal retention of calcium.[9,10] The tumors that most commonly cause HHM are listed in Table 1, but essentially any tumor may cause this syndrome. Some lymphomas secrete the active form of vitamin D, 1,25-dihydroxyvitamin D ($1,25(OH)_2D$), causing hypercalcemia as a result of the combination of enhanced osteoclastic bone resorption

Table 1. Types of Hypercalcemia Associated with Cancer.*

Type	Frequency (%)	Bone Metastases	Causal Agent	Typical Tumors
Local osteolytic hypercalcemia	20	Common, extensive	Cytokines, chemokines, PTHrP	Breast cancer, multiple myeloma, lymphoma
Humoral hypercalcemia of malignancy	80	Minimal or absent	PTHrP	Squamous-cell cancer, (e.g., of head and neck, esophagus, cervix, or lung), renal cancer, ovarian cancer, endometrial cancer, HTLV-associated lymphoma, breast cancer
$1,25(OH)_2D$-secreting lymphomas	<1	Variable	$1,25(OH)_2D$	Lymphoma (all types)
Ectopic hyperparathyroidism	<1	Variable	PTH	Variable

* PTH denotes parathyroid hormone, PTHrP PTH-related protein, $1,25(OH)_2D$ 1,25-dihydroxyvitamin D, and HTLV human T-cell lymphotrophic virus.

and enhanced intestinal absorption of calcium.[1,2,11] Finally, ectopic secretion of authentic PTH is a rare cause of hypercalcemia, having been well documented in only eight patients to date.[1,2,12]

STRATEGIES AND EVIDENCE

Diagnosis

Although clinical laboratories generally measure the total serum calcium level, it is occasionally valuable to measure the serum level of ionized calcium, because increases or decreases in the albumin level may cause misleading increases or decreases, respectively, in the total serum calcium level. In addition, in rare patients with myeloma in whom calcium-binding immunoglobulins are produced,[13] measurement of total serum calcium may substantially overestimate the serum ionized calcium level. There are formulas with which to calculate the serum ionized calcium level or to "correct" the total calcium level (e.g., add 0.8 mg per deciliter to the total calcium level for every 1.0 g per deciliter of serum albumin below the level of 3.5 g per deciliter), but they are not precise or always reliable.[14] Thus, measurement of serum ionized calcium should be considered whenever there is doubt about the validity of the measurement of total calcium. The test can be performed rapidly in most hospital laboratories or neonatal intensive care units.

If the calcium level is elevated, a further evaluation should consider not only the mechanisms that are potentially related to the cancer but also causes of the elevation of the calcium level that are unrelated to the cancer (e.g., primary hyperparathyroidism, the use of thiazide diuretics, and granulomatous disease, among other causes).[15-18] The tumors present in hypercalcemia associated with malignant disease are generally large and readily apparent[1-4]; notable exceptions are small neuroendocrine tumors (such as islet tumors and pheochromocytomas). The levels of intact PTH should be measured routinely. Although ectopic hyperparathyroidism is extremely rare in hypercalcemia associated with cancer, concomitant primary hyperparathyroidism is not (we found that in 8 of 133 patients with cancer and hypercalcemia, primary hyperparathyroidism was the cause).[18] Although most patients with typical HHM (Table 1) have increased levels of circulating PTHrP, the diagnosis is usually obvious on clinical grounds; PTHrP should therefore be measured in the occasional cases in which the diagnosis of HHM cannot be made on clinical grounds or when the cause of hypercalcemia is obscure. Plasma $1,25(OH)_2D$ should be measured when sarcoidosis, other granulomatous disorders, or the $1,25(OH)_2D$ lymphoma syndrome is considered in the differential diagnosis. A bone scan (or a skeletal survey, in the case of myeloma) is useful to assess the skeletal tumor burden in patients with cancer and hypercalcemia, if the test was not previously performed for tumor staging.

Therapeutic Considerations

In planning therapy for patients with hypercalcemia associated with malignant disease, antihypercalcemic therapy should be considered an interim measure, one with no ultimate effect on survival.[5] Thus, it is imperative that antitumor therapy be implemented promptly: control of the serum calcium level merely buys time in which such therapy can work. Another critical point is that when all the available therapies have failed, withholding antihypercalcemic therapy (which will eventually result in coma and death) may be an appropriate and humane approach. In cases in which treatment is considered appropriate, an assessment of the severity of the hypercalcemia is needed to guide therapy.

Although there are no formal guidelines, I consider mild hypercalcemia to be a serum calcium level of 10.5 to 11.9 mg per deciliter (2.6 to 2.9 mmol per liter), moderate hypercalcemia a level of 12.0 to 13.9 mg per deciliter (3.0 to 3.4 mmol per liter), and severe hypercalcemia a level of 14.0 mg per deciliter (3.5 mmol per liter) or greater. In general, the neurologic and renal complications of hypercalcemia worsen with increasing severity of hypercalcemia, but other factors also influence the response to hypercalcemia. For example, the rate of the ascent of the serum calcium level is important — a rapid increase to moderate hypercalcemia frequently results in marked neurologic dysfunction, whereas chronic severe hypercalcemia may cause only minimal neurologic symptoms. Similarly, older patients with preexisting neurologic or cognitive dysfunction may become severely obtunded in the presence of mild hypercalcemia, whereas younger patients with moderate-to-severe hypercalcemia may remain alert. Finally, the concomitant administration of sedatives or narcotics may worsen the neurologic response to hypercalcemia.

The optimal therapy for hypercalcemia associated with cancer is one that is tailored both to the degree of hypercalcemia and to its underlying cause. True hypercalcemia (i.e., an elevated serum level of ionized calcium) occurs through three basic mechanisms: enhanced osteoclastic bone resorption (in local osteolytic hypercalcemia, HHM, $1,25(OH)_2D$-secreting lymphomas, and the rare case of ectopic hyperparathyroidism); enhanced renal tubular reabsorption of calcium (in HHM and ectopic hyperparathyroidism); and enhanced intestinal absorption of calcium (in $1,25(OH)_2D$-secreting lymphomas and possibly ectopic hyperparathyroidism). Therapy should be targeted accordingly.

General Supportive Measures

The important general supportive measures include the removal of calcium from parenteral feeding solutions (a measure often overlooked); discontinuation of the use of oral calcium supplements in enteral feeding solutions or as calcium tablets; discontinuation of medications that may independently lead to hypercalcemia (e.g., lithium, calcitriol, vitamin D, and thiazides); an increase in the weight-bearing mobility of the patient, if possible; and discontinuation of the use of sedative drugs, including analgesic drugs, if possible, to enhance the patient's mental clarity and promote weight-bearing ambulation.

Hypophosphatemia develops in most patients with hypercalcemia associated with cancer at some point during the course of the disease, regardless of the underlying cause, because of decreased food intake, saline diuresis, the use of loop diuretics, the phosphaturic effects of PTHrP, the hypercalcemia itself, and treatment with calcitonin or antacids. In general, the presence of hypophosphatemia increases the difficulty of treating the hypercalcemia, and in animal models hypophosphatemia has been shown to cause hypercalcemia.[19] Phosphorus should be replaced orally or administered through a nasogastric tube as neutral phosphate.[20] The serum phosphorus and creatinine levels should be followed closely, in an effort to keep the phosphorus level in the range of 2.5 to 3.0 mg per deciliter (0.98 to 1.0 mmol per liter), the serum creatinine level in the normal range, and the calcium–phosphorus product below 40, ideally in the range of 30 (when both are expressed in milligrams per deciliter). Intravenous phosphorus replacement should not be given except in dire circumstances, when oral or nasogastric administration is impossible, because its use can result in severe hypocalcemia, seizures, and acute renal failure.[21] These general support measures alone may be sufficient to treat patients with mild hypercalcemia.

Table 2. Pharmacologic Therapy for Hypercalcemia Associated with Cancer.*

Intervention	Dose	Adverse Effect
Hydration or calciuresis		
Intravenous saline	200–500 ml/hr, depending on the cardiovascular and renal status of the patient	Congestive heart failure
Furosemide	20–40 mg intravenously, after rehydration has been achieved	Dehydration, hypokalemia
Phosphate repletion		
Oral phosphorus (if serum phosphorus ≤3.0 mg/dl)†	For example, 250 mg Neutraphos orally, four times daily until serum phosphorus level >3.0 mg/dl or until serum creatinine level increases	Renal failure, hypocalcemia, seizures, abnormalities of cardiac conduction, diarrhea
First-line medications		
Intravenous bisphosphonates‡		
Pamidronate	60–90 mg intravenously over a 2-hr period in a solution of 50–200 ml of saline or 5% dextrose in water§	Renal failure, transient flu-like syndrome with aches, chills, and fever
Zoledronate	4 mg intravenously over a 15-min period in a solution of 50 ml of saline or 5% dextrose in water	Renal failure, transient flu-like syndrome with aches, chills, and fever
Second-line medications		
Glucocorticoids¶	For example, prednisone, 60 mg orally daily for 10 days	Potential interference with chemotherapy; hypokalemia, hyperglycemia, hypertension, Cushing's syndrome, immunosuppression
Mithramycin	A single dose of 25 µg/kg of body weight over a 4-to-6-hour period in saline	Thrombocytopenia, platelet-aggregation defect, anemia, leukopenia, hepatitis, renal failure‖
Calcitonin	4–8 IU per kilogram subcutaneously or intramuscularly every 12 hr	Flushing, nausea
Gallium nitrate	100–200 mg/m² of body-surface area intravenously given continuously over a 24-hr period for five days	Renal failure

* Many of the recommendations in this table are based on historical precedent and common practice rather than on randomized clinical trials. There are data from randomized trials comparing bisphosphonates to the other agents listed and to one another.

† The use of intravenous phosphorus should be avoided except in the presence of severe hypophosphatemia (serum phosphorus level <1.5 mg per deciliter [0.48 mmol per liter]) and when oral phosphorus cannot be administered. If intravenous phosphorus is used, it should be used with extreme caution and with careful observation of the levels of serum phosphorus and creatinine.[20,21] To convert values for phosphorus to millimoles per liter, multiply by 0.3229.

‡ Pamidronate and zoledronate are approved by the Food and Drug Administration. Ibandronate and clodronate are available in continental Europe, the United Kingdom, and elsewhere. Bisphosphonates should be used with caution if at all when the serum creatinine level exceeds 2.5 to 3.0 mg per deciliter (221.0 to 265.2 µmol per liter).

§ Pamidronate is generally used at a dose of 90 mg, but the 60-mg dose may be used to treat patients of small stature or those with renal impairment or mild hypercalcemia.

¶ These drugs have a slow onset of action, as compared with the bisphosphonates; approximately 4 to 10 days are required for a response.

‖ These effects have been reported in association with higher-dose regimens used to treat testicular cancer (50 µg per kilogram of body weight per day over a period of five days) and in patients receiving multiple doses of 25 µg per kilogram; they are not expected to occur with a single dose of 25 µg per kilogram unless preexisting liver, kidney, or hematologic disease is present.

Saline Hydration and Calciuresis

Patients with hypercalcemia associated with cancer are substantially dehydrated as a result of a renal water-concentrating defect (nephrogenic diabetes insipidus) induced by hypercalcemia and by decreased oral hydration resulting from anorexia and nausea, vomiting, or both. The dehydration leads to a reduction in the glomerular filtration rate that further reduces the ability of the kidney to excrete the excess serum calcium. First, therefore, parenteral volume expansion should be initiated, with the administration of normal saline. Although there are no randomized clinical trials to guide this therapy, in general practice normal saline is administered at a rate of 200 to 500 ml per hour, depending on the baseline level of dehydration and renal function, the patient's cardiovascular status, the degree of mental impairment, and the severity of the hypercalcemia. These factors must be assessed with the use of careful clinical monitoring for physical findings that are consistent with fluid overload. The goals of treatment are to increase the glomerular filtration rate, thus increasing the filtered load of calcium that passes through the glomerulus into the tubular lumen, and to inhibit calcium reabsorption in the proximal nephron (because saline itself is calciuretic). Increasing the glomerular filtration rate to or above the normal range (within safe limits) also permits the use of loop diuretics (Table 2) to increase the renal excretion of calcium (loop diuretics block calcium reabsorption in the loop of Henle and make possible increased administration of saline, which induces further calcium excretion). Loop diuretics should not be administered until after full hydration has been achieved, because these agents can cause or worsen dehydration, leading to a decline in the glomerular filtration rate and the filtered load of calcium. In contrast to loop diuretics, thiazide diuretics should not be administered, since they stimulate, rather than inhibit, renal calcium reabsorption.

Medications

Intravenous bisphosphonates are by far the best studied, safest, and most effective agents for use in patients with hypercalcemia associated with cancer. These drugs work by blocking osteoclastic bone resorption.[22-33] Because they are poorly absorbed when given orally (approximately 1 to 2 percent of an oral dose is absorbed), only intravenously administered bisphosphonates are used for this indication. In the United States, the two drugs that are approved by the Food and Drug Administration (FDA) and are currently considered the agents of choice in the treatment of mild-to-severe hypercalcemia associated with cancer are pamidronate[22,24,25] and zoledronate.[22,23,26,27] In continental Europe, the United Kingdom, and other countries, ibandronate[22,28,29] and clodronate[22,30-32] are also widely used. Etidronate, which was the first to be used for this indication,[22] has been replaced by these more potent bisphosphonates. A number of randomized clinical trials comparing bisphosphonates to saline and diuretics alone, to other bisphosphonates, and to other antiresorptive agents such as calcitonin have confirmed the superiority of bisphosphonates.[22,27,28,33]

Bisphosphonate therapy should be initiated as soon as hypercalcemia is discovered, because a response requires two to four days, and the nadir in serum calcium generally occurs within four to seven days after therapy is initiated.[22-33] Approximately 60 to 90 percent of patients have normal serum calcium levels within four to seven days, and responses last for one to three weeks.[22-33] As compared with pamidronate, zoledronate has the advantage of rapid and simpler administration (15 minutes vs. 2 hours for infusion), whereas pamidronate is less expensive. Although a direct comparison of the two drugs in a randomized clinical trial showed a statistically significant increase in the efficacy of zoledronate,[27] the difference in control of calcemia was small (mean nadir serum calcium level, 9.8 mg per deciliter [2.4 mmol per liter] with zoledronate and 10.5 mg per deciliter [2.6 mmol per liter] with pamidronate; the proportion of patients in whom a corrected serum calcium level of 10.8 mg per deciliter [2.7 mmol per liter] was achieved by day 10 was 88 percent and 70 percent, respectively). Thus, the differences are of arguable clinical importance, and the choice is largely one between convenience and cost. Either pamidronate or zoledronate is acceptable therapy.

In animal models, bisphosphonates have been associated with azotemia[22,23] and thus, their use in patients with renal failure is a potential concern. However, because hypercalcemia is a frequent cause of renal dysfunction in patients with hypercalcemia associated with cancer, effective treatment of the hypercalcemia associated with cancer often improves renal function.[25,34] The manufacturer and the American Society of Clinical Oncology[35] do not recommend the use of a reduced dose of pamidronate or zoledronate for patients with serum creatinine values of less than 3.0 mg per deciliter (265.2 μmol per liter), but they do advise that the recommended duration of the infusion not be shortened. Pamidronate and zoledronate have been reported to cause or exacerbate renal failure, but this effect has generally occurred in patients receiving multiple doses.[36] In patients whose condition fails to respond to a low initial dose of bisphosphonates, the use of a second, larger dose (an approach that has not been approved by the FDA) or a second-line agent may be considered.

Other Pharmacologic Agents

Several agents commonly used before the advent of bisphosphonates are now used infrequently, usually when bisphosphonates are ineffective or contraindicated (Table 2). Glucocorticoids[37,38] may still have a role in the treatment of some patients, such as those with lymphomas resulting in elevated levels of $1,25(OH)_2$ vitamin D. Calcitonin may result in a more rapid reduction in serum calcium levels than do other agents (the maximal response occurs within 12 to 24 hours), but its value is questionable because the reductions are small (approximately 1.0 mg per deciliter [0.25 mmol per liter]) and transient.[37,39] Mithramycin, which was the mainstay of therapy for hypercalcemia associated with cancer before the bisphosphonates became available,[40] remains effective, but its use is limited by potential adverse effects (Table 2). Gallium nitrate is also approved for treatment,[41] but the need for continuous intravenous administration over a period of five days limits its use.

Dialysis

In patients who have cancers that are likely to respond to therapy but in whom acute or chronic renal failure is present, aggressive saline infusion is not possible, and other therapies such as bisphosphonates should be used with caution, if at all. In these circumstances, dialysis against a dialysate containing little or no calcium is a reasonable and highly effective option for selected patients.[42,43] There are no specific guidelines with regard to how low the glomerular filtration rate must be for dialysis to be a rational choice in treating hypercalcemia, but in general, when the rate falls below 10 to 20 ml per minute, or when the presence of congestive heart failure contraindicates an adequate administration of saline, or both, dialysis should be considered.

AREAS OF UNCERTAINTY

The receptor activator of nuclear factor-κB ligand (RANKL) system is the molecular pathway that leads to osteoclast recruitment and differentiation and bone resorption in hypercalcemia associated with cancer. Agents that interfere with the system, such as recombinant osteoprotegerin (a decoy receptor for RANKL) or monoclonal antibodies directed against RANKL, have been proposed as novel treatments for hypercalcemia associated with malignant disease, as have monoclonal antibodies, which neutralize PTHrP. Preliminary data from studies in animals or small studies involving women with osteoporosis indicate reductions in bone resorption with these approaches.[44-46] Whether these agents will prove to be safe and effective in humans with hypercalcemia associated with cancer, whether they can be produced commercially at a cost competitive with that of bisphosphonates, and whether they can reverse hypercalcemia more effectively than the potent bisphosphonates remain unknown.

GUIDELINES

No guidelines are available from the major professional societies for the treatment of hypercalcemia associated with cancer.

RECOMMENDATIONS

The patient described in the vignette, who has breast cancer and a large, obvious tumor burden, is typical of patients with hypercalcemia associated with cancer in general and with HHM in particular. As in all cases of hypercalcemia in patients with cancer, other causes of the hypercalcemia need to be carefully considered. Coexisting primary hyper-parathyroidism should routinely be ruled out by measurement of the level of immuno-reactive parathyroid hormone. In the patient described, HHM is the most likely cause of the hypercalcemia; thus, immunoreactive parathyroid hormone would be suppressed and circulating PTHrP would be elevated (however, I do not routinely measure PTHrP unless the diagnosis is uncertain).

When a patient presents with hypercalcemia associated with cancer, the physician should first consider whether treatment is appropriate according to an assessment of the overall prognosis. The cornerstones of successful antihypercalcemic therapy are vigorous rehydration (with the use of normal saline at 200 to 500 ml per hour, depending on the patient's cardiovascular status and renal function); aggressive calciuresis with the use of loop diuretics, after normovolemia has been restored; and inhibition of bone resorption with the use of intravenous bisphosphonates (in the United States, the administration of either pamidronate [an infusion of 60 to 90 mg over a 2-hour period] or zoledronate [4 mg over a 15-minute period]). Pamidronate is at present less expensive, whereas zoledronate is more convenient to use and results in slightly greater mean reductions in the serum calcium level, although the differences are small. The expectation with the use of either regimen is that the serum calcium level will begin to fall within 12 hours after the therapy is initiated and will reach the nadir within approximately four to seven days. The serum calcium level generally will remain in the normal or near-normal range for one to three weeks, allowing time to institute other treatments for the malignant disease responsible for the hypercalcemia.

Supported by a grant (DK 51081) from the National Institutes of Health.

This article first appeared in the January 27, 2005, issue of the New England Journal of Medicine.

REFERENCES

1.
Stewart AF, Broadus AE. Malignancy-associated hypercalcemia. In: DeGroot L, Jameson LJ, eds. Endocrinology. 5th ed. Philadelphia: Saunders, 2006:1555-65.

2.
Horwitz MJ, Stewart AF. Humoral hypercalcemia of malignancy. In: Favus MF, ed. Primer on the metabolic bone diseases and disorders of mineral metabolism. 5th ed. Washington D.C.: American Society for Bone and Mineral Research, 2003:246-50.

3.
Roodman GD. Mechanisms of bone metastasis. N Engl J Med 2004;350:1655-64.

4.
Clines GA, Guise TA. Hypercalcemia in hematologic malignancies and in solid tumors associated with extensive localized bone destruction. In: Favus MJ, ed. Primer on the metabolic bone diseases and disorders of mineral metabolism. 5th ed. Washington D.C.: American Society for Bone and Mineral Research, 2003:251-6.

5.
Ralston SH, Gallagher SJ, Patel U, Campbell J, Boyle IT. Cancer-associated hypercalcemia: morbidity and mortality: clinical experience in 126 treated patients. Ann Intern Med 1990;112:499-504.

6.
Guise TA, Yin JJ, Taylor SD, et al. Evidence for a causal role of parathyroid hormone-related protein in the pathogenesis of human breast cancer-mediated osteolysis. J Clin Invest 1996;98:1544-9.

7.
Stewart AF, Vignery A, Silvergate A, et al. Quantitative bone histomorphometry in humoral hypercalcemia of malignancy: uncoupling of bone cell activity. J Clin Endocrinol Metab 1982;55:219-27.

8.
Nakayama K, Fukumoto S, Takeda S, et al. Differences in bone and vitamin D metabolism between primary hyperparathyroidism and malignancy-associated hypercalcemia. J Clin Endocrinol Metab 1996;81:607-11.

9.
Bonjour J-P, Philippe J, Guelpa G, et al. Bone and renal components in hypercalcemia of malignancy and response to a single infusion of clodronate. Bone 1988;9:123-30.

10.
Horwitz MJ, Tedesco MB, Sereika SM Hollis BW, Garcia-Ocaña A, Stewart AF. Direct comparison of sustained infusion of human parathyroid hormone-related protein-(1-36) [hPTHrP-(1-36)] versus hPTH-(1-34) on serum calcium, plasma 1,25-dihydroxyvitamin D concentrations, and fractional calcium excretion in healthy human volunteers. J Clin Endocrinol Metab 2003;88:1603-9.

11.
Seymour JF, Gagel RF, Hagemeister FB, Dimopoulos MA, Cabanillas F. Calcitriol production in hypercalcemic and normocalcemic patients with non-Hodgkin lymphoma. Ann Intern Med 1994;121:633-40.

12.
Nussbaum SR, Gaz RD, Arnold A. Hypercalcemia and ectopic secretion of parathyroid hormone by an ovarian carcinoma with rearrangement of the gene for parathyroid hormone. N Engl J Med 1990;323:1324-8.

13.
John R, Oleesky D, Issa B, et al. Pseudohypercalcaemia in two patients with IgM paraproteinaemia. Ann Clin Biochem 1997;34:694-6.

14.
Ladenson JH, Lewis JW, McDonald JM, Slatopolsky E, Boyd JC. Relationship of free and total calcium in hypercalcemic conditions. J Clin Endocrinol Metab 1978;48:393-7.

15.
Stewart AF. Normal physiology of bone and mineral homeostasis. In: Andriole TE, ed. Cecil essentials of medicine. 5th ed. Philadelphia: Saunders, 2004:683-94.

16.
LeBoff MS, Mikulec KH. Hypercalcemia: clinical manifestations, pathogenesis, diagnosis, and management. In: Favus MJ, ed. Primer on the metabolic bone diseases and disorders of mineral metabolism. 5th ed. Washington D.C.: American Society for Bone and Mineral Research, 2003:225-30.

17.
Bilezikian JP, Silverberg SJ. Asymptomatic primary hyperparathyroidism. N Engl J Med 2004;350:1746-51.

18.
Godsall JW, Burtis WJ, Insogna KL, Broadus AE, Stewart AF. Nephrogenous cyclic AMP, adenylate cyclase-stimulating activity, and the humoral hypercalcemia of malignancy. Recent Prog Horm Res 1986;42:705-50.

19.
Jara A, Lee E, Stauber D, Moatamed F, Felsenfeld AJ, Kleeman CR. Phosphate depletion in the rat: effect of bisphosphonates and the calcemic response to PTH. Kidney Int 1999;55:1434-43.

20.
Lentz RD, Brown DM, Kjellstrand CM. Treatment of severe hypophosphatemia. Ann Intern Med 1978;89:941-4.

21.
Goldsmith RS, Ingbar SH. Inorganic phosphate treatment of hypercalcemia of diverse etiologies. N Engl J Med 1966;274:1-7.

22.
Fleisch H. Bisphosphonates: mechanisms of action. Endocr Rev 1998;19:80-100.

23.
Cheer SM, Noble S. Zoledronic acid. Drugs 2001;61:799-805.

24.
Nussbaum SR, Younger J, Vandepol CJ, et al. Single-dose intravenous therapy with pamidronate for the treatment of hypercalcemia of malignancy: comparison of 30-, 60-, and 90-mg dosages. Am J Med 1993;95:297-304.

25.
Berenson JR, Rosen L, Vescio R, et al. Pharmaco-kinetics of pamidronate disodium in patients with cancer with normal or impaired renal function. J Clin Pharmacol 1997;37:285-90.

26.
Body JJ, Lortholary A, Romieu G, Vigneron AM, Ford J. A dose-finding study of zoledronate in hyper-calcemic cancer patients. J Bone Miner Res 1999;14:1557-61.

27.
Major P, Lortholary A, Hon J, et al. Zoledronic acid is superior to pamidronate in the treatment of hypercalcemia of malignancy: a pooled analysis of two randomized, controlled clinical trials. J Clin Oncol 2001;19:558-67.

28.
Pecherstorfer M, Steinhauer EU, Rizzoli R, Wetterwald M, Bergstrom B. Efficacy and safety of ibandronate in the treatment of hypercalcemia of malignancy: a randomized multicentric comparison to pamidronate. Support Care Cancer 2003;11:539-47.

29.
Ralston SH, Thiebaud D, Herrmann Z, et al. Dose-response study of ibandronate in the treatment of cancer-associated hyper-calcaemia. Br J Cancer 1997;75:295-300.

30.
Jacobs TP, Siris ES, Bilezikian JP, Bauiran DC, Shane E, Canfield RE. Hypercalcemia of malignancy: treatment with intra-venous dichloromethylene diphosphonate. Ann Intern Med 1981;94:312-6.

31.
Shah S, Hardy J, Rees E, et al. Is there a dose-response relationship for clodronate in the treatment of tumor-induced hypercalcaemia? Br J Cancer 2002;86:1235-7.

32.
Jung A. Comparison of two parenteral diphosphonates in hypercalcemia of malignancy. Am J Med 1982;72:221-6.

33.
Gucalp R, Ritch P, Wiernik PH, et al. Comparative study of pamidronate disodium and etidronate disodium in the treatment of cancer-related hypercalcemia. J Clin Oncol 1992;10:134-42.

34.
Machado CE, Flombaum CD. Safety of pamidronate in patients with renal failure and hypercalcemia. Clin Nephrol 1996;45:175-9.

35.
Hillner BE, Ingle JN, Chlebowski RT, et al. American Society of Clinical Oncology 2003 update on the role of bisphosphonates and bone health issues in women with breast cancer. J Clin Oncol 2003;21:4042-57. [Erratum, J Clin Oncol 2004;22:1351.]

36.
Markowitz GS, Fine PL, Stack JI, et al. Toxic acute tubular necrosis following treatment with zoledronate (Zometa). Kidney Int 2003;64:281-9.

37.
Binstock ML, Mundy GR. Effect of calcitonin and glu-cocorticoids in combination on the hypercalcemia of malignancy. Ann Intern Med 1980;93:269-72.

38.
Watson L, Moxham J, Fraser P. Hydrocortisone suppression test and discriminant analysis in differential diagnosis of hyper-calcaemia. Lancet 1980;1:1320-5.

39.
Wisneski LA, Croom WP, Silva OL, Becker KL. Salmon calcitonin in hypercalcemia. Clin Pharmacol Ther 1978;24:219-22.

40.
Perlia CP, Gubisch NJ, Wolter J, Edelberg D, Dederick MM, Taylor SG III. Mithramycin treatment of hypercalcemia. Cancer 1970;25:389-94.

41.
Leyland-Jones B. Treatment of cancer-related hypercalcemia: the role of gallium nitrate. Semin Oncol 2003;30:Suppl 5:13-9.

42.
Cardella CJ, Birkin BL, Rapoport A. Role of dialysis in the treatment of severe hypercalcemia: report of two cases successfully treated with hemodialysis and review of the literature. Clin Nephrol 1979;12:285-90.

43.
Koo WS, Jeon DS, Ahn SJ, Kim YS, Yoon YS, Bang BK. Calcium-free hemodialysis for the management of hy-percalcemia. Nephron 1996;72:424-8.

44.
Bekker PJ, Holloway D, Nakanishi A, Arrighi M, Leese PT, Dunstan CR. The effect of a single dose of os-teoprotegerin in postmeno-pausal women. J Bone Miner Res 2001;16:348-60.

45.
Bekker PJ, Holloway DL, Rasmussen AS, et al. A single-dose placebo-controlled trial of AMG 162, a fully human monoclonal antibody to RANKL, in post-menopausal women. J Bone Miner Res 2004;19:1059-66.

46.
Sato K, Onuma E, Yocum RC, Ogata E. Treatment of ma-lignancy-associated hyper-calcemia and cachexia with humanized anti-parathyroid hormone-related protein antibody. Semin Oncol 2003;30:Suppl 16:167-73.

Rosacea

FRANK C. POWELL, F.R.C.P.I.

A 47-year-old white woman reports facial redness and flushing. Her eyes are itchy and irritated. She thinks she may have rosacea and is worried that she will have a "whiskey nose." On examination, multiple erythematous papules, pustules, and telangiectasias are observed on a background of erythema of the central portion of her face. How should her case be managed?

THE CLINICAL PROBLEM

A constellation of clinical symptoms and signs are included under the broad rubric of rosacea. These consist of facial flushing, the appearance of telangiectatic vessels and persistent redness of the face, eruption of inflammatory papules and pustules on the central facial convexities, and hypertrophy of the sebaceous glands of the nose, with fibrosis (rhinophyma).[1] Ocular changes are present in more than 50 percent of patients and range from mild dryness and irritation with blepharitis and conjunctivitis (common symptoms) to sight-threatening keratitis (rare).[2] Patients with rosacea may report increased sensitivity of the facial skin[3] and may have dry, flaking facial dermatitis, edema of the upper face,[4] or persistent granulomatous papulonodules.[5] There is often an overlapping of clinical features, but in the majority of patients, a particular manifestation of rosacea dominates the clinical picture. As a useful approach to the guidance of therapy, the disease can thus be classified into four subtypes — erythematotelangiectatic (subtype 1), papulopustular (2), phymatous (3), and ocular (4)[6] — with the severity of each subtype graded as 1 (mild), 2 (moderate), or 3 (severe).[7] The psychological, social, and occupational effects of the disease on the patient should also be assessed and factored into treatment decisions.

The onset of rosacea usually occurs between the ages of 30 and 50 years.[8] The course of the disease is typically chronic, with remissions and relapses. Some patients identify exacerbating factors, particularly in regard to flushing, such as heat, alcohol, sunlight, hot beverages, stress, menstruation, certain medications, and certain foods.[9] Rosacea is

Table 1. Classification, Features, and Treatment of Rosacea.*

Subtype	Clinical Features	Severity†	
		Grade	Features
Erythematotel-angiectatic (subtype 1)	Persistent erythema of the central face. Flushing; telangiectasias often present; easily irritated facial skin. Patient may report stinging or burning of the face and have symptoms of ocular rosacea. Rhinophyma occasionally coexists.	1	Occasional mild flushing; faint persistent erythema; occasional telangiectasias.
		2	Frequent troublesome flushing; moderate persistent erythema; several distinct telangiectasias.
		3	Frequent severe flushing; pronounced persistent erythema; possible edema; many prominent telegiectasias.
Papulopustular (subtype 2)	Persistent erythema of the central face; dome-shaped erythematous papules; small pustules surmount some papules. Flushing, telangiectasias, ocular inflammation, and phymatous skin changes may be present.	1	Few papules or pustules; mild persistent erythema; no plaques.
		2	Several papules or pustules; moderate persistent erythema; no plaques.
		3	Many or extensive papules or pustules; pronounced persistent erythema; inflammatory plaques or edema may be present.
Phymatous (subtype 3)	Thickened skin with prominent pores. May affect nose (rhinophyma — most common type), chin (gnathophyma), forehead (metophyma), ears (otophyma), and eyelids (blepharophyma). May occur in isolation or with other skin changes of rosacea (flushing, erythema, edema, telangiectasias, papules, pustules in a nasal or central-facial distribution) or with ocular rosacea.	1	For rhinophyma: slight puffiness of nose; slight prominence of follicular orifices (patulous follicles); no clinically apparent hypertrophy of connective tissue or sebaceous glands; no change in nasal contour.
		2	For rhinophyma: bulbous nasal swelling; moderately dilated patulous follicles; clinically apparent mild hypertrophy of the sebaceous glands or connective tissue, with change in nasal contour but without nodular component.
		3	For rhinophyma: marked nasal swelling; large dilated follicles; distortion of nasal contour due to hypertrophy of the sebaceous glands or connective tissue, with nodular component.
Ocular (subtype 4)	Sensation of foreign body in the eye; telangiectasia and erythema of lid margins, often with scaling. Conjunctival injection; recurrent chalazion or hordeolum. Keratitis, episcleritis or scleritis, and iritis may occur, though rarely. May precede, follow, or occur simultaneously with cutaneous changes. Both eyes are usually affected.	1	Mild itch, dryness, or grittiness of eyes; fine scaling of lid margins; telangiectasia and erythema of lid margins; mild conjunctival injection (mild congestion of conjunctival vessels).
		2	Burning or stinging of eyes; crusting or irregularity of lid margins, with erythema and edema; definite conjunctival hyperemia or injection; formation of chalazion or hordeolum.
		3	Pain, photosensitivity, or blurred vision; severe lid changes, with loss of lashes; severe conjunctival inflammation; corneal changes, with potential loss of vision; episcleritis or scleritis; iritis.

*Adapted from Wilkin et al.[6,7]

†In general, 1 denotes mild disease, 2 moderate disease, and 3 severe disease, but grades of severity are not always clearly defined. Patients may have more than one subtype, and the grade of severity should be assessed in each of these. Patients should also be asked to grade the psychological, social, and occupational effects of their disease on a similar scale. For example, in grade 1 (mild), the patient is conscious of the condition, but it does not cause embarrassment or inhibit social functioning; in grade 2 (moderate), the patient is constantly aware of the rosacea during social situations and it regularly causes embarrassment; in grade 3 (severe), the patient is constantly thinking about the condition and avoids social interaction because of it. Such grading on the part of the patient facilitates evaluation of the overall effect of the disease on him or her and guides assessment of the efficacy of therapy.

Therapeutic Approach	Comments
Reduce flushing and redness and minimize skin irritation. Topical medications recommended for papulopustular rosacea are not indicated and may cause irritation. Systemic treatments used for papulopustular rosacea may reduce erythema if significant inflammation is present. Ablative therapy of prominent vessels for grade-2-to-3 disease.	Difficult to treat satisfactorily.
Topical or systemic medications for grade-1-to-2 disease; systemic medications for grade 3.	Response to treatment is usually good. Maintenance therapy is usually required to maintain remission.
Rhinophyma (grades 2 and 3) may respond well to surgical or laser therapy. Other phymatous skin changes are very difficult to treat but may improve with treatment of inflammatory skin lesions, if present.	All phymatous skin changes are rare. The most common form (rhinophyma) occurs predominantly in men.
Topical medication for grade 1; systemic medication for grade 2. Refer patients with persistent grade 1 or 2 disease or suspected grade 3 disease to ophthalmologist.	May occur in the majority of rosacea cases, but not often diagnosed. Vision-threatening ocular inflammation is rare.

Table 2. General Nonpharmacologic Guidelines for the Management of Rosacea.

Reassure patients about the benign nature of the disorder and the rarity of rhinophyma (particularly in women).

Direct patients to Web sites such as those of the National Rosacea Society (www.rosacea.org) and the American Academy of Dermatology (www.aad.org), where patient-related information can be accessed.

Advise patients to keep a daily diary to identify precipitating or exacerbating factors.

Suggest a daily application of combined ultraviolet-A–protective and ultraviolet-B–protective sunscreen (with a sun-protection factor of 15 or greater). Sunscreen may be incorporated into moisturizer or topical medication. Vehicle formulations with dimethicone and cyclomethicone may be less irritating than others. Sun-blocking creams containing titanium dioxide and zinc oxide are usually well tolerated.

Suggest a daily application of soap-free cleansers, silicone facial foundations, and liquid film-forming moisturizers.

Suggest cosmetic coverage of excess redness with brush application; matte-finish, water-soluble facial powder containing inert green pigment helps neutralize erythema.

Advise patients to avoid potentially exacerbating factors:
    Overly strenuous exercise, hot and humid atmosphere, emotional upset, alcohol, hot beverages, spicy foods, and large hot meals.
    Exposure to sun or to intense cold or harsh winds.
    Perfumed sunscreens or those containing insect repellents.
    Astringents and scented products containing hydroalcoholic extracts or sorbic acid.
    Cleansers containing acetone or alcohol.
    Abrasive or exfoliant preparations.
    Vigorous rubbing of the skin.
    Toners or moisturizers containing glycolic acid.
    If possible, medications that may exacerbate flushing (e.g., vasodilative drugs, nicotinic acid and amyl nitrite, calcium-channel–blocking agents, and opiates).

more common in women than in men, but men with rosacea are more prone to the development of thickening and distorting phymatous skin changes. Rosacea has been anecdotally reported to be associated with seborrheic dermatitis (this association is likely), with migraine headaches in women[10] (possible), and with *Helicobacter pylori* infection[11] (controversial). A rosacea-like eruption can be induced by the topical application of fluorinated corticosteroids[12] and tacrolimus ointment[13] to the face. In two European population studies, the prevalence of rosacea was reported to be 1.5 percent[14] and 10 percent,[15] but estimates are complicated by the difficulty of distinguishing between chronic actinic damage and erythematotelangiectatic rosacea. Although rosacea can occur in all racial and ethnic groups, white persons of Celtic origin are thought to be particularly prone to the disorder,[16] and it is uncommon in persons with dark skin. Up to 30 percent of patients report a family history of rosacea.[17] The common misconception that both the facial red-

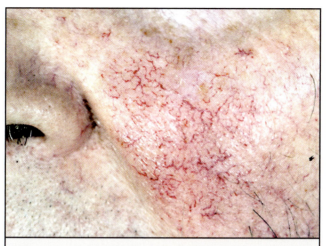

Figure 1. Erythematotelangiectatic (Subtype 1) Rosacea.

Prominent telangiectasias and erythema of the medial cheek are evident in this example of grade 2 disease. As the erythema subsides, the telangiectasias often become more evident. This patient, who has fair skin and works outside, reported sensitive, easily irritated skin and frequent flushing.

ness and the rhinophyma associated with rosacea are due to excessive alcohol consumption makes rosacea a socially stigmatizing condition for many patients.

STRATEGIES AND EVIDENCE

The diagnosis of rosacea is a clinical one. There is no confirmatory laboratory test. Biopsy is warranted only to rule out alternative diagnoses, since histopathological findings are not diagnostic.[18]

The differential diagnosis and therapy vary according to subtype (Table 1). Rosacea that is manifested predominantly by flushing is difficult to treat, but the condition may improve with the management of other manifestations and the avoidance of provoking or triggering factors. Inflammatory changes in the skin are usually responsive to medical therapies and heal without scarring, whereas telangiectasias and phymatous changes often require laser or surgical intervention. Ocular rosacea is usually mild and responsive to lid hygiene, tear replacement, and topical or systemic antibiotics, but patients with persistent or severe ocular disease should be referred to an ophthalmologist. All patients should be advised in regard to protection from climatic influences (both heat and cold), avoidance of factors that trigger or exacerbate flushing or that irritate the often-sensitive skin, appropriate care of the facial skin (Table 2), and a strategy for maintenance of remission when the

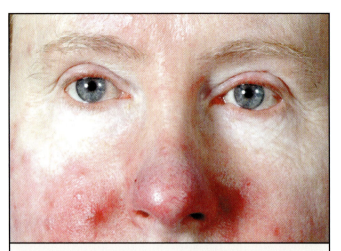

Figure 2. Papulopustular (Subtype 2) and Ocular (Subtype 4) Rosacea of Moderate Severity.

In this example of grade-2-to-3 disease, the typical distribution of papules and pustules on a background of inflammatory erythema is seen over the convexities of the central portion of the face, with sparing of the periocular area. Grade-1-to-2 ocular rosacea (erythema and edema of the upper eyelids) is also present.

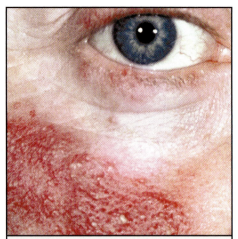

Figure 3. Severe Papulopustular Rosacea with Moderate Ocular Involvement.

In this patient with grade 3 papulopustular disease, inflammatory lesions have coalesced into an erythematous plaque below the eye. Note the multiple small, studded pustules on the surface of the plaque and the inflammatory lesions on the lower eyelid (grade 2 ocular rosacea).

condition improves. The choice of medications, dosages, and duration of therapy is often based on clinical experience. Off-label prescription-drug use is common.[19]

Subtype 1

Flushing, with persistent central facial erythema (erythematotelangiectatic rosacea), is probably the most common presentation of rosacea.[6] Although it has been suggested that rosacea is essentially a cutaneous vascular disorder,[20] facial flushing is not always a feature; patients who report flushing as their only symptom should not receive a diagnosis of "prerosacea," since, in many such patients, rosacea never develops. Common causes of flushing (e.g., psychosocial factors or anxiety, food, alcohol or drugs, or menopause) should become apparent when a medical history is taken. Prolonged episodes of severe flushing accompanied by sweating, flushing that is not limited to the face, and, especially, systemic symptoms such as diarrhea, wheezing, headache, palpitations, or weakness indicate the need for investigations to rule out rare conditions that may be characterized by flushing (e.g., the carcinoid syndrome, pheochromocytoma, or mastocytosis).[21]

Telangiectatic vessels are usually prominent on the cheeks and nose in grades 2 and 3 of subtype 1 rosacea (Figure 1) and contribute to the facial erythema. Erythematotelangiec-

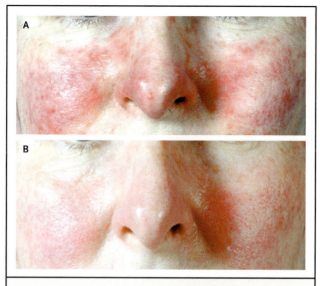

Figure 4. Response to Treatment in a Patient with Papulopustular Rosacea.

This patient with grade-2-to-3 papulopustular rosacea (Panel A) was given oral antibiotics for six weeks, followed by topical maintenance therapy, as well as continuous application of a sunscreen with a sun-protection factor of 15 or greater. Eight weeks after the initiation of therapy (Panel B), the inflammatory papules and pustules had cleared, although some residual erythema persisted.

tatic rosacea is difficult to distinguish from the effects of chronic actinic damage, which may coexist. Since the management of the two conditions is similar, this distinction is not essential for patient care. Erythematotelangiectatic rosacea may occasionally mimic facial contact dermatitis, the "butterfly rash" of lupus erythematosus, or photosensitivity; if the diagnosis is uncertain, skin biopsies, serologic screening for antinuclear and anticyto-plasmic autoantibodies, or other investigations may be indicated.

Subtype 1 rosacea is poorly responsive to treatment. The measures outlined in Table 2 are particularly relevant for patients with subtype 1, who often have sensitive, easily irritated skin. There are few studies of the effectiveness of medical treatments for flushing in patients with rosacea. Beta-blockers in low doses (e.g., nadolol, 20 to 40 mg daily)[22] as well as clonidine and spironolactone have been used to treat flushing in patients with rosacea, but evidence from randomized trials is lacking to support the effectiveness of these agents. Endoscopic transthoracic sympathectomy has been used successfully to treat socially disabling blushing[23]; however, its use as a treatment for rosacea is not

Table 3. Treatment of Papulopustular Rosacea.*

Medication	Properties and Actions	Dosage and Duration†	Contraindications and Side Effects‡	Comments
Topical				
Metronidazole (0.75% gel or cream; 1% cream)	Antibacterial; antiinflammatory.	Applied once or twice daily. Can be used as initial treatment to clear inflammatory lesions or as indefinite maintenance therapy after clearance with systemic therapy.	Contraindications: women of childbearing age not on oral contraception should use with caution because of possibility of absorption and mutagenic effects. Side effects: gel preparation may be irritating to skin. Transient watering of eyes may occur when applied to periocular skin.	Gel and cream and both concentrations appear to be equally effective.
Azelaic acid (20% cream; 15% gel)	Antibacterial; antiinflammatory.	Applied twice daily. Can be used as initial or indefinite maintenance therapy.	Side effects: may cause mild burning or stinging sensation when applied initially. Pruritus, dryness, or scaling can occur. Rarely, contact dermatitis or facial edema may occur.	May be used in women of childbearing age and during pregnancy.
10% Sodium sulfacetamide and 5% sulfur in cream or lotion. Preparations may include 10% urea; sunscreen; green tint.	Antibacterial; keratolytic (sulfur); hydrating (urea).	Applied twice daily. Can be used as initial or indefinite maintenance therapy. Cleanser preparation available.	Contraindications: hypersensitivity to sulphonamide or sulfur. Side effects: rarely, systemic hypersensitivity reactions. May cause redness, peeling, and dryness of skin.	Sulfur component may help accompanying seborrheic dermatitis. Sunscreen or tinted preparations may reduce number of topical preparations needed.
Erythromycin (2% solution)	Antibacterial; antiinflammatory.	Applied twice daily. Can be used as initial or indefinite maintenance therapy.	Side effects: local irritation or dryness.	May be used in pregnancy. Alcohol in solution may reduce tolerance.
Tretinoin (0.025% cream or lotion; 0.01% gel)	Alters epidermal keratinization. May improve photoaging changes.	Applied at night. Can be used as initial or indefinite maintenance therapy.	Contraindications: teratogenic; women of childbearing age not on oral contraceptives should use with caution. Side effects: Irritating and poorly tolerated by some patients. May cause photosensitivity. Use on damaged skin and contact with eyes should be avoided.	Theoretically useful for actinically damaged skin (common in rosacea).
Systemic				
Oxytetracycline	Antibacterial; antiinflammatory.	250 to 500 mg twice daily for 6 to 12 weeks to achieve remission. Intermittent low-dose therapy may prevent relapse.	Contraindications: should be avoided by women who are pregnant, contemplating pregnancy, or lactating and by persons with impaired renal or hepatic function. Side effects: gastrointestinal upset; candida; photosensitivity; benign intracranial hypertension. May reduce effectiveness of oral contraceptives. May cause tooth discoloration or enamel hypoplasia. Poor absorption if taken with food, milk, or some medications.	

Table 3. (Continued.)*

Medication	Properties and Actions	Dosage and Duration†	Contraindications and Side Effects‡	Comments
Doxycycline	Antibacterial; antiinflammatory.	50 to 100 mg once or twice daily for 6 to 12 weeks.	Same as for oxytetracycline.	May be taken with food.
Minocycline	Antibacterial; antiinflammatory.	50 to 100 mg twice daily or sustained-action formulation once daily for 6 to 12 weeks.	Contraindications: pregnancy or lactation. Persons with hepatic impairment should use with caution. Side effects: gastrointestinal upset (but less than with tetracycline); allergic reactions. Hyperpigmentation of the skin may occur. Long-term use should be avoided (hepatic damage or systemic-lupus-erythematosus–like syndrome may be induced). Drug interactions with antacids, mineral supplements, anticoagulants.	Randomized, clinical trials to support its use in rosacea are lacking, but clinical impression is of equal efficacy to oxytetracycline. Unlike oxytetracycline, can be taken with food.
Erythromycin	Antibacterial; antiinflammatory.	250 to 500 mg once or twice daily for 6 to 12 weeks.	Contraindications: severe hepatic impairment. Side effects: gastrointestinal upset; headache or rash. Drug interactions (many).	Alternative to oxytetracycline or minocycline as first-line systemic treatment. Useful if systemic therapy necessary in oxytetracycline-intolerant or pregnant or lactating patients.
Metronidazole	Antibacterial; antiinflammatory.	200 mg once or twice daily for 4 to 6 weeks.	Contraindications: pregnant or lactating women should use with caution. Side effects: gastrointestinal upset; leukopenia; neurologic effect (seizures or peripheral neuropathy). Drug interactions with alcohol, anticoagulants, or phenobarbital.	Side-effect profile limits its use to resistant cases for short periods.

* Topical treatment alone is usually effective for mild-to-moderate (grade-1-to-2) papulopustular rosacea. Topical metronidazole, combination 10 percent sodium sulfacetamide and 5 percent sulfur, and 15 percent azelaic acid have been approved by the Food and Drug Administration for the treatment of rosacea; however, several other topical medications are used off label. For patients with moderate-to-severe papulopustular rosacea (grade 2 to 3), oral medication is usually indicated. These patients may not tolerate topical medications initially, owing to inflamed skin, but topical therapy may be added as the inflammation subsides and is used to maintain remission after cessation of oral therapy.

† Dosage ranges relate to published reports and reflect the lack of uniformity in the approach to the treatment of papulopustular rosacea.

‡ Contraindications and side effects are selected examples rather than a comprehensive summary.

recommended, owing to rare but serious complications such as pneumothorax and pulmonary embolism, as well as postoperative increases in episodes of abnormal sweating.

If the telangiectatic component is prominent, as it is in grade-2-to-3 disease, ablation of vessels by laser can be helpful. A nonblinded, uncontrolled study of 16 patients who had erythematotelangiectatic rosacea and were treated with pulsed-dye–laser therapy showed a significant improvement in erythema and quality of life after treatment.[24] Although topical and systemic therapies, as outlined for papulopustular rosacea below, are often used to treat patients with erythematotelangiectatic rosacea, there is little evidence of the efficacy of these agents. In addition, topical therapy may irritate the sensitive skin of patients with subtype 1 rosacea.

Subtype 2

Small, dome-shaped erythematous papules, some of which have tiny surmounting pustules, on the convexities of the central portion of the face, with background erythema (Figure 2), typify papulopustular rosacea.[6] In grade 3 disease, plaques can form from the coalescence of inflammatory lesions (Figure 3). Telangiectatic vessels, varying degrees of edema, ocular inflammation, and a tendency to flush are present in some patients. The differential diagnosis includes acne vulgaris, perioral dermatitis, and seborrheic dermatitis. Patients with acne vulgaris have less erythema, are often younger, and have oily skin with blackheads and whiteheads (comedones), larger pustules and nodulocystic lesions, and a tendency to scarring. In patients with perioral dermatitis, micropustules and microvesicles around the mouth or eyes and dry, sensitive skin may follow the inappropriate use of topical corticosteroids. Seborrheic dermatitis may accompany rosacea and contribute to the facial erythema, but it is distinguished from rosacea by a prominence of yellowish scaling around the eyebrows and alae nasi, together with troublesome dandruff.

Management   Systemic or topical antibiotics, or both, are the mainstays of therapy for subtype 2 rosacea (Table 3), and the response is often satisfactory (Figures 4A and 4B). Moderate-to-severe (i.e., grade 2 or 3) papulopustular rosacea may require systemic therapy to achieve clearance of inflammatory skin lesions, whereas milder (grade 1 and some cases of grade 2) disease can often be treated with topical medications alone.[25] Although data are lacking to support the combined use of topical and systemic therapies, many clinicians recommend such a combination for the treatment of moderate-to-severe disease.[20,25]

On the basis of an analysis that pooled data from two randomized trials, van Zuuren and colleagues concluded that there was strong evidence of the efficacy of topical metronidazole and azelaic acid cream.[26] Sixty-eight of 90 patients (76 percent) treated with topical metronidazole for eight or nine weeks considered their rosacea to be improved, as

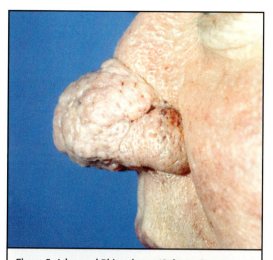

Figure 5. Advanced Rhinophyma (Subtype 3).

In grade 3 rhinophyma, enlargement and distortion of the nose occur, with prominent pores and thickened skin due to hyperplasia of the sebaceous glands and fibrosis of the connective tissue. There is follicular prominence and a distorted nodular appearance. In this patient, the rhinophyma was accompanied by mild papulopustular rosacea, which responded well to topical medications.

compared with 32 of 84 patients (38 percent) in the placebo group.[26] Significant reductions in the number of inflammatory lesions and in erythema were reported in two large placebo-controlled, double-blind studies of a 15 percent azelaic acid gel applied twice daily.[27] A double-blind, randomized, parallel-group trial involving 251 patients with papulopustular rosacea[28] demonstrated the superiority of 15 percent azelaic acid gel over 0.75 percent metronidazole gel applied twice daily for 15 weeks. In a double-blind study of 103 patients, a lotion containing 10 percent sodium sulfacetamide and 5 percent sulfur reduced inflammatory lesions by 78 percent, as compared with a reduction of 36 percent in the placebo group.[29] An investigator-blinded study involving 63 patients that compared the combination of 10 percent sodium sulfacetamide and 5 percent sulfur lotion with 0.75 percent metronidazole showed a significantly greater clearance of lesions among the patients treated with sodium sulfacetamide and sulfur.[30] An uncontrolled study showed a reduction in erythema, papules, and pustules in 13 of 15 patients (87 percent) who were treated with topical erythromycin applied twice daily for four weeks.[31]

Evidence of the efficacy of oral metronidazole and tetracycline was also reported by van Zuuren et al.[26] Of 73 patients who were treated with tetracycline for four to six weeks, 56 (77 percent) were considered to have improvement, as compared with 28 of 79 (35 percent) in the placebo group.[26] Among 14 patients treated with 200 mg of metronidazole twice daily for six weeks, 10 were considered to have improvement, as compared with 2 of 13 patients (15 percent) who received placebo pills.[32] A double-blind trial that compared 200 mg of metronidazole twice daily with 250 mg of tetracycline twice daily for 12 weeks among 40 patients showed that the two agents were equally effective.[33] Although both minocycline and erythromycin are frequently used in the systemic treatment of rosacea, there are few data available on the effectiveness of these agents. On the basis of clinical experience, some investigators have suggested that intermittent low-dose antibiotic treatment (250 mg of tetracycline on alternate days) may be as effective as multiple daily doses.[34] An uncontrolled study of 10 patients with moderate or severe rosacea that had responded poorly to treatment were prescribed 250 mg of azithromycin three times per week; moderate or marked improvement was observed in all patients after four weeks of therapy.[35]

Oral isotretinoin in low doses has been reported to be effective in the control of rosacea that was otherwise resistant to treatment, but the ocular and cutaneous drying effects of this agent are poorly tolerated, and its potential for serious adverse effects (including teratogenic effects) contradicts its use in routine care. Topical tretinoin has been reported to be as effective as oral isotretinoin after 16 weeks of treatment[36] and may be helpful in the treatment of patients with papulopustular rosacea who also have oily skin.[37]

Anecdotal reports have suggested that *Cucumis sativus* (cucumber), applied in a cooled yogurt paste, is helpful in reducing facial edema of rosacea that is otherwise resistant to treatment[38] and that facial massage involving rotatory movements of the fingers from the central to the peripheral face may improve papulopustular and edematous skin changes.[39] However, data that support the effectiveness of either of these treatments are lacking.

Maintenance Therapy   Because relapse occurs in about one quarter of patients within weeks after the cessation of systemic therapy,[40] topical therapy is usually used in an effort to maintain remission.[41] The required duration of maintenance therapy is unknown, but a period of six months is generally advised.[42] After this time, some patients report that they can keep their skin free of papulopustular lesions with topical therapy applied on alternate days or twice weekly, whereas others require repeated courses of systemic medication.

Subtype 3

Phymatous rosacea is uncommon. The most frequent phymatous manifestation is rhinophyma (known familiarly as "whiskey nose" or "rum blossom"). In its severe forms (grade 3), rhinophyma is a disfiguring condition of the nose resulting from hyperplasia of both the sebaceous glands and the connective tissue (Figure 5). Rhinophyma occurs much more often in men than in women (approximate ratio, 20:1),[43] and a number of clinico-pathologic variants have been described.[44] Although rhinophyma is often referred to as "end-stage rosacea," it may occur in patients with few or no other features of rosacea. The diagnosis is usually made on a clinical basis, but a biopsy may be necessary to distinguish atypical, or nodular, rhinophyma from lupus pernio (sarcoidosis of the nose); basal-cell, squamous-cell, and sebaceous carcinomas; angiosarcoma; and even nasal lymphoma.[45]

Data from randomized trials of therapies for rhinophyma and long-term follow-up studies of recurrence rates are lacking. Clinical experience suggests that grades 2 and 3 rhinophyma respond well, at least initially, to surgical excision, electrosurgery, or carbon dioxide–laser therapy. A case series of 30 patients who were treated with carbon dioxide lasers and followed for one to three years showed good cosmetic results in almost all the patients.[46]

Subtype 4

Ocular rosacea is common but often not recognized by the clinician.[47] It may precede, follow, or occur simultaneously with the skin changes typical of rosacea. In the absence of accompanying skin changes, ocular rosacea can be difficult to diagnose, and there is no test that will confirm the diagnosis. Patients usually have mild, nonspecific symptoms, such as burning or stinging of the eyes. A sensation of dryness is common, and tear secretion is frequently decreased.[48] Mild-to-moderate ocular rosacea (including blepharoconjunctivitis, chalazia, and hordeola) occurs frequently, whereas serious (grade 3) disease with the potential for visual loss, such as that which results from keratitis, occurs rarely.

Artificial tears, eyelid hygiene (i.e., cleaning the lids with warm water twice daily), fucidic acid, and metronidazole gel applied to lid margins are treatments that are frequently used to treat mild ocular rosacea. Systemic antibiotics are often additionally required for grade-2-to-3 disease, although limited data are available to support these approaches. In a double-blind, placebo-controlled trial, 35 patients with ocular rosacea who received 250 mg of oxytetracycline twice daily for six weeks had a significantly higher rate of remission than did patients who received a placebo (65 percent vs. 28 percent).[49] In an uncontrolled study of 39 patients with cutaneous rosacea (28 with ocular symptoms), 100 mg of doxycycline daily for 12 weeks improved symptoms of dryness, itching, blurred vision, and photosensitivity.[50] After ocular symptoms subside, the maintenance of lid hygene and the use of artificial tears are usually recommended. However, such treatment may be inadequate for moderate-to-severe ocular rosacea, and patients with persistent or potentially serious ocular symptoms should be referred to an ophthalmologist.

AREAS OF UNCERTAINTY

The causes and pathogenesis of rosacea remain poorly understood.[4,51] Data from randomized, clinical trials on the efficacy and optimal duration of many of the therapies, including complementary therapies that are frequently used by patients,[52] are lacking. The possibility of emergence and carriage on the skin of resistant organisms is a concern with regard to the prolonged use of topical and systemic antibiotics.

GUIDELINES

There are no specific guidelines for the management of rosacea.

SUMMARY OF RECOMMENDATIONS

"Rosacea" is a diagnostic term applied to a spectrum of changes in the skin and eyes. Until the causes and pathogenesis are better understood, the classification of rosacea by its predominant features and grading according to severity (Table 1) are recommended to guide management. The emotional effect of rosacea on the patient must also be considered in the management of this condition, and advice on improving the cosmetic appearance of the skin is an important aspect of overall care.

The woman described in the vignette should be reassured that inflammatory papules and pustules usually respond to therapy and resolve without scarring and that rhinophyma rarely develops in women. She should be advised to apply a sunscreen daily that provides protection against both ultraviolet A and ultraviolet B irradiation and to avoid using irritating topical products. Treatment should be initiated with 100 mg of doxycycline or 100 mg of minocycline daily for a period of 6 to 12 weeks. This should be followed by maintenance therapy with azelaic acid, topical metronidazole, or a sodium sulfacetamide–sulfur preparation applied twice daily for six months and then gradually discontinued, as outlined above. Laser therapy should be considered for residual, prominent telangiectatic vessels. The oral antibiotic is likely to help the patient's ocular symptoms, and she should also be advised to clean her eyelids with warm water twice daily and to use artificial tears. Referral to an ophthalmologist should be considered if her ocular symptoms persist.

Dr. Powell reports having received speaking fees from Galderma Laboratories, Bradley Pharmaceuticals, and Dermik Laboratories.

This article first appeared in the February 24, 2005, issue of the New England Journal of Medicine.

REFERENCES

1.
Wilkin JK. Rosacea. Int J Dermatol 1983;22:393-400.

2.
Starr PA. Oculocutaneous aspects of rosacea. Proc R Soc Med 1969;62:9-11.

3.
Lonne-Rahm SB, Fischer T, Berg M. Stinging and rosacea. Acta Derm Venereol 1999;79:460-1.

4.
Crawford GH, Pelle MT, James WD. Rosacea: I. Etiology, pathogenesis, and subtype classification. J Am Acad Dermatol 2004;51:327-41.

5.
Helm KF, Menz J, Gibson LE, Dicken CH. A clinical and histopathologic study of granulomatous rosacea. J Am Acad Dermatol 1991;25:1038-43.

6.
Wilkin J, Dahl M, Detmar M, et al. Standard classification of rosacea: report of the National Rosacea Society Expert Committee on the Classification and Staging of Rosacea. J Am Acad Dermatol 2002;46:584-7.

7.
Wilkin J, Dahl M, Detmar M, et al. Standard grading system for rosacea: report of the National Rosacea Society Expert Committee on the Classification and Staging of Rosacea. J Am Acad Dermatol 2004;50:907-12.

8.
Sobye P. Aetiology and pathogenesis of rosacea. Acta Derm Venereol 1950;30:137-58.

9.
Kligman AM. A personal critique on the state of knowledge of rosacea. Dermatology 2004;208:191-7.

10.
Ramelet AA. Rosacea: a reaction pattern associated with ocular lesions and migraine? Arch Dermatol 1994;130:1448.

11.
Diaz C, O'Callaghan C, Khan A, Ilchyshyn A. Rosacea: a cutaneous marker of Helicobacter pylori infection? Results of a pilot study. Acta Derm Venereol 2003;83:282-6.

12.
Litt JZ. Steroid-induced rosacea. Am Fam Physician 1993;48:67-71.

13.
Antille C, Saurat JH, Lubbe J. Induction of rosaceiform dermatitis during treatment of facial inflammatory dermatoses with tacrolimus ointment. Arch Dermatol 2004;140:457-60.

14.
Lomholt G. Prevalence of skin diseases in a population — a census study from the Faroe Islands. Dan Med Bull 1964;11:1-7.

15.
Berg M, Liden S. An epidemiological study of rosacea. Acta Derm Venereol 1989;69:419-23.

16.
Plewig G, Kligman AM. Acne and rosacea. 2nd ed. Berlin: Springer-Verlag, 1993.

17.
Rebora A. The red face: rosacea. Clin Dermatol 1993;11:225-34.

18.
Powell FC. The histopathology of rosacea: 'where's the beef'? Dermatology 2004;209:173-4.

19.
Sugarman JH, Fleischer AB Jr, Feldman SR. Off-label prescribing in the treatment of dermatologic disease. J Am Acad Dermatol 2002;47:217-23.

20.
Wilkin JK. Rosacea: pathophysiology and treatment. Arch Dermatol 1994;130:359-62.

21.
Greaves MW, Burova EP. Flushing: causes, investigation and clinical consequences. J Eur Acad Dermatol Venereol 1997;8:91-100.

22.
Wilkin JK. Effect of nadolol on flushing reactions in rosacea. J Am Acad Dermatol 1989;20:202-5.

23.
Drott C, Claes G, Olsson-Rex L, Dalman P, Fahlen T, Gothberg G. Successful treatment of facial blushing by endoscopic transthoracic sympathicotomy. Br J Dermatol 1998;138:639-43.

24.
Tan R, Tope WD. Pulsed dye laser treatment of rosacea improves erythema, symptomology, and quality of life. J Am Acad Dermatol 2004;51:592-9.

25.
Del Rosso JQ. Medical treatment of rosacea with emphasis on topical therapies. Expert Opin Pharmacother 2004;5:5-13.

26.
van Zuuren EJ, Graber MA, Hollis S, Chaudhry M, Gupta AK. Interventions for rosacea. Cochrane Database Syst Rev 2004;1:CD003262.

27.
Thiboutot D, Thieroff-Ekerdt R, Graupe K. Efficacy and safety of azelaic acid (15%) gel as a new treatment for papulopustular rosacea: results from two vehicle-controlled, randomized phase III studies. J Am Acad Dermatol 2003;48:836-45.

28.
Elewski BE, Fleischer AB Jr, Pariser DM. A comparison of 15% azelaic acid gel and 0.75% metronidazole gel in the treatment of papulopustular rosacea: results of a randomized trial. Arch Dermatol 2003;139:1444-50.

29.
Sauder D, Miller R, Gratton D, et al. The treatment of rosacea: the safety and efficacy of sodium sulfacetamide 10% and sulfur 5% lotion (Novacet) is demonstrated in a double-blind study. J Dermatol Treat 1997;8:79-85.

30.
Lebwohl M, Medansky RS, Russo CL, Plott RT. The comparative efficacy of sodium sulfacetamide 10% sulphur 5% (Sulfacet R) lotion and metronidazole 0.75% gel (Metrogel) in the treatment of rosacea. J Geriatr Dermatol 1995;3(6):183-5.

31.
Mills OH Jr, Kligman AM. Topically applied erythromycin in rosacea. Arch Dermatol 1976;112:553-4.

32.
Pye RJ, Burton JL. Treatment of rosacea by metronidazole. Lancet 1976;1:1211-2.

33.
Saihan EM, Burton JL. A double-blind trial of metronidazole versus oxytetracycline therapy for rosacea. Br J Dermatol 1980;102: 443-5.

34.
Jansen T, Plewig G. Rosacea: classification and treatment. J R Soc Med 1997;90: 144-50.

35.
Fernandez-Obregon A. Oral use of azithromycin for the treatment of acne rosacea. Arch Dermatol 2004;140: 489-90.

36.
Erlt GA, Levine N, Kligman AM. A comparison of the efficacy of topical tretinoin and low-dose oral isotretinoin in rosacea. Arch Dermatol 1994;130:319-24.

37.
Pelle MT, Crawford GH, James WD. Rosacea: II. Therapy. J Am Acad Dermatol 2004;51:499-512.

38.
Powell FC. Rosacea. In: Katsambas AD, Lotti TM, eds. European handbook of dermatological treatments. 2nd ed. Berlin: Springer-Verlag, 2003.

39.
Sobye P. Treatment of rosacea by massage. Acta Derm Venereol 1951;31:174-83.

40.
Knight AG, Vickers CFH. A follow-up of tetracycline-treated rosacea: with special reference to rosacea keratitis. Br J Dermatol 1975;93: 577-80.

41.
Dahl MV, Katz HI, Krueger GG, et al. Topical metronidazole maintains remissions of rosacea. Arch Dermatol 1998;134:679-83.

42.
Wilkin JK. Use of topical products for maintaining remission in rosacea. Arch Dermatol 1999;135:79-80.

43.
Roberts JO, Ward CM. Rhinophyma. J R Soc Med 1985;78:678-81.

44.
Aloi F, Tomasini C, Soro E, Pippione M. The clinico-pathologic spectrum of rhinophyma. J Am Acad Dermatol 2000;42:468-72.

45.
Murphy A, O'Keane JC, Blayney A, Powell FC. Cutaneous presentation of nasal lymphoma: a report of two cases. J Am Acad Dermatol 1998;38:310-3.

46.
el-Azhary RA, Roenigk RK, Wang TD. Spectrum of results after treatment of rhinophyma with the carbon dioxide laser. Mayo Clin Proc 1991;66:899-905.

47.
Kligman AM. Ocular rosacea: current concepts and therapy. Arch Dermatol 1997;133:89-90.

48.
Gudmundsen KJ, O'Donnell BF, Powell FC. Schirmer testing for dry eyes in patients with rosacea. J Am Acad Dermatol 1992;26:211-4.

49.
Bartholomew RS, Reid BJ, Cheesbrough MJ, Macdonald M, Galloway NR. Oxytetracycline in the treatment of ocular rosacea: a double-blind trial. Br J Ophthalmol 1982;66:386-8.

50.
Quarterman MJ, Johnson DW, Abele DC, Lesher JL Jr, Hull DS, Davis LS. Ocular rosacea: signs, symptoms, and tear studies before and after treatment with doxycycline. Arch Dermatol 1997;133: 49-54.

51.
Powell FC. What's going on in rosacea? J Eur Acad Dermatol Venereol 2000;14:351-2.

52.
Ernst E. The use of complementary therapies by dermatological patients: a systematic review. Br J Dermatol 2000;142:857-61.

Pertussis — Not Just for Kids

ERIK L. HEWLETT, M.D., AND KATHRYN M. EDWARDS, M.D.

Six weeks ago, a 45-year-old woman noticed a scratchy feeling in her throat that has now progressed to more than 20 episodes of severe, spasmodic coughing per day. Her coughing spells are worse at night and are sometimes associated with gagging and vomiting. Her adolescent son and several of his friends, who received all of their childhood immunizations on schedule, had similar illnesses involving cough several weeks before the onset of her symptoms, and they continue to cough. How should the patient be assessed for possible pertussis? Should she be treated and, if so, how? Could this illness have been prevented?

THE CLINICAL PROBLEM

Despite rates of immunization for pertussis of more than 80 percent among young children, the number of cases of pertussis reported annually in the United States has increased by a factor of six since 1980, with 11,647 cases reported in 2003 (Figure 1). The reported incidence rates probably substantially underestimate the true burden of disease because of incomplete reporting and a lack of recognition of the illness on the part of physicians.[1-4] The diagnosis of pertussis is frequently missed, often because of misconceptions that whooping cough is solely a pediatric illness that has been controlled by routine childhood immunizations and that immunity resulting from pertussis disease or immunization is lifelong. In addition, residual immunity from prior vaccination may modify the clinical presentation of pertussis in adolescents and adults and make the diagnosis even more difficult.

Clinical Presentation and Complications

Anyone who has heard the frightening paroxysmal cough of a child with classic pertussis would question how the diagnosis of pertussis could be overlooked. The illness begins, however, less dramatically, with the catarrhal phase, which consists of nonspecific symptoms such as coryza, conjunctival irritation, and, occasionally, a slight cough, none of

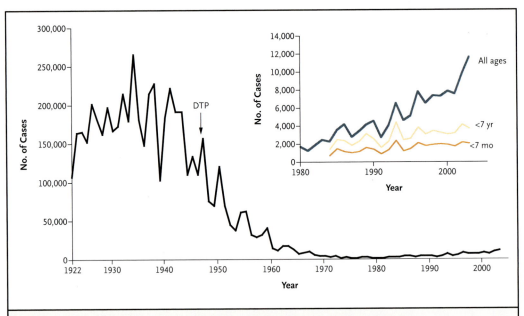

Figure 1. Annual Reported Cases of Pertussis in the United States from 1922 through 2003.

The inset shows changes in the number of reported pertussis cases since 1980 according to age group (<seven months, <seven years, and all ages). DTP denotes diphtheria, tetanus toxoids, and pertussis vaccine. Unpublished data are from the Centers for Disease Control and Prevention, by permission of Dr. Trudy Murphy and Dr. Margaret Cortese.

which suggest pertussis as the primary diagnosis. After 7 to 10 days, the characteristic cough heralds the onset of the paroxysmal phase. After several weeks, the intensity and frequency of the cough may begin to decrease, but the convalescent phase, which can include episodes of exacerbated paroxysmal coughing brought on by unrelated upper airway infections, can last for weeks to months.

The typical paroxysmal cough in a child who is not immunized consists of a series of rapid, forced expirations, followed by gasping inhalation, which can result in the typical whooping sound. Post-tussive vomiting is common. These symptoms often occur in the absence of fever. Asymptomatic intervals occur between coughing spells. Very young infants may present with apnea or cyanosis in the absence of cough and are at greater risk than are older children for death or severe complications, including pneumonia (*Bordetella pertussis* infection or infection with another pathogen), pneumothorax, severe pulmonary hypertension, seizures, or encephalopathy.[5-9]

The current pertussis-related mortality rate among infants in the United States is 2.4 deaths per 1 million, and fatal cases in infants account for more than 90 percent of all deaths from pertussis. These numbers highlight the need for new approaches to protect infants, who are too young to be immunized according to the current vaccination schedule.[2,10,11]

Among immunized patients, especially adolescents and adults, a prolonged cough may be the only manifestation of pertussis.[3] A number of studies have documented that between 13 and 32 percent of adolescents and adults with an illness involving a cough of six days' duration or longer have serologic evidence of infection with B. pertussis.[12-17] The symptoms and complications of pertussis infection reported in these studies are often quite different from those seen in children.[14-18] For example, scratchy throat and other pharyngeal symptoms occur in about one third of adults with pertussis, and episodes of sweating are reported by 40 to 50 percent of persons over the age of 30 years. Although 70 to 99 percent of adolescents and adults with pertussis are reported to have paroxysmal cough, the reported frequencies of other symptoms are more variable, with whoop in 8 to 82 percent and post-tussive vomiting in 17 to 50 percent.[6] Because adolescents and adults often do not seek medical care until several weeks after the onset of their illness, the differential diagnosis includes other causes of chronic cough, such as asthma, gastroesophageal reflux disease, postviral bronchospasm, chronic sinusitis with postnasal drip, tuberculosis, chlamydia or mycoplasma infections, other chronic lung diseases, and malignant conditions. Almost 80 percent of adults with confirmed pertussis have an illness involving a cough of at least 3 weeks' duration, and 27 percent still had a cough after 90 days.[18,19] Complications of pertussis, which are similar in adolescents and adults, include pneumonia (in 2.1 to 3.5 percent of patients), seizures (0.3 to 0.6 percent), and encephalopathy (0.1 percent). Some complications, such as cough-induced urinary incontinence, increase with age. Unusual complications that have been reported anecdotally in older patients include a herniated intervertebral disc, the sudden onset of hearing loss, angina, and carotid-artery dissection.[6,18-24]

Epidemiology, Incidence, and Burden of Disease

Although multiple reports have highlighted the role of pertussis as an important cause of persistent cough in adolescents and adults, the actual burden of disease in these groups is difficult to determine.[4,6,12-25] This seemingly simple task is complicated by the biology of B. pertussis and the difficulty in detecting the organism.[4] Most pathogens of the respiratory tract have short incubation periods, are easy to culture, cause illness for a relatively short period, and are rapidly eliminated. B. pertussis is different in that the incubation period is measured in days to weeks, the organism exhibits fastidious behavior in culture, and it has the ability to cause, as the Chinese term it, a "cough of 100 days." The organism can be recovered from patients only during the first three to four weeks of illness and is particularly difficult to isolate in previously immunized persons.[25] These factors result in outbreaks that span months and that can be difficult to track epidemiologically.[26]

Table 1. Recommended Immunization Schedules for Pertussis in Canada, France, Germany, and the United States.

Country	Type of Vaccine*	Ages at Vaccination	Ages at Booster†
Canada	DTaP†	2, 4, and 6 mo	18 mo; 4–6 and 14–16 yr
France	DTP‡	2, 3, and 4 mo	
	DTaP		16–18 mo; 11–13 yr
Germany	DTaP	3, 4, and 5 mo	11–14 mo; 9–17 yr
United States	DTaP	2, 4, and 6 mo	18 mo; 4–6 yr

* DTaP denotes diphtheria, tetanus toxoids, and acellular pertussis vaccine. There are multiple formulations of this vaccine, with each formulation containing one to four antigens, and multiple manufacturers; therefore, no two vaccines are identical. Commonly recognized side effects include swelling, redness, and tenderness at the site of injection; fever; and secondary febrile convulsions.

† Canada, France, and Germany have initiated the use of a booster dose in adolescents at the ages indicated. In France, a DTaP booster is used after the primary series with DTP. In Canada and Germany, the adolescent booster is dTap, reflecting a reduced dose of diphtheria and acellular pertussis.

‡ DTP denotes diphtheria, tetanus toxoids, and pertussis vaccine. Side effects include anaphylaxis; swelling, redness, and tenderness at the site of injection; prolonged or inconsolable crying; fever; and secondary febrile convulsions.

Before vaccination was available, pertussis was responsible for more than 270,000 cases of severe illness involving cough and 10,000 deaths annually in the United States.[27] The introduction of whole-cell pertussis vaccine into the general population during the 1940s was associated with a 99 percent reduction in the incidence of the disease, with a nadir of 1010 reported cases in 1976. Since that time, the absolute number of reported cases has increased, with the 11,647 cases in 2003 approaching the highest total since 1964 (Figure 1).[1] The routine immunization of young children in the United States according to the schedule shown in Table 1 has markedly reduced the rates of reported pertussis in children. However, striking increases in rates of disease have been seen among adolescents and adults during the past 10 years (Figures 1 and 2). In the United States, from 1997 to 2000 there were 8273 cases of pertussis reported in patients 10 to 19 years of age and 5745 cases in those older than 19 years.[1] There are probably multiple reasons for this increase, and they include the increased recognition of the disease (with the use of serologic testing for diagnosis) and the limited duration of protection from vaccine.[28]

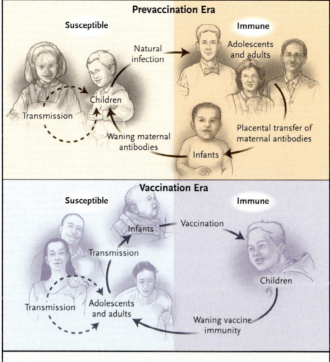

Figure 2. Epidemiologic "Life Cycles" of *B. pertussis* before and after the Generalized Use of Pertussis Vaccine.

In the prevaccination era, the majority of pertussis cases occurred in children. Adults who had had pertussis as children had their acquired immunity boosted by recurrent exposures in the population, and mothers then passed protection to infants through the placental transfer of antibodies. After the use of pertussis vaccine has been established in a population, the newly immunized pediatric group is protected; an increasing proportion of cases occur in adolescents and adults, who have lost their vaccine-induced immunity, and in infants, who receive fewer passive antibodies than did infants in the prevaccination era and who are too young to be immunized according to the current immunization schedule (Table 1).

STRATEGIES AND EVIDENCE

The critical elements involved in the diagnosis and treatment of pertussis, as with other infectious diseases, are its inclusion in the differential diagnosis, the availability of reliable and rapid laboratory tests for confirmation, and the prompt and appropriate use of the resultant information.

Diagnostic Methods

Three laboratory tests have been used to detect *B. pertussis* or related bordetella species in the respiratory secretions of patients suspected of having pertussis: direct fluorescent antibody staining, bacterial culture, and polymerase chain reaction (PCR).[29] Because the direct fluorescent antibody technique has low sensitivity and specificity in comparison with culture and PCR, this method is not currently recommended.[29,30] A positive culture of nasopharyngeal secretions (preferably an aspirate) on selective Regan–Lowe medium is the gold standard for the diagnosis of pertussis. The sensitivity of culture is limited by the fastidious nature of *B. pertussis* and the loss of viability between the site of collection and the clinical laboratory. The yield is lower from dilute specimens, specimens from patients who have had a long duration of illness, and specimens obtained after antibiotic therapy. Nonetheless, when carried out appropriately, culture continues to be recommended in patients who present within three weeks after the onset of cough. Although antibiotic resistance is rare, isolation of the causative organism, as recommended by the Centers for Disease Control and Prevention (CDC), allows for characterization of antigenic variation and antibiotic sensitivity.[31]

The use of PCR-based diagnostic assays with one or more primers, available in many health departments and clinical laboratories, is an alternative approach. These assays have been reported to detect fewer than 10 organisms, which do not need to be viable to be detected, and thus the tests have significantly greater sensitivity than does culture.[29,32] PCR assays with multiple primers can be used to identify and distinguish among several bordetella species (i.e., *B. pertussis*, *B. parapertussis*, and *B. bronchiseptica*).[29,33,34] Although the period during which the organism can be identified is longer with PCR than for culture, false positive PCR results have been a problem.[35] For these reasons, the National Immunization Program of the CDC recommends the use of culture and PCR assays during the period in which patients could be infectious — at least three weeks after the onset of cough or four weeks after the appearance of any symptoms.[36] Standardized procedures and reagents and rigid quality control of PCR assays are needed to ensure accurate diagnoses and to minimize false positive results.[35,37,38]

An alternative method of diagnosing pertussis in adolescents and adults is the measurement of antibody to specific components of *B. pertussis* with the use of enzyme-linked immunosorbent assays. Since the diagnosis of pertussis is often not considered during the period when organisms can still be detected, the demonstration of increased antibody titers between the acute phase of illness (i.e., in serum obtained within the first week after the onset of symptoms) and the convalescent phase (in serum collected four to six weeks later) may be necessary. Alternatively, a single serum antibody titer (that exceeds a diagnostic cutoff point for the level of IgG against pertussis toxin or another antigen) obtained at least three weeks into the illness may be required to confirm the diagnosis.[29,38-40] However, the lack of a widely available serologic test with an established cutoff point, the limited diagnostic value of commercial tests, and the delay in obtaining results limit the usefulness of serologic testing in practice.[6,41] As a result, the CDC recommends that combinations of diagnostic tests be used to identify persons with pertussis more effectively.[29,38] Within the first four weeks after the onset of symptoms (when cough has been present for three weeks), the use of culture and PCR is appropriate for diagnosis; when cough has been present for three to four weeks, PCR and serologic tests can both be used; and after four weeks of cough, serologic tests alone are most likely to provide a diagnosis.

Treatment

Antibiotics should be administered to patients with pertussis to hasten clearance of the organism and to limit transmission to susceptible contacts. Although controversial, it appears that treatment can sometimes reduce the duration or severity of symptoms, or both, but a benefit is unlikely when treatment is initiated after the first week of symptoms.[36] Adolescents and adults with sporadic cases frequently present during the paroxysmal phase, which occurs at least a week after the onset of symptoms, and in such cases, antibiotics rarely affect the course of the disease. However, viable organisms can be recovered from untreated patients for three weeks after the onset of the cough. Thus, the routine administration of antibiotics during the first four weeks of illness is justified. For patients who are likely to be in contact with high-risk persons, such as infants, women in the third trimester of pregnancy (who might continue to be infectious after delivery), and health care workers, treatment is recommended even six to eight weeks after the onset of illness.[36]

The National Immunization Program recommends erythromycin for the treatment of pertussis.[42] However, the newer macrolides azithromycin and clarithromycin have been demonstrated in head-to-head trials to be similar in efficacy to erythromycin, with fewer side effects and more convenient administration.[43-45] Dosages, common side effects, and contraindications are summarized in Table 2.[46,47] An alternative treatment for patients who cannot tolerate macrolides is trimethoprim–sulfamethoxazole. Although B. pertussis strains are sensitive in vitro to fluoroquinolones and ketolides, there are no clinical data to support the use of these agents.[48]

Treatment also involves supportive care, which is most important for infants and small children, since they are vulnerable to dehydration and malnutrition from post-tussive vomiting and an inability to eat. None of the pharmacologic or immunologic interventions that have been tested, such as corticosteroids, salbutamol, diphenhydramine, and pertussis immune globulin, have been documented to be effective in reducing the symptoms or controlling the cough of pertussis.[49]

Table 2. Choice of Antibiotic Agents for the Treatment of Pertussis.

Drug	Dosage	Regimen	Side Effects	Contraindications
Erythromycin	Children, 40–50 mg/kg/day Adults, 1–2 g/day	4 divided doses for 14 days*	Gastrointestinal irritation, abdominal cramps, nausea, vomiting; hypertrophic pyloric stenosis has been reported in infants	Known sensitivity to any macrolide antibiotic; should be used with caution in infants because of association with hypertrophic pyloric stenosis[46]
Azithromycin	10 mg/kg (maximum, 500 mg) as a single dose on day 1; 5 mg/kg (maximum, 250 mg) thereafter[43]‡	Lower dose once daily for 4 additional days	Allergic reaction and hepatic toxicity	Known sensitivity to any macrolide antibiotic
Clarithromycin	20 mg/kg/day (maximum, 1 g/day)	Two divided doses daily for 7 days	Allergic reaction and hepatic toxicity	Known sensitivity to any macrolide antibiotic
Trimethoprim–sulfamethoxazole†	Trimethoprim, 8 mg/kg/day (maximum, 320 mg/day); sulfamethoxazole, 40 mg/kg/day (maximum, 1600 mg/day)	Two divided doses daily for 7 days	Rash, kernicterus in newborns	Known allergy to sulfonamides or trimethoprim; should not be given to pregnant women shortly before delivery, breast-feeding mothers, or infants <2 mo old, because of the risk of kernicterus

* A 7-day regimen has been shown to be similar in efficacy to a 14-day regimen.[54]
† Trimethoprim–sulfamethoxazole should be prescribed as an alternative to the macrolides in patients who cannot tolerate them.
‡ The *2003 Red Book* recommendation is for 10 to 12 mg per kilogram per day once daily for five days.

Prophylaxis after Exposure

The same agents and regimens used for the treatment of patients with established pertussis are recommended for chemoprophylaxis in contacts. These modes of treatment are expected to be effective in the protection of persons exposed to patients with active pertussis, when administered before the onset of symptoms in the contact. Because infectiousness declines with the increasing duration of illness, prophylaxis for contacts needs to be initiated only if the interval since the onset of cough in the index case is three weeks or less. Prophylaxis is generally recommended only if the contact was exposed within the previous three weeks,[50] but for persons at high risk or those who are likely to come into contact with high-risk persons, prophylaxis may be warranted for up to six to eight weeks after exposure.

Prevention

The mainstay for control of pertussis is vaccination, and this is recommended routinely for infants and young children according to the schedules shown for several countries in Table 1. Whole-cell vaccines consisting of killed organisms are highly effective but have been associated with frequent local and systemic reactions.[27] In the 1980s and early 1990s, new acellular vaccines, which contain one or more purified pertussis components, were demonstrated to be immunogenic, associated with fewer local and systemic reactions than whole-cell vaccines, and efficacious in the prevention of culture-confirmed pertussis disease in infants and young children.[51] These acellular vaccines have replaced whole-cell vaccines in the United States and elsewhere.

Given the recognition that immunity wanes after vaccination early in life, repeated vaccination in adolescence or adulthood has been proposed. A large, randomized clinical trial evaluated the efficacy of a three-component acellular pertussis vaccine (containing pertussis toxoids, filamentous hemagglutinin, and pertactin) in nearly 3000 healthy subjects 15 to 65 years of age. Active surveillance for pertussis was conducted every two weeks for two years. With the use of culture or PCR and serologically confirmed disease as end points, preliminary data from this study indicated that there was a 92 percent efficacy rate for the vaccine (95 percent confidence interval, 32 to 99 percent).[52]

A recently published cost-benefit analysis that assumed that the incidence of pertussis was the same as that observed in the above-mentioned trial led to the conclusion that an additional booster dose of pertussis vaccine would be cost-effective.[53] Of the scenarios considered in the analysis, vaccination of adolescents was considered to be the least expensive, the easiest to implement, and the most acceptable. In light of the greater recognition of disease in adolescents and adults, some countries, such as Germany, France, and Canada, now recommend the routine vaccination of adolescents with acellular pertussis vaccine boosters (Table 1). Although there are no formulations of pertussis vaccine currently licensed in the United States for use in persons over the age of six years, advisory groups are considering the routine use of acellular vaccines in this population once vaccines are approved and become available.

AREAS OF UNCERTAINTY

Despite extensive research on the toxins, adhesions, and other factors related to the virulence of B. pertussis, little is known about the mechanisms by which these factors cause the illness of pertussis. For example, although it is clear that pertussis toxin causes the characteristic lymphocytosis and other abnormalities associated with the disease, the mechanism responsible for the severe and prolonged cough remains unknown.

Vaccination of pregnant women has been proposed as a strategy to protect infants from pertussis passively before they receive active vaccination. The potential for such a strategy to work is based on observations that maternal antibody titers to pertussis antigens are low but that, when present, antibodies are actively transported in cord blood.[55] However, data to support the safety and efficacy of maternal vaccination are lacking. An alternative or complementary approach would be the active immunization of newborns with acellular pertussis vaccines; such approaches are being studied.

GUIDELINES

The CDC recommends that for all patients with presumed pertussis, culture be performed to identify the etiologic agent during the time when patients are likely to be infectious, regardless of which other diagnostic tests are used.[36] The CDC and the Food and Drug Administration are currently working on standardization of PCR and serologic methods for the diagnosis of pertussis. Patients seen early in the course of their illness (i.e., during the first three weeks after cough begins) should be evaluated with the use of culture and PCR; PCR and serologic tests can be used when cough has been present for three to four weeks; and serologic tests should be used for patients who present with cough that has persisted for longer than four weeks.

The CDC also recommends the treatment of presumed or confirmed cases of pertussis with erythromycin but acknowledges the limitations of this treatment due to side effects. In cases in which the patient presents after the onset of paroxysmal cough, antibiotic treatment is unlikely to affect the clinical course but will preclude transmission to susceptible hosts beginning five days after the onset of therapy.

CONCLUSIONS AND RECOMMENDATIONS

For the patient described in the vignette, whose symptoms started six weeks ago, single-sample serologic testing is the only method that could yield the diagnosis. Given the duration of the symptoms, treatment with antibiotics would not affect the course of the patient's illness, and we would not recommend it at this point. If, however, the diagnosis of pertussis had been made two or more weeks earlier, it would have been appropriate to treat the patient in order to prevent further spread of the infection. If pertussis had been documented (by culture, PCR, or both) in the patient's son during the first three weeks of his illness, it would have been appropriate to consider her a contact and to treat her, whether or not she became symptomatic, with either azithromycin or clarithromycin, according to the regimen in Table 2. With this approach, even if her condition did progress to clinical pertussis, the antibiotic treatment would have the potential to reduce the duration and severity of her illness.

Pertussis vaccines are highly efficacious, but in many countries, including the United States, they are administered only to a small subgroup of the population — namely, children younger than six years of age. The control of pertussis requires an increase in the immunity of all age groups. We believe that the vaccination of adolescents (with a suitable formulation of acellular pertussis vaccine) should be added to the current immunization schedule for pertussis in order to reduce the risk of the disease later in life as well as the transmission to infants.

We are indebted to Dr. Trudy Murphy and Dr. Margaret Cortese of the National Immunization Program, CDC, for their review of the manuscript; to Dr. Emily Wong and Mr. Alan Wong for their contribution to Figure 2; and to Ms. Candace Green and Mrs. Sarah Baugher for their assistance in the preparation of the manuscript.

This article first appeared in the March 24, 2005, issue of the New England Journal of Medicine.

REFERENCES

1.
Pertussis — United States, 1997–2000. MMWR Morb Mortal Wkly Rep 2002;51: 73-6.
2.
Vitek CR, Pascual FB, Baughman AL, Murphy TV. Increase in deaths from pertussis among young infants in the United States in the 1900s. Pediatr Infect Dis J 2003;22:628-34.
3.
Deeks S, De Serres G, Boulianne N, et al. Failure of physicians to consider the diagnosis of pertussis in children. Clin Infect Dis 1999;28:840-6.
4.
Crowcroft NS, Stein C, Duclos P, Birmingham M. How best to estimate the global burden of pertussis? Lancet Infect Dis 2003;3:413-8.
5.
Casano P, Odena MP, Cambra FJ, Martin JM, Palomeque A. Bordetella pertussis infection causing pulmonary hypertension. Arch Dis Child 2002;86:453.
6.
von Konig CH, Halperin S, Riffelmann M, Guiso N. Pertussis of adults and infants. Lancet Infect Dis 2002;2:744-50.
7.
Smith C, Vyas H. Early infantile pertussis: increasingly prevalent and potentially fatal. Eur J Pediatr 2000;159: 898-900.

8.
Goulin GD, Kaya KM, Bradley JS. Severe pulmonary hypertension associated with shock and death in infants infected with Bordetella pertussis. Crit Care Med 1993;21:1791-4.
9.
McEniery JD, Delbridge RG, Reith DM. Infant pertussis deaths and the management of cardiovascular compromise. J Paediatr Child Health 2004;40:230-2.
10.
Edwards KM. Pertussis: an important target for maternal immunization. Vaccine 2003;21:3483-6.
11.
Tanaka M, Vitek CR, Pascual FB, Bisgard KM, Tate JE, Murphy TV. Trends in pertussis among infants in the United States, 1980-1999. JAMA 2003;290: 2968-75.
12.
Mink CM, Cherry JD, Christenson P, et al. A search for Bordetella pertussis infection in university students. Clin Infect Dis 1992;14: 464-71.
13.
Cattaneo LA, Reed GW, Haase DH, Wills MJ, Edwards KM. The seroepidemiology of Bordetella pertussis infections: a study of persons ages 1-65 years. J Infect Dis 1996;173:1256-9.
14.
Schmitt-Grohe S, Cherry JD, Heininger U, Uberall MA, Pineda E, Stehr K. Pertussis in German adults. Clin Infect Dis 1995;21:860-6.

15.
Birkebaek NH, Kristiansen M, Seefeldt T, et al. Bordetella pertussis and chronic cough in adults. Clin Infect Dis 1999;29:1239-42.
16.
Nennig ME, Shinefield HR, Edwards KM, Black SB, Fireman BH. Prevalence and incidence of adult pertussis in an urban population. JAMA 1996;275:1672-4.
17.
Wright SW, Edwards KM, Decker MD, Zeldin MH. Pertussis infection in adults with persistent cough. JAMA 1995;273:1044-6.
18.
Postels-Multani S, Schmitt HJ, Wirsing von Konig CH, Bock HL, Bogaerts H. Symptoms and complications of pertussis in adults. Infection 1995;23:139-42.
19.
Thomas PF, McIntyre PB, Jalaludin BB. Survey of pertussis morbidity in adults in western Sydney. Med J Aust 2000;173:74-6.
20.
Trollfors B, Rabo E. Whooping cough in adults. Br Med J (Clin Res Ed) 1981;283:696-7.
21.
De Serres G, Shadmani R, Duval B, et al. Morbidity of pertussis in adolescents and adults. J Infect Dis 2000;182: 174-9.
22.
Skowronski DM, De Serres G, MacDonald D, et al. The changing age and seasonal profile of pertussis in Canada. J Infect Dis 2002;185:1448-53. [Erratum, J Infect Dis 2002;185:1696.]

23.
Skowronski DM, Buxton JA, Hestrin M, Keyes RD, Lynch K, Halperin SA. Carotid artery dissection as a possible severe complication of pertussis in an adult: clinical case report and review. Clin Infect Dis 2003;36: e1-e4.
24.
Halperin SA, Marrie TJ. Pertussis encephalopathy in an adult: case report and review. Rev Infect Dis 1991;13:1043-7.
25.
Strebel P, Nordin J, Edwards K, et al. Population-based incidence of pertussis among adolescents and adults, Minnesota, 1995-1996. J Infect Dis 2001;183: 1353-9.
26.
Kurt TL, Yeager AS, Guenette S, Dunlop S. Spread of pertussis by hospital staff. JAMA 1972;221:264-7.
27.
Cherry JD, Brunell PA, Golden GS, Karzon D. Report of the task force on pertussis and pertussis vaccine. Pediatrics 1988;81: Suppl:939-84.
28.
Cherry JD. The science and fiction of the "resurgence" of pertussis. Pediatrics 2003;112:405-6.
29.
Muller FM, Hoppe JE, Wirsing von Konig CH. Laboratory diagnosis of pertussis: state of the art in 1997. J Clin Microbiol 1997;35:2435-43.
30.
Ewanowich CA, Chui LWL, Paranchych MG, Peppler MS, Marusyk RG, Albritton WL. Major outbreak of pertussis in northern Alberta, Canada: analysis of discrepant direct fluorescent-antibody and culture results by using polymerase chain reaction methodology. J Clin Microbiol 1993;31:1715-25.

31.
Mastrantonio P, Spigaglia P, van Oirschot H, et al. Antigenic variants of Bordetella pertussis strains isolated from vaccinated and unvaccinated children. Microbiology 1999;145: 2069-75.

32.
Edelman K, Nikkari S, Ruuskanen O, He Q, Viljanen M, Mertsola J. Detection of Bordetella pertussis by polymerase chain reaction and culture in the nasopharynx of erythromycin-treated infants with pertussis. Pediatr Infect Dis J 1996;15:54-7.

33.
Cloud JL, Hymas WC, Turlak A, et al. Description of a multiplex Bordetella pertussis and Bordetella parapertussis LightCycler PCR assay with inhibition control. Diagn Microbiol Infect Dis 2003;46:189-95.

34.
Farrell DJ, McKeon M, Daggard G, Loeffelholz MJ, Thompson CJ, Mukkur TK. Rapid-cycle PCR method to detect Bordetella pertussis that fulfills all consensus recommendations for use of PCR in diagnosis of pertussis. J Clin Microbiol 2000;38:4499-502.

35.
Lievano FA, Reynolds MA, Waring AL, et al. Issues associated with and recommendations for using PCR to detect outbreaks of pertussis. J Clin Microbiol 2002;40: 2801-5.

36.
Guidelines for the control of pertussis outbreaks. Atlanta: National Immunization Program, 2000. (Accessed January 31, 2006, at http://www.cdc.gov/nip/publications/pertussis/guide.htm.)

37.
Meade BD, Bollen A. Recommendations for use of the polymerase chain reaction in the diagnosis of Bordetella pertussis infections. J Med Microbiol 1994;41:51-5.

38.
Fry NK, Tzivra O, Li YT, et al. Laboratory diagnosis of pertussis infections: the role of PCR and serology. J Med Microbiol 2004;53:519-25.

39.
Hallander HO. Microbiological and serological diagnosis of pertussis. Clin Infect Dis 1999;28:Suppl 2: S99-S106.

40.
Heininger U, Schmidt-Schlapfer G, Cherry JD, Stehr K. Clinical validation of a polymerase chain reaction assay for the diagnosis of pertussis by comparison with serology, culture, and symptoms during a large pertussis vaccine efficacy trial. Pediatrics 2000; 105(3):E31.

41.
Kosters K, Riffelmann M, Dohrn B, Konig CHW. Comparison of five commercial enzyme-linked immunosorbent assays for detection of antibodies to Bordetella pertussis. Clin Diagn Lab Immunol 2000;7: 422-6.

42.
Bergquist SO, Bernander S, Dahnsjo H, Sundelof B. Erythromycin in the treatment of pertussis: a study of bacteriologic and clinical effects. Pediatr Infect Dis J 1987;6:458-61. [Erratum, Pediatr Infect Dis J 1987;6: 1035.]

43.
Langley JM, Halperin SA, Boucher FD, Smith B. Azithromycin is as effective as and better tolerated than erythromycin estolate for the treatment of pertussis. Pediatrics 2004;111: e96-e101.

44.
Aoyama T, Sunakawa K, Iwata S, Takeuchi Y, Fujii R. Efficacy of short-term treatment of pertussis with clarithromycin and azithromycin. J Pediatr 1996;129: 761-4.

45.
Summaries of infectious diseases: pertussis. In: Pickering L, ed. 2003 Red book: report of the Committee on Infectious Diseases. 26th ed. Elk Grove Village, Ill.: American Academy of Pediatrics, 2003:472-86.

46.
Mahon BE, Rosenman MB, Kleinman MB. Maternal and infant use of erythromycin and other macrolide antibiotics as risk factors for infantile hypertrophic pyloric stenosis. J Pediatr 2001;139: 380-4.

47.
Ray W, Murray K, Meredith S, Narasimhulu S, Hall K, Stein C. Oral erythromycin and the risk of sudden death from cardiac causes. N Engl J Med 2004;351:1089-96.

48.
Hoppe JE, Bryskier A. In vitro susceptibilities of Bordetella pertussis and Bordetella parapertussis to two ketolides (HMR 3004 and HMR 3647), four macrolides (azithromycin, clarithromycin, erythromycin A, and roxithromycin), and two ansamycins (rifampin and rifapentine). Antimicrob Agents Chemother 1998;42: 965-6.

49.
Pillay V, Swingler G. Symptomatic treatment of the cough in whooping cough. Cochrane Database Syst Rev 2003;4:CD003257.

50.
Steketee RW, Wassilak SGF, Adkins WN Jr, et al. Evidence for a high attack rate and efficacy of erythromycin prophylaxis in a pertussis outbreak in a facility for the developmentally disabled. J Infect Dis 1988;157:434-40.

51.
Edwards KM, Decker MD. Combination vaccines. Infect Dis Clin North Am 2001;15:209-30.

52.
Ward J. Acellular pertussis vaccines in adolescents and adults. In: Program and abstracts of the 41st Interscience Conference on Antimicrobial Agents and Chemotherapy, Chicago, December 16–19, 2001. Washington, D.C.: American Society for Microbiology, 2001:520. abstract.

53.
Purdy KW, Hay JW, Botteman MF, Ward JI. Evaluation of strategies for use of acellular pertussis vaccine in adolescents and adults: a cost-benefit analysis. Clin Infect Dis 2004;39: 20-8.

54.
Halperin SA, Bertolussi R, Langley JM, Miller B, Eastwood BJ. Seven days of erythromycin estolate is as effective as fourteen days for the treatment of Bordetella pertussis infections. Pediatrics 1997;100:65-71.

55.
Healy CM, Munoz FM, Rench MA, Halasa NB, Edwards KM, Baker CJ. Prevalence of pertussis antibodies in maternal delivery, cord, and infant serum. J Infect Dis 2004;190: 335-40.

ADDENDUM

The proceedings of a conference on the Global Pertussis Initiative, at which experts from 17 countries analyzed the status of pertussis disease worldwide and evaluated potential immunization strategies, have been published.[1] The recommendations included increased protection of infants and toddlers by immunization of groups at the highest risk of transmitting *Bordetella pertussis* to them; development of a better understanding of the epidemiology and transmission of pertussis; and improved surveillance, diagnosis, and education. A recently published multicenter placebo-controlled randomized trial in the United States involving subjects ages 15 to 65 years demonstrated that acellular pertussis vaccination conferred 92 percent protection (95 percent confidence interval, 32 to 99 percent) against pertussis infection.[2] Another recent study using a cost–benefit analysis of tetanus, diphtheria, and acellular pertussis (Tdap) booster immunization in the United States projected that vaccinating all adolescents (persons 10 to 19 years of age) would prevent 0.4 to 1.8 million cases of pertussis and save from $0.3 to $1.6 billion in medical care costs over 10 years.[3]

Since publication of our article, we have been informed that in addition to those countries noted in Table 1, Australia has added a booster dose of acellular pertussis vaccine for adolescents 15 to 17 years of age.[4] This dose replaces the 18-month booster and, on the basis of computer simulation, is anticipated to reduce the overall incidence of pertussis.[5]

1. Plotkin S. The Global Pertussis Initiative: process overview. Pediatr Infect Dis J 2005;24:Suppl 5:57-9.
2. Ward JI, Cherry JD, Chang S-J, et al. Efficacy of an acellular pertussis vaccine among adolescents and adults. N Engl J Med 2005;353:1555-63.
3. Hay JW, Ward JI. Economic considerations for pertussis booster vaccination in adolescents. Pediatr Infect Dis J 2005;24: Suppl 6:S127-S133.
4. The Australian Immunisation Handbook. 8th ed. Canberra: Australian Government Department of Health and Ageing, 2003:205-20.
5. Hethcote HW, Horby P, McIntyre P. Using computer simulations to compare pertussis vaccination strategies in Australia. Vaccine 2004;22:2181-91.

INDEX

Page numbers followed by italic f or t denote figures or tables, respectively.